No Margin For Error

A Surgeon's Struggle Repairing Hypospadias

Warren Snodgrass, MD

OH PRESS

ISBNs: 979-8-9894235-1-4 (pbk)
979-8-9894235-0-7 (hc)
979-8-9894235-2-1 (ebook)

Cover and book design by Mayfly Design

Library of Congress Catalog Number: 2023920455
First Printing: 2024
Printed in the United States of America

Praise for *No Margin for Error*

"This memoir tells the story of one surgeon's passion to study, understand, improve, and teach hypospadias surgery – one of the most technically demanding operations in pediatric urology. The book is filled with feisty anecdotes from his roller-coaster ride of success and rejection by colleagues, administrators and businessmen as he worked to increase public awareness of hypospadias and improve the results of surgery to correct it."

—Dr. Richard Hurwitz, pediatric urologist, Los Angeles

"Dr. Snodgrass's memoir is an inspiring story of a pair of surgeons on a mission to change the mindset of an entire profession. My husband and I enjoyed reading it!"

—Jaye Ryan, a concerned parent, Montreal

"The book combines evidence, experience, and the perspectives of patients and their families to encourage surgeons to strive for excellence repairing hypospadias."

—Dr. Martin Koyle, former Chief of Pediatric Urology, SickKids Hospital, Toronto

"This could have been my story of worry and guilt when my son was born with hypospadias and then had complications after his surgery. Every parent of a boy with hypospadias should read Dr. Snodgrass's book."

—Laura H, hypospadias mother, New York

"It was embarrassing going through childhood and into adulthood having hypospadias. I didn't really know what the condition was, only that I was different from other boys. I feel much better about myself now that it has been repaired, and I hope this book will help others so little boys don't have to go through life with hypospadias."

—Michael Rogers, adult with hypospadias, Michigan

"It made me mad to read that most surgeons do not know their own results from hypospadias operations they do on our sons. That explains a lot…"

—Charles K, hypospadias father, St. Louis

"I have seen how my grandson, my daughter, and their entire family have been affected by his hypospadias. It was surprising to learn that this is so common, since none of us had ever heard of it before. This wonderful book by Dr Snodgrass really helped us understand hypospadias better."

— Mary A, grandmother, Florida

For the patients and all their loved ones affected by hypospadias,
and for the surgeons committed to repairing it better.

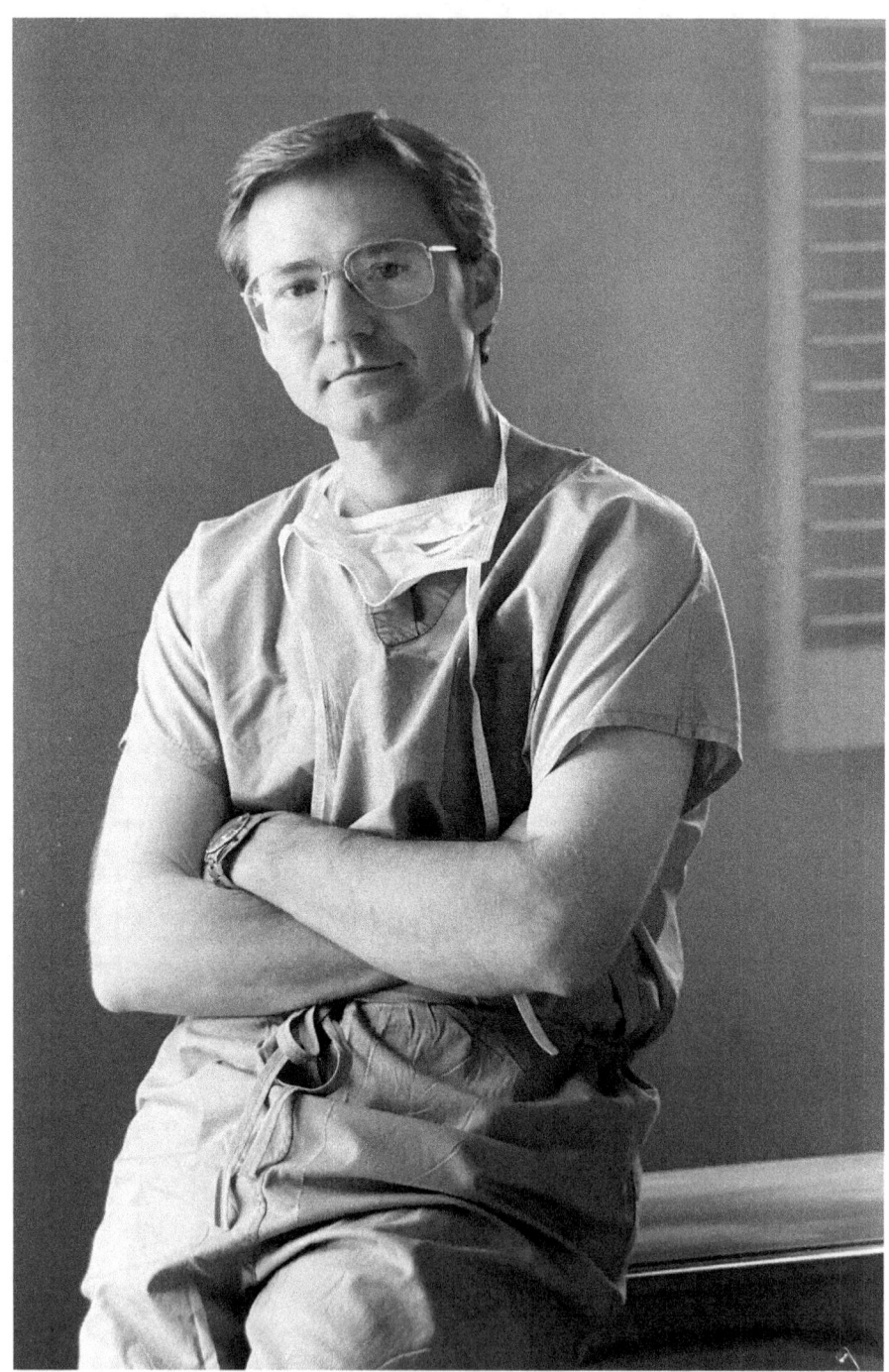

I was driven to teach others what hypospadias taught me.

Contents

TIP Repair
Children's Medical Center Dallas

STAG Repair
Three Corporotomies
PARC Urology

STAC Repair
Hypospadias Specialty Center

Foreword

Hypospadias is a common birth defect. Every day in the United States twenty-seven boys are born with the condition, compared to sixteen children with Down's syndrome and twelve with a cleft lip. But if you are not a doctor, or a patient, or a parent of a son with hypospadias you likely have never heard of it. Because it affects the penis.

And because it is the penis, hypospadias is hidden by embarrassment, concealed by worries over privacy, shrouded by a prudish reluctance to discuss what is just another body part. So, parents, and patients as they get older, often feel ashamed and isolated, wondering if anyone else has a penis like this. A penis with the opening lower than normal and prone to spray urine outside the toilet and down the pants, a foreskin that does not enclose the head and looks neither natural nor circumcised, and a shaft which is sometimes bent, making intercourse difficult.

A birth defect made worse because the penis is special. A symbol of both maleness and manliness, representing strength and virility. An organ whose daily function can be taken for granted, even as it is revered for the immense pleasures it gives to both the man and his lover. Will the newborn with hypospadias grow up to view himself fully a man if he must sit to pee, or worries what a new lover will think of his bent and different-looking penis?

There is surgery to transform hypospadias into a normal penis. Many surgeons can do that, but too many others cannot because they lack the temperament and skills, or they are capable but refuse to do the best operations, or they choose the best operations but fail to do the key steps in the best way, or they try to do the best operations in the best ways but do not repair hypospadias often enough to become adept. Most do not realize they need to do better, because few surgeons know their own results for the operations they do, and only assume they are as good as what the experts publish.

The history of hypospadias repair dates to the late 1800s, to the beginnings of elective surgeries. The first surgeons excised tissues they thought bound the penis down to make it straight, and then extended the urinary channel using various skin flaps and grafts. They retired to succeeding generations, who modified those techniques and innovated new ones until more than 200 operations had been tried and discarded over time. That process continued into a recent era dominated by a tall, gregarious surgeon at a leading children's hospital in Philadelphia who condensed the choices to three operations of his own making. And then to current times when a surgeon from a small city on the plains of West Texas upended that algorithm with his own new trilogy.

This is his story, and the story of the struggle for change to make hypospadias surgery better.

Influenced by my father, I grew up with no other plan but to become a doctor. More precisely, a surgeon. I still remember going to the operating room for the first time as a teenager. How Gradine, the grandmotherly head nurse, showed me the way to scrub and then enter the OR backward through the door protecting my clean hands, as surgeons do. How she tied my gown from behind while the tech gloved me, and then led me to the table to stand next to my dad while he operated.

Years later a professor of Internal Medicine at the University of Texas Medical Branch told medical student Snodgrass that, in more than twenty years of teaching, he had never encountered a student already specialized in only his third year. But anyone who observes a group of medical students knows that most sort into medicine or surgery naturally. I just revealed my future early.

I almost missed that opportunity. It is possible that I had the lowest MCAT score of my class, but I could not bring myself to spend the summer before my senior year at Texas Tech behind a desk refreshing my memory of freshman chemistry and sophomore biology to raise it. I just assumed my score would be good enough. And even though my final college transcript reported just a couple of Bs hardly visible in the thicket of As, the first week of medical school so overwhelmed me with a mountain of information to commit to memory that I very nearly quit on Friday afternoon.

Looking back, I still regret not lugging my boxes of lecture notes and piles of syllabuses to a photography studio to have my picture shot standing in my short white medical school coat with each arm resting on a stack of all I somehow managed to learn sufficiently well to finish AOA.[1]

I was surprised to open my envelope on Match Day[2] and learn I was not moving up the freeway from Galveston to Houston, even though the Chief of Surgery at Hermann Hospital promised to rank me number one. But then I learned he made that same commitment to several other applicants. It was just as well since that chief left the next year under murky circumstances. Instead, I spent my two years of general surgery residency at the Ochsner Clinic in New Orleans and would have gladly stayed on for another three to become a general surgeon if I did not already have a position to train with the Urology Department at the Baylor College of Medicine.

That department was led by Gene Carlton, Jr, a visionary recruited from private practice who pioneered subspecialization among the faculty. I trained with world experts managing urologic cancers, kidney stones, male infertility, erectile dysfunction, and pediatric urology, and finished those four years ready to use all the knowledge and skills I gleaned from my mentors.

Then I returned to Lubbock, to a private practice standing on the opposite side of the operating room table across from my father.

I did some of almost everything a urologist is credentialed to do during those twelve years. I also raised three kids, designed and built my dream house, shared my home with several foreign exchange students, taught myself to speak and read German, wrote a book on the fall of communism in East Germany, taught Sunday School for adults, served as Chief of Staff at Methodist Hospital, and invented a new operation

---

1. *AOA* is the Alpha Omega Alpha honorary medical society, which selects the top students for membership.
2. Senior medical students across the US learn where they have been selected for postgraduate residency training on *Match Day*.

for hypospadias. Then I left this life and moved to UT Southwestern Medical Center and the Children's Medical Center of Dallas to learn more about that penis condition, because even a common birth defect does not happen very often.

I named the new operation the TIP repair, but others renamed it the "Snodgrass." And that name became one of the best known in all of urology. I was made a celebrity, at least within the small community of pediatric urologists, and invited around the world to lecture and operate.

But I was content in my first life and mourned selling the house I built just seven years after moving in. I did not want to live in a big city or work in a large university. I was uneasy lecturing at meetings and shocked that so many gathered to hear me speak, especially in the early years before I really knew much to tell. I never became comfortable with being projected onto large screens in auditoriums while colleagues watched me operate.

Their respect was less a tribute to my knowledge or skill than a sign of how difficult it is to repair hypospadias. There is no margin for error in an operation when dissection a few millimeters in the wrong direction can lead to disastrous complications. But using my repair surgeons could, for the first time, reliably fix distal hypospadias into a normal penis.

Everywhere I was invited, I prepared new lectures. In fact, despite my many travels, I never gave the same lecture twice. Several times each year I reviewed my databases to update information. I made new slides and revamped others, changing the fonts and the background colors, and I even translated the text into Spanish when I started traveling to Latin America. I was never satisfied that a lecture clearly and convincingly spoke my message.

Of the many lessons I taught the most important was self-assessment, how every surgeon should review his or her own work to be certain it is as good as it could be. The 3Ps, Prospective data collection, Periodic review of the results, and Practice changes to get better, which I first applied to myself before recommending it to others.

Meanwhile, I was not sure how to respond when someone argued there were limitations to TIP that my data could not find. Or wanted to modify TIP without showing their results from doing it differently.

Or encouraged others to cling to older ways when this new way was better. Maybe it is not possible to persuade some without unsettling others, especially those who heard arrogance in the passion I brought to debates.

There are types of hypospadias that TIP cannot repair, the severe forms when the penis is bent down with "chordee."[3] Even though I learned the most up-to-date operations for these cases during residency, I found that they did not work either. I was not sure what to do. How should I make the curved penis straight? What was the best way to extend the urine opening from the scrotum out to the tip of the head?

I moved to Dallas to find the boundaries of TIP. Then I had to learn the best way to repair hypospadias when TIP could not be done. I heard a plastic surgeon lecture on how to make a urethra from skin grafts, but had to devise a new way to straighten penile curvature so that I could use them. Combining these eventually led to a new operation called STAG. Then, with more experience, I realized that it was usually better to separate the straightening from the grafting, and that evolved into another procedure I named STAC.

Together, TIP, STAG, and STAC created a new algorithm to consistently transform hypospadias into a normal penis.

In the midst of this work, I was forced out of the university back into private practice. I left with a partner willing to share the uncertainties of exploring frontiers, and together we built a new practice doing general pediatric urology that featured complex hypospadias repair.

Her insights polished the STAG and suggested the STAC, which we both soon realized was the most important innovation since TIP repair. It was Nicol Bush who found the goniometer to accurately measure how bent a penis is. She studied how to best manage the skin of the penis that hypospadias left deficient on the underside. It was her idea to use hyperbaric oxygen to rejuvenate tissues damaged from unsuccessful surgeries when I had a patient whose wounds would not heal.

And it was Bush who envisioned us doing *only* hypospadias, work-

---

3. *Chordee* refers to the bending of the penis.

ing together as a surgical team in a specialized center. I did not think that would be possible when she first mentioned it, knowing that it had never been done before. But social media referred so many new patients to us that we soon had no time to see children with other problems.

It was not only boys who filled our practice, but also men still troubled by the penis defect they were born with. Some had been told their hypospadias was so minor that it did not need to be repaired, while others struggled with damage from unsuccessful operations. Soon Bush and I were managing the consequences of hypospadias in more men than any other practice in the US, and possibly anywhere in the world. These patients taught us lessons that pediatric urologists could never learn treating only boys. I was surprised when some of those colleagues did not want to hear them.

A practice devoted exclusively to hypospadias also taught me that this birth defect is much more than the surgical challenge that was my primary focus as a professor. How the condition affects not only the boy born with it and the man he will become, but also his parents, siblings, and lovers, most of whom had never heard of hypospadias before. Once I made time to listen, I found the stories these people told me heartbreaking.

But a surgical practice for boys and men did not fit into either a children's or a general hospital. That left us little choice but to create our own center, the Hypospadias Specialty Center, to welcome patients of all ages from all around the world. This Shangri-La came with some thorns, but five-star reviews from parents and patients confirmed we had made the right decision.

TIP REPAIR

Children's Medical Center of Dallas Urology

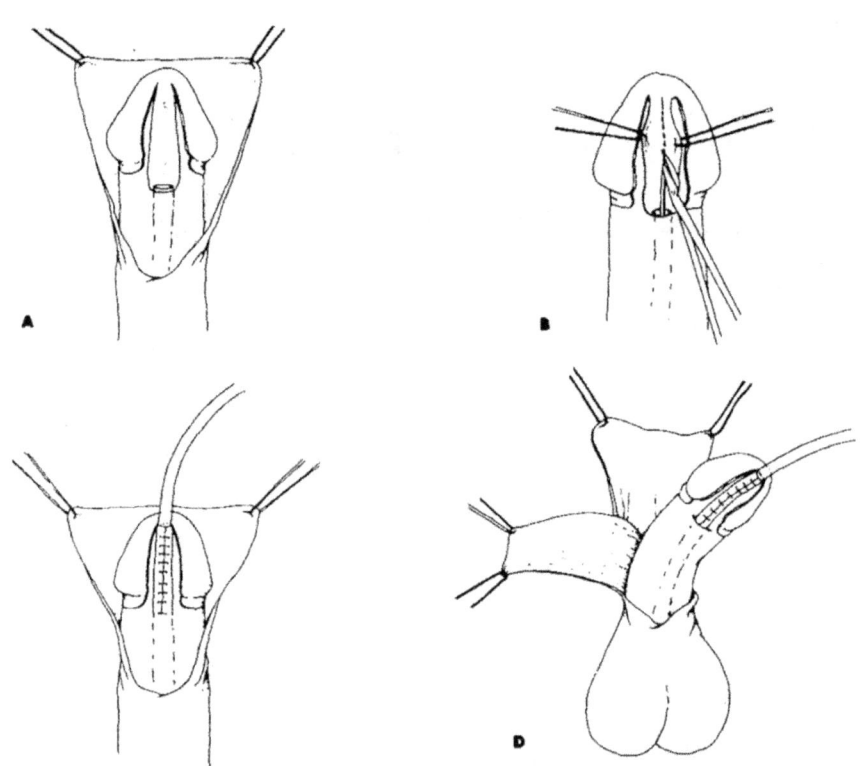

The first diagram of the TIP repair for distal hypospadias, published in 1994.

◀ CHAPTER 1 ▶

Chance Favors the Prepared Mind

I am not sure what to do.

I study the wound again, then take forceps in each hand and stretch the edges apart, measuring the incision with my eyes, sensing the give of the tissues. My nurse stands on the other side of the table watching. She glances up from the operation and I feel her search my face half hidden behind a mask. She does not say a word, and after a moment looks back down, knowing she has not seen this step before.

"I don't remember how far it said to incise," I explain to no one, the words exhaled in a sigh.

I do not hear the anesthesia bellows marking time with each breath the patient takes. I do not see the circulating nurse off in a corner studying a takeout menu for lunch. I shift my weight and try to recall the exact description of this key maneuver, realizing, finally, that I cannot.

Only my nurse, and the scrub tech, know the operation has stopped. I have said nothing to cause the anesthesiologist to look over the drape to see if something is wrong, or to disturb the concentration of the circulator planning her break. Nor have I paused long enough to worry the routine in the operating room with my silence.

I release the tissues, toss the forceps off to the side and squeeze my eyes closed, focusing on the drawing in the article, comparing it to the real life before me. I take a deep breath and sigh again.

A decision must be made. Cut more, or not. In my mind, every complexity becomes a binary choice.

"Tenotomies," I command, reaching my left hand toward the scrub tech for the scissors while keeping my eyes on the incision. "Pick up opposite me," I tell my nurse, who knows to hold the tissues just like I do.

With a cut of the scissors, I extend the small incision I have already made in the urethral plate, the strip of tissue running from where the urine opening is to the end of the head where it should be. I re-grab the edges a little farther back and snip again, making it wider, continuing until the scissors reach into the urinary channel. Then I cut deeper back in the other direction toward where I began and see the plate opening even wider. Counter-traction from my forceps and the nurse's pulling away from each other exposes more wisps of tissue to divide, back and forth up and down the entire length of the plate, until I feel the tips of the scissors butting against solid structures underneath and know I cannot incise any deeper. This will either work, or it won't.

No other surgeon has seen this view. Later, some will worry the incision I have just made to create a normal-caliber urethra will instead scar it closed, but that thought does not occur to me.

I only see that the urethral plate has widened and deepened enough that I can roll it directly into a tube to extend the urinary channel to the tip of the head of the penis. I do not need the rectangular flap of skin on the shaft that I would ordinarily sew onto the plate to make the new urethra. That is a relief, because in this boy the edge of that flap is dotted with tiny hair follicles that might sprout a beard from the urinary opening when he begins puberty. I snip it off.

Next, I slide a catheter down the channel, tie it into place, and start sewing the edges of the urethral plate around it.

When that is done, I pause again, studying the tube I have created. Tiny stitches run along its top, and I worry they might join other stitches that will close the skin above the new urethra and make a leak. So I fashion a protective layer from tissue under the foreskin and cover it over the tube to keep the sutures apart.

Soon I am done, the final steps to close the head and skin of the penis a familiar routine.

I drive back to the office, and, in the time remaining before clinic begins, flip back through the article that sparked this idea and read that the incision those other surgeons made went through only the far end rather than the entire urethral plate, as mine did. And they did not say how deep to cut. Then I pull down textbooks from my father's collection and thumb through diagrams sketching a history of hypospadias surgery reaching back over a hundred years. I cannot find a drawing of the repair I just did.

It was the beginning of 1990, and I had been in practice as a general urologist with my father for nearly four years treating a variety of ailments afflicting the kidneys, bladder, and genitals. I cut out cancers, basketed out stones, and cored out enlarged prostates. Occasionally, I repaired a distal hypospadias.[4] I lived in Lubbock, a small city isolated on the high plains of the Texas panhandle, confident I could manage whatever walked through my door because I was well trained, and young.

Of all those various operations I did, the one with the least margin for error was correcting hypospadias. In the future I would warn trainees that dissection just one millimeter into the wrong plane is still in the wrong plane, and sometimes enough to complicate the entire operation. In that future, patients with complications would travel from around the world for my hands to heal what others' maimed, and I would learn how very deep the scars from failed repairs penetrate their lives.

I would also tell younger colleagues how confusing it was in the 1980s, when I was a resident, trying to decide which hypospadias repair to do from the half dozen then in vogue. How one of my faculty teachers began each operation by examining the patient and then sketching options to repair the anatomy he saw, using marking pens on the surgical drapes until they were covered in nearly indecipherable hieroglyphics. How the dominant surgeon of that era organized courses where he showed invited experts photographs of hypospadias and asked which operation they would do, stoking their disagreements into a blood sport of controversy for the entertainment of the audience.

Nevertheless, I graduated from residency in 1986 with a repertoire of three operations my mentors taught could repair every type and variation of hypospadias. And to be certain that I did each one right, I wrote

---

4. *Distal hypospadias* refers to a urine opening near or just on the head of the penis and is the most common variety of hypospadias.

down the key steps, and the instruments and sutures needed to do them, on five-by-seven index cards that I carried into private practice.

My first patient with hypospadias was the infant son of a pathologist at the hospital, which prompted the unspoken thought that doctors' kids always seem to have complications! After the boy was asleep with anesthesia, I studied his penis, magnified 2.5 times by surgical loupes,[5] and recognized David Gibbon's sketches on the OR drapes showing the ideal anatomy for a MAGPI.[6] I was pleased that the boy's penis looked normal when he returned for a checkup after surgery, and relieved that my first hypospadias repair was a success.

The next did not fare as well.

Several months later another boy was brought to me with distal hypospadias, but my examination found subtle differences in anatomy that recommended a Mathieu "flip-flap"[7] instead of a MAGPI. Following my notes precisely, I outlined a rectangle of skin below the abnormal urinary opening and then "flipped" this flap up and over, like a mousetrap slowly snapping closed. Before sewing it, I slid a catheter into the bladder so that he would not pee through the fresh surgery. Then I stitched the edges of the flap to the urethral plate to make the urinary channel longer and bring the new opening to the tip of the head of his penis, called the glans.

My nurse removed the catheter a week later, and Mom brought her son for his first postoperative assessment by me after another month of healing had passed.

"How's he doing?" I asked, as Mom opened his diaper.

"OK, I guess," she answered, a little hesitant, "but I don't really know what it's supposed to look like. I'm curious to hear what you think."

I felt her scrutinizing my face while I studied her son's penis. The opening was in the correct location at the end of the glans, and there was no leak or wound separation. I pointed out these features of a successful repair to her matter-of-factly.

---

5. Surgeons repairing hypospadias commonly wear *loupes,* a type of magnifying glasses.

6. The name *MAGPI* was derived from the key steps in the operation, Meatoplasty and Glanuloplasty, which was published by John Duckett in 1981.

7. The *Mathieu* operation was described by the French surgeon Paul Mathieu in 1932 and is known by both his name and as the "flip-flap," the key step in the procedure.

"So it looks OK?" she persisted.

Maintaining a noncommittal gaze, I continued the evaluation. *Maybe it looks OK,* I thought, *but it certainly does not look normal.* I was not sure why. What exactly was not right? I stared at it for a few moments longer, while she kept her eyes locked on me. Then I realized the problem: the meatus was round, like the mouth of a fish, and not the usual slit. Such a minor difference, yet so important!

"I think it'll be fine," I declared, not knowing what else to say.

I waved to signal the exam was over and Mom could close the diaper as I turned to wash my hands. I pulled out a few paper towels and began drying them while I turned back to her.

"I'll need to see him back in six months," I said, tossing the wadded towels into the trash.

Over the next year I only saw another three boys with distal hypospadias, and each of them also fit the criteria for a Mathieu flip-flap. Although all of them healed without a complication, I was disappointed to see that none of them looked quite right. What should I say to their moms when they asked if the surgery was a success?

I looked up articles written about the Mathieu and read the authors describe "satisfactory," or even "good," cosmetic results. Not convinced, I asked a few colleagues from training if they noticed the same problem with the urinary opening, called the meatus, and one of them summarized the response of them all.

"If the meatus is at the tip, and there aren't any complications, the operation was a success. You can't expect to make something *look* normal that wasn't *made* normal in the first place."

But was that really the final answer? Was mom consoled that her son had no fistula, or dehiscence, or stricture[8] when his penis still did not look right? Can hypospadias repair be declared a success when the penis does not look normal?

They say that chance favors the prepared mind. When I saw a new

---

8. *Fistula* is a urine leak; *dehiscence* means a wound has come apart; a *stricture* is a scar inside the urethra that narrows it.

article that described "hinging" the urethral plate,[9] promising to significantly improve the cosmetic results of flip-flaps, I read it enthusiastically and resolved to try this maneuver during my next case.

But I did more than hinge, more than just cut a short distance into the distal end of the plate as the illustration showed. Instead, I incised the entire urethral plate, cutting from within the hypospadias opening all the way to near the tip of the glans, and deeply through its surface all the way down to the underlying structures. Which changed the operation from Mathieu's flip-flap into something very different—a repair that relied only on urethral tissues to make the urethra without adding a flap of skin from the penis. And in that process, also created a slit meatus.

Six weeks later, I did not have to hide my opinion behind a dispassionate face. If this mom was scrutinizing my reaction, she needed only to see my smile stretching from ear to ear to know the operation was a success. I did not have to point out that the meatus was at the tip and that there was no complication. Now it was sufficient to say her son's penis was normal.

Almost nine months would pass before I could try this operation again. Birth defects are, after all, rare, and even though hypospadias is one of the most common, it happens only in one boy of every 200 born. On the sparse plains of West Texas that meant I would never see more than a handful of new patients each year even if I saw all the newborns there with it.

So I was excited when the next patient came for surgery, and thrilled to see that the new repair worked again to make his penis look normal. So natural, in fact, that if the parents took their son to a new pediatrician that unknowing provider would never suspect that he once had hypospadias.

When subsequent boys all had the same result, I realized it was not a fluke. This innovation reliably changed a penis born with abnormal anatomy to look normal. And the boys seemed fine afterward, peeing straight and strong with no fistulas or worries from a stricture blocking

---

9. "Hinging the Urethral Plate in Hypospadias Meatoplasty" was published by the *Journal of Urology* in 1989.

their new urethra. Even though I was in private practice with no academic obligations, I knew these results had to be published.

I happened to mention that one evening to my neighbor, a general surgeon who worked at the same hospital. We were sitting outside on his front porch while the sun fell beyond the treeless plains. He stopped strumming his guitar and looked at me, clearly perplexed.

"You want to write a paper? Like a research paper when we were in college?"

But I was not deterred. I studied other articles describing other hypospadias repairs and concluded I would need at least fifteen cases to submit a report. Yet even that low number was a high threshold to reach when I saw only four or five new patients with hypospadias each year. It would take at least another three years to gather enough experience.

During each of those operations, I could not help but wonder if some other surgeon somewhere else who repaired hypospadias more often had made the same observation that I did. Month by month I watched for the next issue of the *Journal of Urology* and scanned the table of contents the moment it was delivered to the office, hoping not to find an article that would scoop the one I was yet to write.

I also realized the new operation needed a name if it was to join the pantheon of other popular repairs of those times. Something like a MAGPI or flip-flap, the GAP, a transverse island, or an onlay flap—a simple name that described the essence of the repair. And a name that was catchy as well, at least to other surgeons.

I no longer recall all the ideas I considered and discarded trying to condense the operation into one or two words. I eventually focused on the key step, which produced the Incised Tubularized Plate repair. I-T-P I said out loud several times, testing the sound, feeling the letters in my mouth. But then I remembered those were already the initials of a blood disease! So I rearranged the title into Tubularized Incised Plate, (TIP) which, though a bit awkward, cleverly explained the operation and hinted at the normal meatus it made at the tip of the glans.

Meanwhile, I worried the new operation was really the old "blank-blank" repair long since abandoned by surgeons, and then forgotten. Having found nothing similar in my father's textbooks, I gave a list of articles to the hospital librarian to track down and copy. When a review of those also uncovered no precedent, I decided to present my preliminary results at a regional meeting of the American Urologic Association to see if any delegate stood to announce the true origin of the repair.

I flew to Houston and rented a car for the drive down to Galveston, the island city where I was born when my father was a medical student at UTMB a generation earlier. My mind filled with memories of earlier passages across the bridge arching high over the bay and then onto Broadway, the main entrance lined with palm trees and pink oleanders that led to the medical school where I also became a doctor. Arriving at the hotel, I pushed these remembrances aside to practice the five-minute lecture I would deliver the next morning, holding each of the Kodachrome slides up to the light one at a time.

The familiarity of the place was lost in the unfamiliarity of the task I was there to perform. The medical student and resident Snodgrass had given the presentations expected of all trainees, but never a summary of my own work before a jury of my peers. Well, not really peers, since the doctors who would hear this first description of the TIP repair were pediatric urologists, specialists dedicated to children, whereas I was a general urologist treating patients of all ages. In fact, I declined the suggestion of my mentor, Edmond Gonzales, Jr, to join their ranks by doing additional fellowship training after residency.

A fellowship in those times usually led to an academic surgical career. And an academic career meant research, as well as teaching pediatric urology to residents. I did not want to limit my practice to children, could not think of any topic I wanted to research, and already anticipated the frustration of working with an ever-changing line of trainees with the same basic, underdeveloped skills as my own surgical abilities improved with time.

I was not a peer among these pediatric urologists, and the best I could do was to feign confidence during my few minutes at the lectern.

My presentation first reviewed the Mathieu operation, emphasizing that while it might deliver the urethra to the tip of the glans, the meatus it created rarely looked natural. Next, I acknowledged the authors whose idea to hinge the urethral plate was the seed of my repair, and explained the major steps in the new operation illustrated by line drawings that my wife, Virginia, sketched. Then I summarized the results for eleven boys and finally concluded that TIP made a urethra as good as a flip-flap in a penis that was better, because it looked normal.

At the end of the session, a moderator commented on each presentation. Coming to mine, Ricardo Gonzalez, a transplant from Argentina, observed in a thick Spanish accent, "This is an interesting idea, but these few patients do not convince me to switch from the flip-flap, which has given me excellent results that I am happy with for many years!"

But I did not go to this meeting to proselytize. From my perspective, the most important comment was the one not made. In a room filled with senior pediatric urologists, no one recognized TIP as an old operation newly renamed. I left the island invigorated, but still needing another year and five more patients to write a report.

I ripped the side tab off the mailer to find a letter from the editor at the *Journal of Urology* and Xeroxed comments from Reviewer 1 and Reviewer 2. "Dear Warren, your manuscript has now been reviewed, and the consensus is that it be returned to you for revision. If you choose to amend your work, changes must be made in bold, and the revised manuscript returned within thirty days . . ."

I read through the comments and laughed at the question from one reviewer asking if the pictures in Figure 2 showing a urethral plate before incision, and then much wider after incision, were from the same patient? That was the most important message in the article, and so I was happy to write more clearly that the TIP incision makes a normal-sized urinary channel without needing to add skin flaps.

But a normal-sized urethra could have an opening made too small if the urethral plate was rolled too far toward its end. Ironically, neither I nor the reviewers realized that the diagram of the operation in the article illustrated exactly how to make this mistake! In the years to come, I would learn that most complications happen because of errors that surgeons make and would warn against tubularizing the urethral plate this far and creating a partial blockage, sometimes showing the original illustration to make that point.

Fortunately, it was not the line drawings but the picture in Figure 3 that made the greatest impression on readers when the article was published in 1994, four years after I did the first TIP repair. A photo that showed the normal appearance of a penis after surgery that I, at least, never achieved with a flip-flap.

Events soon proved that other surgeons were also quietly frustrated trying to make a penis born with hypospadias look normal. Generally, surgeons are a conservative lot, many clinging with determination to the lessons taught by mentors they continue to revere long after passing through training, and long after their teachers have passed on to their eternal rewards. But this operation proved exceptional, spreading like a prairie wildfire out of Lubbock, across the US, and then all around the world.

In hindsight, what stoked this fire was neither the name of the operation that I labored to perfect, nor the picture of perfection shown in Figure 3, but rather my response to a question at a national meeting not long after the article was published.

"Dr. Snodgrass, isn't this like a urethrotomy[10] for stricture, which we all know doesn't work?" someone in the audience asked. "How do you *know* this incision in the urethral plate doesn't scar closed?"

I had not imagined a connection between the TIP incision into a healthy urethral plate and a urethrotomy incision made into an unhealthy, scarred urethra. But judging from the murmur of nodding heads in the audience, many others had. So I walked totally unprepared to a microphone and gave just the right answer.

"I know it doesn't stricture because I checked every one of those patients with a sound[11] postoperatively." *Just like I wrote in the paper.*

Meanwhile, after the article was published, Richard Ehrlich called Marty Koyle and asked if he had seen it. Koyle answered that he first heard about the operation during a meeting in Galveston a couple of years earlier and started using it soon afterward. Not only that, but he had also spread the word to a few other friends, including Tony Caldamone in Rhode Island, Rick Hurwitz in California, and Giantonio Manzoni in Italy, convincing them to give it a try.

---

10. A *urethrotomy* is a cut to open a stricture made with a small knife fitted onto the end of a scope.
11. A *sound* is a metal instrument used to calibrate the size of the urethra.

In the time before email, Koyle, a balding socialite who stood a head taller than most pediatric urologists, wrote me a letter saying the five of them had collected their results, and were inviting me to add in my own and then present the combined work at the next American Academy of Pediatrics Urology congress.[12] I pointed out that I was in private practice and had no experience on a national stage, suggesting instead that Koyle should represent the group. However, he persisted and reassured me that he could help make the presentation acceptable.

So I made drafts of the slides and faxed them to Koyle, who marked them up like a schoolteacher might and sent them back for revisions. Back and forth we faxed, until those revisions became tweaks and then minor style adjustments.

Once during this process I called Koyle, who was out of the office changing his summer tires before winter arrived in Denver. His secretary offered to take a message, and then, after a lingering pause, asked, "Dr. Snodgrass? THE Dr. Snodgrass?"

"Well, *a* Dr. Snodgrass," I answered, puzzled.

"THE Dr. Snodgrass of the hypospadias operation?" she clarified.

"Well, yeah. That's what I need to talk to Dr. Koyle about. But how do you know about the hypospadias repair?"

"I know your name because I post his surgeries, including the 'Snodgrass repair,'" she explained.

"The 'Snodgrass repair?'"

"Yes, that's what he calls it."

I hung up and immediately recalled the many hours I'd spent thinking of a name for the new operation. Koyle was the first to ignore the title I suggested, and soon others everywhere followed his lead and simply called it the Snodgrass.

Except not me. To this day I have never called the "TIP" a "Snodgrass." But I have to smile at the irony that my name, mercilessly ridiculed on the playgrounds of my youth, became the preferred title of a new operation.

When the presentation was finalized, I had slides made and imagined

---

12. The American Academy of Pediatrics Section on Urology meeting was, at that time, the largest gathering of pediatric urologists and held once a year.

the words I would say with each. Then I rehearsed out loud to better simulate the lecture, knowing there is a difference between thinking words and speaking them. Finally, like an athlete before a competition, I visualized the entire event: sitting near the stage, counting down the talks before mine, hearing my name called, climbing the steps to the lectern, pushing the button to advance the first slide, speaking the opening sentence.

I practiced every day until the day finally came, and my moment finally arrived, when John Duckett, the moderator, announced my name and I went up the steps and brought up the first slide and spoke the first sentence, and then relaxed as the following sentences spilled out effortlessly. I did not embarrass myself, or my co-authors, who lent their reputations to promote my idea.

After speaking, I took my place at a table on the stage, waiting for the remaining presentations to end so that members of the audience could ask questions or make comments. I anticipated several possible questions and prepared succinct answers for each. But all these years later the only comment I still recall was the one made by my mentor, who walked to a microphone in the center of the conference hall right in front of the stage.

"Warren's been talking about this operation for a few years now, but at Texas Children's we've not found it necessary to do it."

That I had not foreseen, nor prepared for. Especially since my teacher was a gentle man who rarely spoke at these meetings, and never critically. The words stung, and to this day I do not understand why he was compelled to say them.

A few years later it was my honor to co-moderate the hypospadias session at another national congress. Which meant I announced the names of the authors chosen to present their work and then called on those in the audience who went to microphones to ask a question or challenge a conclusion afterwards.

As the session came to its end, the other moderator covered our microphone with his hand, turned to me, and whispered, "Watch this."

Then a grinning Bill Cromie called for everyone in the audience using the Snodgrass repair to raise their hand. A swarm of hands filled the air.

He turned back to me still smiling. "I thought you should see this. Maybe no other operation has ever been accepted by so many surgeons so fast."

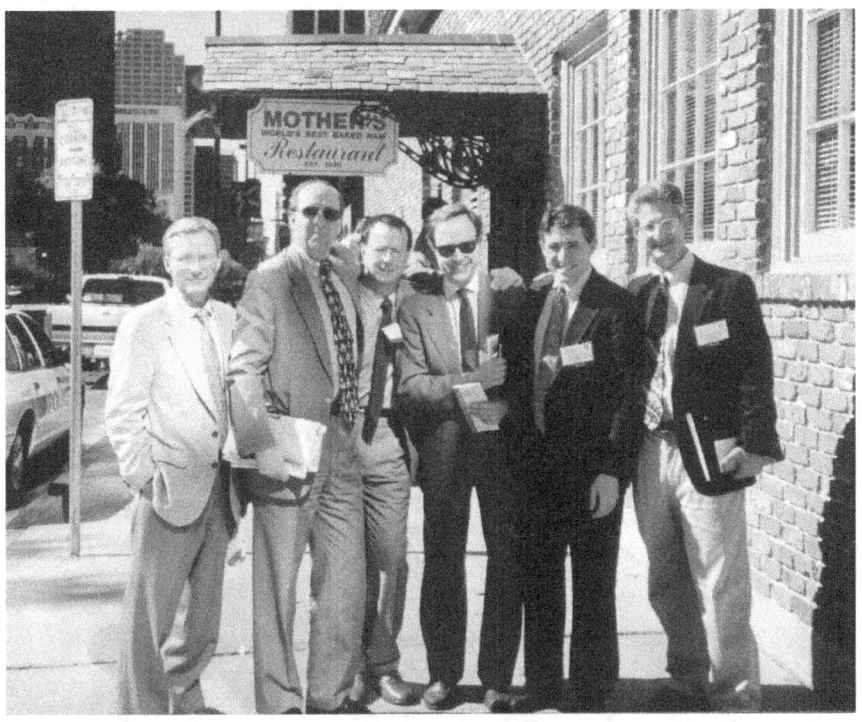

I am standing on the far left with four of the original five surgeons who first promoted TIP. Marty Koyle, another pediatric surgeon Emilio Merlini, Giantonio Manzoni, Tony Caldamone, and Rick Hurwitz. Missing is Richard Erlich.

◀ CHAPTER 2 ▶

You Have One Year to Become an Expert

The boy had proximal hypospadias; his meatus opening down on the shaft of the penis was a short distance above the scrotum. If hypospadias is uncommon, proximal cases are quite rare, found in just *one tenth of one half percent* of newborn boys. And this boy's case was even more unusual because, unlike most others with proximal hypospadias, his penis stood straight during erections.

Three and a half years after I did the first TIP to repair a distal hypospadias, I examined this patient in the office and did not consider that an option.

"Most likely, I'll do an onlay flap," I told the parents as I sketched a rough diagram of the procedure on the exam table paper.

That referred to the last of a troika of operations developed by John Duckett, the repair which sewed a rectangle of foreskin onto the urethral plate which seemed perfect for this occasion.

But after making the opening incisions, I examined the tissues again and worried the urethral plate was too narrow just below the glans.

"I think it might stricture here," I said to my nurse, Tracey Long, while my forceps tested the width.

"Maybe you should make that TIP incision in it," Tracy ventured.

I stretched the plate again; then I told her to hold the opposite side, took scissors, and made an incision through the narrowed region. Seeing it widen, I continued cutting up and down the entire plate just as I had in the first TIP repair until it looked the same—only three times longer. I smiled and then inserted a catheter, sewed the long plate into a tube with one continuous stitch zigzagging back and forth, covered the new urethra tissue from under the skin, sewed the glans together over this new urinary channel, and finished with a circumcision. Steps like a distal TIP, but done the first time for severe hypospadias.

Well, not *very* severe hypospadias, when one considers more extreme forms where the urine opening emerges between the scrotum and the anus, the penis curves down more than ninety degrees, and the testicles dangle beside the glans on either side.

Fortunately, no boys with perineal hypospadias came to me during the remaining five years of my Lubbock practice. In fact, I repaired only five more patients with any variety of proximal hypospadias during that time, which seemed a frustratingly small number. More than a decade would pass before the Board of Urology discovered that half of all the full-time pediatric urologists in the US operate on just one or two a year.

The penis was straight in one of those five boys. But the other four had varying degrees of chordee, meaning the penis bent down during an erection. I cannot say how much curvature they each had, since in those days no one I knew actually measured it. Nor did most surgeons give much thought to why the penis was bent, the word chordee efficiently lumping the various reasons into a single explanation.

The practical concern was how to make the bent penis straight. In the beginning, nineteenth century surgeons took their knives, cut right across the bend, and then removed "contracted structures" they imagined running under the skin from the hypospadias opening to the glans. They dissected down to the surface of the corpora, those paired erection cylinders that comprise most of the penis, and declared success when it was "clean and glistening white." The tissues they removed became known as chordee some fifty years later, when surgeons began using that word to mean both curvature and the structures they thought caused it.

Yet the most meticulous dissection might not suffice to make the penis straight. A few surgeons warned the penis could still be bent despite a thorough chordee excision, but their voices drowned in a sea of protests from others defending the common wisdom.

Not until 1974 was a way devised to simply check during surgery if the penis is straight. Looking back, it is surprising that it took so long for someone to poke a needle into one of the erection cylinders and inject saline, which then flows through internal connections into the other cylinder to make them both hard.

Using this artificial erection test, Duckett, a big Texan cut from the same boisterous cloth as John Wayne, proved the dogma passed through generations of surgeons wrong. Rather than straightening most bent penises, chordee excision left most of them still curved. Not only that, but he argued the presumedly scarred and contracted chordee tissues surgeons cut away were actually healthy and did not have to be removed. In fact, Duckett renamed the visible band extending from the hypospadias opening to the end of the glans the "urethral plate" and urged surgeons to keep and use it while making the new urinary channel.

But the penis still had to be straightened. If chordee on the surface of the erection cylinders did not restrict their expansion and cause the penis to bend, then the erection cylinders themselves were bent. Or, more precisely, the sheath enclosing the erectile tissues to make the penis hard developed shorter on the underside than on the topside. Other surgeons had reached this conclusion before Duckett and then considered the options. They could make the short side of the penis longer or the longer side of the penis shorter. Certainly, it seemed easier to pull the penis straight with a few stitches into its longer side. Reed Nesbit described that technique in the 1960s, and Duckett devised his own variation of "Nesbit plications" twenty years later to straighten the penis while conserving the urethral plate.

I followed Duckett's advice and did Nesbit plications in those four boys with proximal hypospadias and a bent penis that I operated on in Lubbock. After making their penises straight while keeping their urethral plates intact, I TIP-ed them too.

But they did not do so good. The entire wound pulled open in one boy, and another returned for follow-up obviously bent again. A third boy never came back for a checkup after surgery. I would eventually document that only one of the four had a good result.

It was difficult to place those results into perspective at the time. That handful of hypospadias repairs I did each year was diluted into a pool filled with several hundred other operations—those surgeries for stones, cancers, and enlarged prostates—that filled my schedule week to week. All I knew was that I was not doing enough to learn the limits of TIP repair. Someone was going to define those, but, if I stayed home in West Texas, it would not be me.

The phone rang in the operating room. I was in the middle of a case and could just hear the anesthesiologist explain to someone that Snodgrass was scrubbed and could not come to the phone. When I asked who called, he said he would tell me later.

I continued operating, doing something that must have been difficult for the anesthesiologist to not want to disturb my concentration. Finally, as I closed the wound, I asked again about the call.

"It was someone calling to tell you that a urologist you know named John Duckett just died."

"What? That's impossible!" I protested. "I skied with him just last week!"

But it was true. The giant of hypospadiology died suddenly. The surgeon whose three operations gave new ways to repair nearly any penis afflicted with the condition. The Duckett who conceived the MAGPI, that sleight of hand which easily moved the meatus and gave surgeons courage to start routinely repairing distal hypospadias. The same Duckett who perfected rolling a tube out of foreskin, and then used this transverse island flap to make the new urethra. The Duckett who next improved his own operation into a flat onlay island flap that he sewed onto the urethral plate as an alternative to the Mathieu flip-flap.

I often marveled that this one man confronted the many hypospadias repairs devised and revised by the many surgeons preceding him and, through the genius of his imagination and the force of his personality, reduced the field to just three operations.

His death left the Children's Hospital of Philadelphia without a plan for succession. While his colleagues attended to the myriad of details that mark a passing—the obituary, letters to his patients, an announcement to the world of pediatric urology, special messages to his closest friends, the funeral—behind the scenes the chairman of surgery weighed options for who would take the helm as the new chief of pediatric urology.

The title was soon granted to a junior faculty member promoted over others more senior. Some months later, the young chief Doug Canning leaned over to me just as a surgical video session began at a convention in Chicago and whispered, "Do you think we could get you to move to Philadelphia?"

It was a big ask. My family lived in Lubbock, and though my father could see retirement on the horizon, we had agreed he could still come to the office to drink coffee and see a few of his favorite patients as far into the future as he wished. In addition, I had already prepared for my own future, designing and building the dream house where I would finish raising my kids, and then, eventually, welcome the grandkids. Was TIP so important that I should leave all this, and the comfort of life in a small city, to move far away to a large city in the cold northeast?

"OK, Doug," I heard myself say when Canning called again a few days later.

"Really, Warren? That's great! Everyone in the group is excited to have you!" Canning nearly shouted into the phone. "I'll start making arrangements to get you up here to do the formal interviews." Then he added, in almost an afterthought, "I just need you to send me a copy of your CV."

I hung up the phone with a smirk. Of course, I did not have a CV, that chronicle of an academic career. No one in private medicine cared where I trained, or if I had ever published anything. I opened a drawer of my desk, found a blank sheet of paper, and scratched out a draft that my receptionist translated into type the next day.

That evening I faxed both sheets of my brand-new CV to Canning. Almost immediately the phone rang again.

"Warren, you left off your fellowship training."

"That's because I didn't do a fellowship."

There was a long pause on the other end. "But didn't you train with Edmond in Houston?"

"I did, but that was just residency. I never did a fellowship."

This time the pause stretched longer, before ending in a sigh.

"Well, let me see what I can do. But I'm not optimistic that I can get you credentialed at CHOP[13] without a fellowship."

---

13. The Children's Hospital of Philadelphia is commonly referred to as *CHOP*.

This proved to be true, although a glimmer of hope strung the conversation along for several frustrating months before it finally faded away.

A few weeks later I heard from Bill Strand, who heard from Canning that I might be available for a job in Dallas.

"OK, Bill, I'll interview there, but let's be clear up front that I didn't do a fellowship. Please don't fly me there to tell me you can't hire me because of that!"

But Bill, an amicable Midwesterner, thought that deficiency could be papered over, and arranged a visit. I arrived early one Friday morning and felt important seeing a chauffeur holding a sign with my name. Then I rode from the airport in a limo to find no one waiting for me at the entrance to the hospital, or in the surgery lounge where I was told to go. Strand was stranded in some operation, and so his guest, his potential partner, sat alone out of place in his suit as surgeons in scrubs strolled in and out. I wondered when a resident would appear to guide me on a tour of the hospital, and when the usual interviews were scheduled to begin. But I had no itinerary and so I sat and waited, watching the minutes tick into hours until, finally, the phone in the lounge rang and John McConnell's secretary asked if I was free for an early lunch.

I wandered alone on an uncertain path out of Children's, through a confusion of hallways deep inside Parkland Hospital,[14] and then down another passageway in a connected office building, asked someone in a white coat for directions, and finally reached the University Doctor's Dining Room. There the Urology Department Chairman, groomed and dressed impeccably, as always, pointed me to the buffet line.

I filled my plate and then sat down, but before I could take one bite, McConnell shook his head and said, "Warren, thanks for coming. I've given this a lot of thought, and I just don't think we can make it work for you here."

He held his gaze on me as he explained, "David Ewalt, you know him, he's in private practice, will go around to all the pediatricians and

---

14. *Parkland* is the county hospital where John Kennedy was taken after he was shot.

say something like, 'Yes, they have a new pediatric urologist. Interestingly, he never did a fellowship . . .'"

Meanwhile, Canning resumed his search, ultimately hiring away a pediatric urologist from Seattle. Which left that program short of faculty too late in the spring to hire a replacement, since, by then, all the graduating fellows already had jobs. But Mike Mitchell, the slender chief of that program, needed help, having already reduced his own workload after surviving a heart attack a few months earlier.

This time it was the hospital operator in Lubbock who found me for a call.

"Doctor, I'm going to patch through a Dr. Mitchell, who wants to speak to you."

"Warren. I hear you need a fellowship," he opened, straight to the point. "Mike Carr is taking a job at CHOP, which leaves me shorthanded. I could use your help this year and you could get your certificate."

And so on that Sunday morning in April, I learned I had two months to close twelve years of practice in Lubbock and fly to Seattle for the seal of approval needed to enter the world of pediatric urology.

A journey I would travel alone, since this stop in Seattle would only last one year before I would take a permanent position somewhere else. Virginia reassured me the family would survive my absence; the separation broken by a handful of visits.

"It'll be over before you know it."

That year, 1998, was filled with contradictions. I was officially a fellow, even though there was a fellow training there already. When Mitchell was in town, I was a trainee requiring supervision, but when Mitchell left town, I was promoted to senior faculty, supervising others. Despite that responsibility, I was paid a fellow's salary, the drastic cut in pay from my practice offset only in part by Mitchell's invitation to live downstairs in his house. Fellow, senior faculty, house guest, only the nurses at the children's hospital found no confusion in these alternating roles—reminding me one day that I needed someone more senior to approve the surgeries I scheduled in clinic, while not hesitating to post the operations I, as senior faculty, scheduled the very next day.

I arrived filled with anticipation for all the interesting cases I was going to see and then was surprised there was not so much work as I expected. I flew more than six hours and two time zones away from my family and my former practice to find I had more free time than the time scheduled in either the clinic or the operating room.

One afternoon a few weeks after starting, I sat in my office staring out the window into a steady drizzle wondering what to do with this surplus of time. Before there was Skype, I could only imagine my teenage daughter dressed in the bright red and yellow cheerleading outfit I saw her wear only once before flying away. Or my two sons tricking on their BMX bikes down ramps they built in the garage.

"What am I doing here?" I asked in a moment of doubt and self-pity, seeing this year stretching far longer than I had imagined.

Suddenly the door cracked open, and Mitchell, a reserved man who never seemed quite at ease, looked in.

"Warren, what're you doing?"

"Nothing, Mike. I don't have anything to do right now."

"Well, everyone sees you as a hypospadias expert. You have one year to read everything you can get your hands on to become that expert!"

And with his advice dispensed, Mitchell disappeared.

The internet was still in its infancy, and before there was a Google or a PubMed, I found information the traditional way, the same way I used nearly a decade earlier searching for an operation that resembled TIP. I read an article, studied the references, then tracked down those which seemed of interest, read them and their references, pulled another series of articles, and repeated the process over and over until the references ran dry. I copied the articles I thought important, starting a collection that rapidly grew to pack a large filing cabinet. It was tedious and time-consuming, but I was rich with free time.

What I really wanted was to do more hypospadias surgery. Although my number of distal repairs slowly increased from four or five a year when I was anxiously accumulating enough to write my manuscript, up to twelve the year I left for Seattle, I was certain this was only a fraction of what I would see in a fellowship training center. Besides, the number of proximal repairs had remained a stagnant one each year in Lubbock.

Yet, during my fellowship in Seattle I would still do only one distal operation each month, and just two proximal repairs all year, if I counted a hypospadias opening on the middle of the penis as proximal.

Nevertheless, I was grateful for that one true proximal case, which was fortuitously scheduled for me to repair in August just weeks after I arrived. I had been invited earlier that year to film a proximal TIP to show in a forum at a national meeting in October. But I had already operated on my one proximal case for that year, and all my worrying to find a second did not bring another patient before I left Lubbock.

As it happened Mitchell had spent the entire discretionary budget, and more, producing his own movie showing the bladder exstrophy repair he was known for. So, I had to work on a shoestring. I borrowed a digital video camera, then appointed a resident to film and literally sandbagged him at the foot of the OR table to steady his hands, since there was no tripod. I did the operation just inches away, somehow managing not to contaminate either the surgical field or the camera lens. Afterward, I took the digital tape downtown to an editing studio and was relieved to hear the cost for making the movie was less than $250.

But as lucky as I was to do that proximal repair, I would eventually learn more from my operation on the other boy, the one with a midshaft opening. I had just begun sewing the urethral plate into a tube when Mitchell slipped into the operating room, one of the very few times he came to observe me working. He stopped slightly behind and to the side, and then watched as I wove a suture back and forth, in and out of the urethral plate from one end to the other.

"You'll have fewer fistulas if you sew that in two layers," Mitchell said, matter-of-factly, and then retreated from the room as quietly as he had entered.

I glanced over my shoulder at the closing door, and then looked across the table at Chad Plaire, the official fellow assisting me.

"You don't have to do two layers," I whispered. "That takes longer, and I can't even remember the last time I saw a leak!"

As the year came to an end, Mitchell and I sat on his balcony looking over Lake Washington.

"I've been surprised at all the redo bladder exstrophy operations you do," I commented, leaving unsaid that I was also surprised we only saw one new baby with exstrophy during my stay.

"Yeah," Mitchell nodded, "everyone takes their shot and then sends the complications somewhere else."

We sat quietly for a moment.

"And that's what your life's going to be like, too, someday," he predicted.

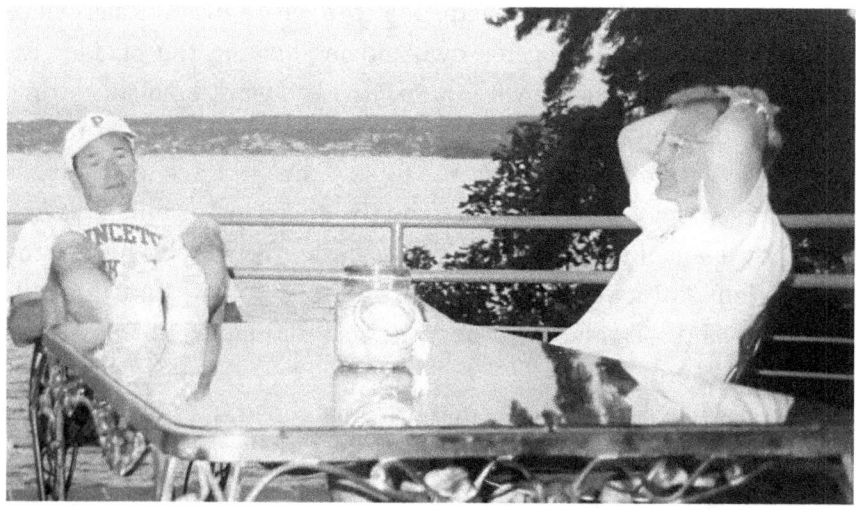

Relaxing with Mitchell on his back porch overlooking Lake Washington in Seattle, 1999.

◀ CHAPTER 3 ▶

You Could Put That Data into an Excel Spreadsheet

The trail that I followed out of Lubbock up to Seattle next looped all the way back down to Dallas. In one sense that seemed right, a Texan relocating to a place where he spoke with no accent and raised no eyebrows when he wore slacks over ostrich skin boots. Though my new home was 350 miles to the east, that was just an afternoon drive for fellow Texans, and I knew at least some of my patients would travel from Lubbock to the Children's Medical Center of Dallas to see me again.

Still, it was unusual that I left private practice and joined a university, weaving my way upstream through the exodus of doctors who usually flowed in the opposite direction. A few who had made that transition warned me what I already knew; I would make less money and forfeit some personal freedoms in the exchange. One colleague who had left another university for private practice sat in a hot tub after skiing in Telluride and listened as I described my plans. The altitude, the skiing, and now this news left him nearly breathless and only able to reply, "Warren, are you *crazy*?"

It was a surprise that it was Dallas. I first met UT Southwestern interviewing for medical school, a blind date that quickly went bad. I remember gathering with all the other candidates in a large auditorium early one Saturday morning, everyone dressed in their Sunday finest and trying to hide their jitters. After we all waited well past the scheduled start, a side door opened and the dean marched in. Without a glance toward his audience, he strode directly to a large blackboard, picked up a piece of white chalk, and wrote in big block letters, EXCEL-LENCE.

Only then did he turn to face us, waited while we absorbed this message, and then announced with a flourish, "If *this* isn't your goal, you're in the wrong place."

Somehow, I repressed an urge to stand up and walk out.

Four years later I returned there, this time to interview for urology residency. But I already had doubts about the small program with only three faculty, and immediately recognized the truth in the gossip that it was just one heart attack away from collapse when I met the portly Type A chairman.

Then there was that disastrous Friday a year earlier when I was invited to interview for a faculty position only to sit alone all morning waiting to be told they could not hire me. Yet here I was, a new associate professor at the UT Southwestern Medical Center. I accepted the position confident there would be enough work to keep me busy, and enough hypospadias surgery to make me the expert I was rumored to be. I also took the job because it was the only one I was offered; the market that year not searching for a mid-career pediatric urologist.

Nevertheless, I moved my family and arrived eager to begin a new life filled with learning, teaching, and writing. Enthusiasm that was only partly dampened by the official contract placed before me at the very last moment, a prenup ending in a no-compete clause that allowed the university to terminate my employment at anytime and for any reason and gave me, in return, the right to move my practice somewhere far away if they did.

McConnell quickly put everything into perspective when I objected. "Warren, if you don't sign it, you won't have a job."

Orientation followed. In the first weeks, experts from the administration instructed how they wanted me to bill for my services (to protect the university from the feds), how they expected me to enroll patients into research projects (to protect the university from HIPPA[15]), and how I should handle animals in the lab, should I ever do animal research (to protect the university from PETA).

---

15. The *HIPPA* Privacy Rule was created to protect personal health information.

But no experts from the university told me how best to mentor the medical students, residents, and fellows who would soon inhabit my world. No experts advised how to design my clinical research to answer questions my curiosity would ask. No one at the university suggested how I could improve my writing and my presentations to better convey discoveries I might make to colleagues.

I moved to the university knowing the lessons I taught trainees would impact patients that I would never see. With time, I also came to realize the errors I might teach would also carry into their practices, multiplying the harm. Yet no experts from the administration ever discussed ways for me or other professors to monitor our work to ensure it met the highest standards.

I wondered if the dean still scrawled EXCELLENCE across a blackboard.

Between these tutorials, I hauled boxes filled with paper charts from my old life into this new career, but the Children's Medical Center record system promptly rejected them all. The clinic nurses studied the situation and decreed my charts would have to be stored separately, filed in a cabinet sequestered in a storage room down the hall well away from the hospital's official records.

As I predicted, over the following months a steady trickle of patients journeyed from Lubbock to see me. Their old records were retrieved, and new ones were made coded with CMC's identity. My notes from these visits went into the new charts, duly filed into the clinic system for easy access at the next appointment. The Lubbock charts faced a less certain fate. Some returned to the security of the Lubbock file cabinet, while others lounged for a time on a nurse's desk, or hid under piles of forms in the clinic, or fell into the narrow crevasse between a trash can and the coffee machine. I caught glimpses of those prodigal charts as I walked through the clinic and worried the data they held would eventually be lost forever.

To this day I cannot remember who suggested the simple remedy of transferring the information from paper to computer. I asked for a laptop as part of my recruitment package, even though I had no idea what to use it for, and a nurse, a resident, or maybe a secretary, told me I could put that data into an Excel spreadsheet.

I sorted through the charts and made a stack of the ones that recorded hypospadias repairs. Then I opened Excel and pecked into the little boxes: the patient's name, his birthdate, surgery date, if he had distal or proximal hypospadias, whether it was a first repair or a reoperation, some technical details of the surgery, the date of his last postoperative follow-up, and if there was a complication such as a fistula, glans dehiscence, or a blockage from meatal stenosis or a stricture.

Although I typed slowly, having dropped a high school typing class because I could see no possible relevance for that skill years before computers arrived, the task was completed in an afternoon or two. I pushed back my chair and admired the work. With just a glance I could see how many patients with hypospadias I had operated, the severity of their condition, and if they had a complication afterward. Even the novice professor could sense the power of this data on the screen before me. I resolved to add the same information on new patients with hypospadias after I operated and when they returned to the clinic for follow-up.

Being a novice, and lacking guidance from the University, I filled that spreadsheet full of words. Readers who know better will immediately see the limitations this imposed. I could add up the total of patients and calculate their rate of complications, but as the numbers grew larger and I began to wonder *why* some developed a fistula or glans dehiscence while others did not, this database was unable to provide an answer.

Nearly a decade would pass before a fellow aspiring to become a hypospadiologist like me took that primitive spreadsheet and converted the words into the zeros and ones that computers speak, tediously dummy coding one little box at a time so that she could run logistic regression to find those answers.

Meanwhile, I also had to learn my way around the hospital, a task made more difficult because I could not even see it from the windows of the pediatric urology department on the top floor of the Bank One office tower maybe a half mile away. Strand promptly left town for Naval Reserve training the day I arrived, trusting me to care for his patients recovering from surgery. Of course, I had no idea where they were. So I called the chief resident and asked her to guide me on rounds to see them.

"I've already made rounds, Dr. Snodgrass," she curtly replied, abandoning me to find the patients myself.

I thought the residents rotating at Children's would be interested in my story, with its insights from years in private practice. But they already had a private practice mentor, and it was immediately made clear that they valued David Ewalt's guidance more than what their academic faculty had to say.

McConnell tried to prevent that fault line from developing as he organized the new pediatric urology group at the university. He recruited not only me, but also Linda Baker to start a research lab and Clanton Harrison to leave his nearby practice to create a four-faculty group led by Strand. But he could not persuade Ewalt, despite handing him a blank sheet of paper to list the terms of a deal. Finally, McConnell proposed a "virtual group" to include everyone, although in two separate practices sharing call and resident teaching.

Not surprising, town/gown[16] frictions arose from the outset, made worse when I insisted the university group adopt private practice ways, such as having the faculty, rather than trainees, answer calls after hours from worried mothers.

"It's the right thing to do," I explained a third time to my new partners. "Residents don't know how to answer their questions and so they call us, and then they have to call the parents back, and maybe us again, going back and forth, and things can get confused or overlooked in all that. We can cut straight to the chase if the calls just come to us first." Which finally convinced them but not the contentious Ewalt, who protested vigorously when the residents stopped screening his calls. He coerced the page operators at the hospital to restore the old system until his subterfuge was discovered.

During all this, I also had to adjust my routine to operate with residents. Fortunately, since I am left-handed and nearly all the trainees were right-handed, we each stood on the side of the table that felt comfortable to do the surgery. But nearly everything else was different. In private practice I operated with my father providing experienced help,

---

16. *Town* refers to private practice doctors, while *gown* are those in academic practice.

or with my nurse giving obedient help. I soon discovered that residents were neither experienced, nor always concerned to retract something or hold something steady or cut something exactly as I instructed.

And they always wanted to do more than I wanted them to do. Even if they had never seen the operation, some expected their faculty teacher to talk them through the steps while they wielded the scalpel or guided the scissors, convinced they were not learning if they were not handling sharp instruments.

Once, during my first year on faculty, a senior resident informed me before surgery to lower a testicle born too high, "Dr. Snodgrass, the group I'm joining does orchiopexies. So, I think *I* should do this case while you watch, and then you can critique me afterward."

Though amazed by his chutzpah, there was no way I was going to turn over responsibility for an operation and stand by observing while a trainee practiced. Which left me irritated with the resident, and the resident irritated with me.

I wrestled with this dilemma throughout that first year, remembering that the gulf between my skills and the basic abilities of trainees was one of the main reasons I once declined a life of academic surgery. How much of an operation could I allow a resident to do before teaching encroached on the obligation to do my best for the child?

I recalled times from my own residency when the scales tipped askew, like the day a faculty surgeon asked his fellow if he had ever seen a Mustarde hypospadias repair? When he replied he had not the decision was made—not because it was the best operation for that boy, especially not *that* operation known for its tendency to scar at the meatus, but only so the trainee could see something he had not seen before.

On another day, my mentor took one look at the OR schedule and wailed that his secretary had scheduled three circumcisions in a row! But then a sudden inspiration to do each operation differently, like a chef preparing shrimp three ways, restored purpose to his work. That day I learned the best way to do a circumcision, but the other two boys were left with erratic scars winding around their penises for life.

After a year of this struggle to do the best for patients while instructing trainees, I asked the department chairman to explain the goal of teaching residents pediatric operations that most would never do again.

"To help them become better surgeons," McConnell replied, without hesitation. "We can always see the difference after a resident rotates on peds. They come back more exact and delicate."

And this I could accept, granting trainees the least demanding parts of an operation to teach them how to operate better. Like making the skin incision precisely with a small scalpel lightly pressed along the line I marked, because every surgeon has to learn how much pressure to apply so that the knife will penetrate the skin but not gash important structures underneath. And later sewing that incision closed with a needle the size of an eyelash placed exactly under the surface, because every surgeon should remember that the scar is what the patient will see forever.

Years later a survey was published confirming that colleagues around the US did much the same, at least during hypospadias repairs, generally limiting residents to opening and closing the wounds.[17] But no one explained this when I arrived at the university, and I grew increasingly anxious that in so many ways I did not fit into this strange new world.

Naturally, these problems went home with me at night. The chief residents who even McConnell admitted were a surly lot, the growing pains of the new group learning to work together, my expectations crashing against the realities of academia, David Ewalt. All new troubles I brought upon myself by leaving my former practice. My wife soon tired of these stories, since it seemed their telling lightened my burdens by shifting them to her.

"Don't you have any *funny* stories from work you can tell me?" Virginia asked one evening.

I looked at her and answered, "I don't work in a funny place."

Then another task came to me without instructions. The chairman summoned me to his office.

Warren, I've decided to make a change in the chief position," McConnell began. "The pediatric group needs new leadership."

I knew my colleagues agreed, though the department chairman did not need our approval.

---

17. "Training Residents in Hypospadias Repair: Variations of Involvement" was published by the *Journal of Urology* in 2008.

"So, I'm curious, who would you choose if you were in my shoes?"

And now the trap was set. I thought through the options and saw no escape.

"Well, you could put Linda in charge."

"Yes, and what do you think about that?"

"That she's too young; she's only been out of fellowship two years, and she's too busy trying to get her lab established."

"That was my thought too."

"Or you could make Clanton chief," I suggested, without conviction, adding before McConnell did, "But he's part time and doesn't want to work that hard."

"That's true," McConnell nodded. "Other thoughts?"

I shrugged my shoulders.

"You could do a national search for a new chief."

"And how do you think that would go?"

"I think you'd probably end up hiring someone from Boston who'd make us all stay in the office until late at night trying to look busy."

McConnell laughed. "Yes, that would be a risk."

Then we sat quietly, taking each other's measure. I finally looked away, and then shook my head at the future I could not escape.

"Dammit, John. I don't want this job."

◀ CHAPTER 4 ▶

I'm Not as Good as I Thought

It was only a matter of time before a boy came into my clinic with proximal hypospadias too severe for a TIP repair. Not because the meatus was too low down on the shaft, but because the penis was too bent to straighten with plications shortening its longer side. I did not see this type of severe hypospadias in either Lubbock or Seattle, and I was not sure how I would repair it when I finally did at Children's. I may have moved to Dallas to find the boundaries of TIP, but hypospadias that fell outside those still had to be fixed.

Certainly, I was not going to do another plication and Duckett transverse island. Not after a very traumatic experience when that repair, which rolled the foreskin into a tube connected to the hypospadias opening, made complications demanding urgent attention almost as soon as the catheter was removed. Apparently, other surgeons were having similar troubles with that operation. I heard murmurs that some of them were turning back to Byars flaps, a 1950s technique I did not see during training and did not have a chance to learn before I flew off to Istanbul.

"Sherif, I don't think we should do this case tomorrow," I declared after a brief examination.

I was beginning to realize that hosts often save their most difficult patients, like this boy with perineal hypospadias, to challenge a visiting professor.

"Why not, professor?" Sherif Ekter asked with a frown. "The audience very much wants to see you do this operation."

"Because I have no special expertise for this degree of hypospadias," I replied. "In fact, I'm sure there will be some in the audience who have much more experience with this than I do!"

Disappointment spread across Ekter's face as I explained, "I can't do a TIP because of the chordee. So, I think we should focus this course on distal repairs to show how versatile TIP is for the most common type of hypospadias."

"But professor, we only have one case of distal hypospadias, plus this one. Everyone will be very disappointed if you don't show us how you do it," Ekter protested, ending the debate.

That night I tossed and turned in bed, visions of demonstrating the Byars flap operation I hardly knew playing over and over in my restlessness. I was confident I could split the hood of foreskin[18] on the top of the penis and move the two strips of skin that created around to the underside to eventually make the urethra. The problem was straightening the curvature, which was the most severe I had ever encountered. Although Duckett taught that nearly all curvature could be made straight with one or several plications shortening the longer side of the penis, this boy, whose penis bent at least ninety degrees, really needed the shorter side of his penis made longer.

I tried to coax images of that ventral lengthening from my past, but found no memory of having seen the maneuver during residency in Houston and knew it was fruitless to search my recollections from Lubbock or Seattle. All I could remember were drawings in articles I had read, copied, and then filed in a cabinet standing thousands of miles away.

I lay in bed imagining the incision I would make across the bend in the erection cylinders so they would straighten, and the tissue I would take from under the skin in the groin through a second incision to patch over it. But the details would not come into focus. How wide should I make the incision across the corpora? How large should I harvest the patch to account for it possibly shrinking? How could I be certain that I made the penis straight, and what would I do if it still was not?

---

18. The foreskin is typically absent on the underside of the penis with hypospadias, leaving a partial *hood* on the topside.

There was little sleep for me that night, and no appetite for breakfast the next morning.

Ekter waited anxiously at the entrance to the hospital, and immediately tugged me back into the exam room to look at the patient again. God blesses the pure in heart, and the boy we examined just last evening arrived for surgery with his genitals covered by an angry red rash—a plague sent to protect, rather than punish.

"Sherif, I'm so sorry, but we obviously can't do this operation today, not with the skin infected with yeast," I said, feigning disappointment as I closed the diaper.

I flew back to Dallas, and more than a year passed before I examined another boy with a proximal hypospadias that I thought needed ventral lengthening and a Byars flap repair. In the meantime, there were another eight that I straightened with a plication and did a proximal TIP. Here was the volume of cases that moved me from Lubbock, but more time had to pass before they had sufficient follow up to see if these operations worked. In the meantime, when a mom asked what the chances were that her son would have a fistula or some other complication after a proximal TIP, I had no idea. So, I extrapolated from other operations and guesstimated 30 percent.

I was shocked when my database finally announced in 2002 that *over half* my proximal TIPs had some type of complication that needed more surgery, including fistulas in one out of every three of them. I really had no idea.

The natural reaction was to protest the figures staring at me from the computer screen, but they remained stubbornly unchanged after I double-checked the tally. I looked away and visualized the operation step by step, seeing my single-layer closure of the urethra stitched the same way I had learned for transverse island repairs and then covered by a blanket of dartos tissues.[19]

Then I recalled Mitchell's advice that day in the OR to sew the urethral plate with two layers of stitches and realized the dartos that covered over it afterward did not protect against sins committed while

19. *Dartos* is the name of tissues under the skin of the penis.

sewing the edges together. Faced with proof of my own mistake, I now resolved to change. Furthermore, I decided the closure would be more exact if I interrupted the first layer—meticulously, tediously, placing and tying one stitch at a time to constantly adjust for subtle variations along the two edges of the plate. Then I would run the second layer over those to ensure the new urethra was watertight.

I inserted additional columns into my spreadsheet to record these technical changes. Having modified the operation, I then used the new method for every subsequent proximal TIP. But another five years passed before there were enough cases to determine if those changes worked. Once again, I scrolled down the database counting the patients and the number of fistulas to calculate the rate had dropped to only 10 percent.

But 10 percent was still a lot—five times more leaks than after my distal TIPs. During this time I also noticed the dartos laid over the urethra in proximal operations was often a little thin, and I wondered if that allowed some leaks to burrow their way through to the surface. Then I remembered an article I once read describing a different blanket created from tissue near the testicles. It was not much more effort to dissect this tunica vaginalis from its attachments and then swing it over onto the penis. This cover certainly appeared more robust than dartos so I resolved to use it instead, adding one new column to the database to track results.

The next time I searched I could not find a single fistula. Not only that, but my overall complications were also much less, falling from the original 54 percent down to a much more respectable 13 percent.

A lecture at a national congress in 2008 affirmed my growing reliance on data, even when it argued against what I thought was right. I recall the large conference hall was not quite large enough to comfortably accommodate all the delegates, leaving me a seat in the middle of the back row when I made my way in after a coffee break. I did not much care, assuming the title "Trauma Lessons From the Second Gulf War" promised little more than twenty minutes of slides showing mangled genitals cobbled back together.

I watched with mild amusement as a nearby door opened and an army officer in full dress uniform marched briskly down the center aisle and decisively up the stairs to the speaker's lectern. I slouched low in my seat, barely able to see the screen at the front of the auditorium.

The colonel began. "Contrary to what we've been taught, whole blood transfusions are better than packed cells and platelets."

Well, that's interesting, I had to admit, since I, and likely everyone else in the audience, had been taught the opposite during trauma rotations in residency. I sat up some and craned my neck to see better.

The colonel moved on to his next example. "Contrary to what we've been taught," he repeated, "tourniquets save lives on the battlefield. The data are so convincing that now all American and British soldiers carry them in their backpacks."

He gave more illustrations, and then drew the bigger picture.

"MASH units started during the Second World War. Everyone knows them from the TV show about the Korean conflict, but we used them in Vietnam, the First Gulf War, and still do today."

He advanced through slides showing an evolution from tents to Quonset huts to complete mobile hospitals, a transition from stretchers balanced on sawhorses to modern operating tables, and from postoperative recovery in open wards to fully equipped surgical ICUs.

"Despite these technologic advances," Colonel Holcomb continued, "25 percent of the soldiers who arrived alive to a MASH unit died from their injuries in WWII, in Korea, in Vietnam, and in the first Gulf War." He advanced the slide again. "But today we've managed to significantly reduce that to just 10 percent. Today a soldier who arrives alive has a 90 percent chance of leaving alive."

Now I sat bolt upright, looking from the slides to the officer with silver birds pinned to his shoulders and rows of multicolored ribbons covering his heart. But my mind flashed back to the memory of "Taps" played every evening over loudspeakers scattered across the air force base where my father served, bringing my baseball games to a halt. And to images from college of the Fightin' Band from Aggieland marching through the same half-time show in the same brown uniforms and tall brown boots every time their team came to Lubbock. And to those precisely sharpened pencils lined up in descending order of length I happened to see in the drawer of a fellow medical student discharged from the service. And to the stories a few of my older classmates told of slithering down into booby-trapped tunnels in Vietnam only because they were ordered to slither down into booby-trapped tunnels even when it was known that the cause was lost. I could not fathom how the tradition-bound military of my youth was now innovating its way to saving lives. How could that be?

"A datasheet is filled out for every single injury, and then entered into a database," Holcomb explained, apparently anticipating my question. "Once a week we link with the battlefield surgeons to review what they are doing and how that's working. If something's not getting good results, we change it and then measure if that does better."

In the chaos of the battlefield, the army had found—no, *made*—time to collect and enter data in real time. The colonel described how in the past this information was collected haphazardly and was then filed away and forgotten in storage unless someone decided to excavate it, whatever lessons it held otherwise lost for years, if not forever. Without data, dogma took hold, like those "expert" opinions dictating that transfusing red blood cells, platelets, and plasma separately was somehow better than the whole blood that soldiers bled. From conflict to conflict over more than fifty years, wounded soldiers were treated in the best way known at the time, yet the best way was not really known. As a result, some died who could have been saved.

"We're able to make these changes because everything we do is driven by data," Colonel Holcomb concluded.

Why don't we do that? I wondered, looking around at my colleagues applauding the colonel.

I thought about my journey with proximal TIPs. How, like the army, I collected data as I worked, entered it into a database, and then reviewed it to see how I was doing. And how, like the army, I changed from the dogma I was taught to the lessons my data proved.

I shook my head at the picture of all those piles of files dumped into storage after a war and saw they resembled the stacks of charts residents are routinely tasked to review. How they struggle to decipher handwriting impossible to read and try not to get frustrated by confusing notes or important information found missing. How the trainees end up knitting together bits and pieces, filling in the gaps, fudging a point or two, all to bring order to disorder so they can write a retrospective review looking backward at what they think was done that concludes a prospective study is needed to accurately capture the facts that answer what should be done.

I realized this process that Holcomb described could be summarized as *Prospective* data collection (to be sure information is recorded accurately), *Periodic* review (to know the results sooner), and *Practice* changes (to do better). I laughed that I and my fellow pee-pee doctors could become 3P surgeons, committed to our own quality improvement.

I added this idea to my lectures and started preaching the 3Ps around the world, using my own example from proximal TIPs to show how it worked and helped the boys I operated. The message was always the same. Whenever I reviewed my own work I learned, "I'm not as good as I thought." I let that confession sink into the audience accustomed to braggart visiting surgeons touting their superior skills. Then I would bring up the next slide, "But I can get better!"

Sometimes I would add, looking directly at the surgeons looking at me, "You're not as good as you think either . . . but you can get better too."

◄ CHAPTER 5 ►

I Had a Dream

───────────────

He was scheduled as a new patient, but when I walked into the exam room, Mom reminded me, "We met in Seattle. You helped Dr. Mitchell with Craig's operation."

I immediately recalled that surgery, Mitchell devising a flap to repair a hypospadias that had already defied several flap repairs. I studied the tiny meatus encased in dense scar where the urine struggled to escape. There was no other choice but to operate again.

Nearly twenty years later I do not remember the details of that operation, except that I made my own version of a skin flap which must have resembled the four previous ones done by four other pediatric urologists that all ended in meatal stenosis. Mine fared better, but only because the entire wound fell apart all the way back to the opening he had at birth, though leaving it large enough to pee through.

"Well, at least he doesn't have meatal stenosis now," I shrugged, looking for something positive amid so much discouragement.

I lingered in the exam, analyzing the wound from every perspective, trying to recall, or conjure up, a different remedy.

"It's time to quit operating on your son," I finally declared, folding my arms decisively across my chest. "He's had five operations by five pediatric urologists who've all done basically the same thing. I don't know anything different to do, and I don't know anyone else who has a better idea, either."

Then I unfolded my arms and put both hands into the pockets of my slacks.

"But he can pee, so there's no urgency to do something. I'll call you if I hear anything new that might work."

I saw the burden fall from Mom's shoulders and realized I had just freed her from continuing her fruitless quest for a surgeon and an operation to heal her son.

Soon after that I noticed a postcard in the mail announcing a live-surgery workshop in Italy. I glanced at it and started to toss it into the trash. But then I saw that it advertised the same workshop that Koyle and Duckett flew off to the day after my speech describing TIP to that congress of pediatric urologists more than five years earlier. The workshop where Duckett was rumored to have said, "This new TIP operation is so simple it's going to ruin hypospadias surgery!"

Of course, I had to attend.

A few weeks later I got a response from Gianantonio Manzoni, the event organizer and one of the surgeons who pooled their results for my speech.

"Warren, if you're going to come, you have to be part of the faculty!" meaning I would give a lecture and do an operation or two for an audience of maybe 150 surgeons.

I thought if Manzoni, who I barely knew, really wanted me on the faculty, he would have invited me to be on the faculty. So I wrote back that I was content to sit at the rear of the auditorium and watch others operate.

But Manzoni insisted.

I was shown to a seat reserved on the front row as Aivar Bracka began his lecture. We had never met, but I had read his article advocating two operations to repair every hypospadias, even the most distal ones opening on the glans. I tossed the journal aside, thinking at the time, *And that's why plastic surgeons shouldn't do hypospadias repairs!*

Bracka, tall and lean with close-cropped graying hair, looked over an audience of skeptical urologists and outlined his argument. The dominant limb of hypospadias surgery creates the new urethra from a skin *flap*, a rectangle of skin left attached to the penis. The scores of operations described over more than a century of surgical trial and error were mostly variations of flaps tailored from the foreskin and swung to the underside of the penis, or raised from the penile shaft near the meatus.

Duckett's transverse island rolled the foreskin into a tube and connected one end to the natural channel, while the other became the new meatus on the glans. Byars flaps followed the same principle but took two operations to do it. For more distal hypospadias, the Mathieu made a rectangle of skin that was flipped up and over the abnormal meatus to supplement the urethra plate.

Meanwhile, a separate lineage used *grafts* to make the urethra, completely detaching the foreskin from the topside of the penis, and its blood supply, and then sewing it back onto the underside. New blood vessels had to grow into the graft, and when that process was complete months later, the foreskin was rolled into the urethral tube.

It seemed unquestionable that preserving the blood supply to a flap would be more reliable than trusting new blood vessels to grow into a graft. And that self-evident truth became the dogma for generations of urologists, who spent their creative energies devising new ways to transform the same skin into different flaps.

Through the eyes of plastic surgeons, however, it was these skin flaps that urologists made which had an uncertain blood supply. Especially at either end, where there were fewer blood vessels. And that meant urologists created new urethras at risk to make strictures where they joined the normal channel and meatal stenosis where they ended on the glans—two problems rarely encountered using grafts.

Bracka sliced to the core of this long-standing debate, speaking his British accent with a slow precision that gave his comments an air of superiority.

"We do not need a MAGPI and a Mathieu, a GAP and an Arap, or a transverse island and an onlay flap. Every hypospadias can be repaired by the two-stage graft technique," explaining how the urethral plate was removed and replaced with a foreskin graft sewn down flat on the penis during the first operation, and then rolled into the urinary channel at the second once new blood vessels had grown in.

Facing the audience, Bracka continued. "Two-stage grafts have few complications, and make a normal meatus—like this one," he said, laser pointing at a photo of a normal-looking teenage penis. Then he advanced another slide. "In exchange for the convenience of a one-stage repair, Duckett flaps make a meatus resembling the puckered arse of a cat!" which, fortunately, he illustrated with a cartoon and not an actual photograph.

Bracka's lecture then moved in traditional fashion from first-time repairs to redo surgeries, as he again extolled the wonders of two-stage grafts. How the surgeon could remove battle-scarred wounds from prior failures and replace them with a healthy strip of tissue from inside the cheek. How he did not have to worry about the nearly choked-off blood supply to a flap fashioned from previously operated skin. How the surgeon could make a penis weary from failure stand proud.

That article I once cast aside said all this, but I did not hear it. Now as I listened and watched, I remembered the boy with several failed flaps and the promise I made to his mother. As Bracka spoke, I pictured that boy's scarred penis with its meatus down on the shaft causing frustration every time he tried to pee standing, and threatening more despair in the future when a lover wished to see it. Now I had found the "new" idea I told Mom was needed before operating again. It had been there all along.

I was not the only urologist slow to hear Bracka's message. There was another boy suffering after a flap repair who was scheduled for reoperation as part of this workshop. X-rays of his urethra showed a twisting, turning passageway leading to a tight exit, a perfect illustration of the imperfect blood supply at the meatus that Bracka had just warned was the downfall of these flaps. But the plastic surgeon was an outsider among urologists, and Manzoni assigned his own mentor to this task.

I stood in the OR watching that well-known surgeon fashion a Duckett onlay flap to rescue the Duckett transverse island flap done earlier, just as Mitchell, and I, had made flaps to save another flap. I knew this operation would fail too.

And, in that moment, I decided I was done with flaps.

"I told you I would call if I found a new idea to help your son," I reminded Mom over the phone. "I just got back from a meeting in Italy, and a plastic surgeon talked about redo operations for situations like his."

"So what would you do?" she asked me a few days later at the clinic.

I explained how I would cut out all the scarred tissues and replace them with a graft taken from inside her son's mouth.

Mom nodded as I spoke, as though she understood each point. When I finished, she immediately asked, "When can we schedule it?"

"Well, we can look," I answered, and reached for my scheduling book.

"Let's do it as soon as you can," she insisted.

I considered this for a moment, hesitated, and then looked back to her.

"It seems you're kind of in a hurry to do this."

"Well, yes, I just want to get it over with."

I thought about that for another moment.

"But I just told you that I've never done this operation before. I haven't even seen it before! Maybe you should fly to England and have that surgeon who's done hundreds of these do it."

"No," she replied firmly, "You can schedule it."

While I flipped through the calendar searching for a time, she stared beyond me into the recent past.

"Last week I had a dream that you were going to call and tell me you found a way to fix my Craig. I woke up and felt such a peace . . . I can't really describe it . . . and a feeling that, if you called, I should just say yes, that everything would work out fine."

My skin crawled as she spoke, and to this day I break into goosebumps whenever I tell this story. But the operation healed her son, the first of many hundreds I would help using it.

Maybe there were other signs of divine intervention at that workshop in Italy. Was it only an accident that I happened to see that postcard in a stack of junk mail? Could it only be coincidence that Bracka was invited and agreed to attend this gathering of urologists?

When I stood to speak, Bracka saw my pictures of penises made normal by TIP and realized his two-stage repair was no longer needed for distal hypospadias to avoid a cat's-puckered-arse meatus. We explored the intricacies of each other's repairs while sightseeing together the day after the meeting. Then he returned to England converted to distal TIP while I flew back to Texas convinced to try two-stage grafts.

◀ CHAPTER 6 ▶

I Can't Visit Everywhere Three Times!

Two months after arriving in Dallas, I flew away to Sweden on my first official trip as a visiting professor, invited to another institution to lecture and demonstrate surgery. But, since I was new at the university and had accrued no vacation time, special approval was required from the department chairman to stay one extra day for sightseeing before flying all the way back home again. Yes, there were administrators who checked such details.

My host, Goren Lackgren, emailed asking what instruments and sutures I would need for the two operations they planned. I read through their list of supplies and made a few additions that I emailed back. Since I am left-handed, and had learned that not all scissors cut the same for me, I decided to take my own tenotomies.

However, when I saw their hypospadias kit laid out on the Mayo stand[20] in the operating room, I instantly realized that "delicate" tissue forceps and "fine" sutures translate quite differently among surgeons. There was almost nothing in their setup that I would ever use. If the goal of a visit is to show surgeons who could not easily travel to Dallas what they would see if they did, it was apparent that the next time I would have to bring the instruments and sutures I normally used.

Both the boys had distal hypospadias, and it happened, by chance, that the first was the child of an immigrant family that wanted him circumcised. I took a surgical marking pen and drew the usual blue line

20. The *Mayo stand* is a flat tray positioned over the operating table where surgical instruments are laid until the scrub tech hands them to the surgeon.

going around the penis in a circle a half-inch below the glans. Then I started the incision, checking that it showed on the closed-circuit TV linked to a conference room where the audience watched.

Immediately, agitated, thickly accented voices poured through speakers and filled the operating room as a stampede of surgeons jostled for the microphone to question me.

"Professor, why are you making that incision?"

"Why are you cutting on the top of the penis?"

"Is this the usual skin incision you make?"

I tried to answer, but it seemed that only added to the confusion. I could not imagine why there were so many questions about this basic first step.

"This is the standard incision," I explained, and then repeated several times before finally adding in exasperation, "If y'all have this many questions about the *skin incision*, I don't think we'll have time to finish the operation!"

My host spoke something in Swedish that calmed the storm. I was relieved to move on to the next step and began peeling the skin down the shaft of the penis. But the voices returned, as loud, and as urgent, and as difficult to understand as before. The TV showed only my hands, so the audience did not see me shake my head and frown, puzzled, and growing frustrated. *I'm just degloving!*[21] I wanted to shout back at the rabble.

The furor finally subsided as I pushed on toward more important steps. The monitor assured me they could see what I was doing, and I spoke slowly to help them understand my drawl. Now the surgery flowed smoothly with only a few more comments from the audience, and was soon finished. I followed Lackgren out of the OR to meet the second patient, still wondering about that initial flurry of questions.

The next family was Swedish and wanted their son to have a natural penis. I told Lackgren that he would have to show me how to save and repair the foreskin since I had never seen the foreskin reconstructed.

After the boy was anesthetized, we adjusted the operating lights and again checked that the camera was centered on the operative field.

---

21. *Degloving* is peeling the skin down toward the base of the penis to gain access to the inside structures.

Then Lackgren marked lines for the skin incision, and the mystery of the first case was solved. There were no questions from the surgeons watching what was familiar to them: a skin incision making a V along the edges of the foreskin and down the underside of the penis, rather than a circle around the glans I made for a circumcision.

I laughed to myself how the situation would be reversed if I started a hypospadias repair the Swedish way with a room full of American urologists watching!

Without distractions from the skin incision, the surgeons in the conference room focused more intently on the actual TIP repair and now asked the questions I expected. As I would do in live surgeries for years to come, I explained where to draw lines to define the urethral plate, showed how to hold the edges of the plate apart while making the TIP incision deep into it, and emphasized where to put the first stitch to tubularize the plate without narrowing the end. Then I sewed it into a tube keeping the needle just under the surface to reduce the chance for a fistula.

Normally, I would raise a blanket of dartos from under the foreskin on the topside of the penis to cover the new urinary channel, but I could not easily reach there through this incision. So I skipped that step and moved on to stitch the glans together.

"Goren, you'll have to close the skin," I reminded my host, and then watched him finish the foreskin repair.

"That's fabulous," the visiting expert declared at the end, pleased to have learned something new himself.

I carried that lesson back to Dallas. From that time on I asked parents what they originally planned for their newborn son, and then repaired the foreskin or did the circumcision they wanted. I was surprised how many preferred their sons to look natural. Once I began offering foreskin reconstruction, one out of every five families requested it.

Doing it that often I discovered there was dartos available to lay over the new urethra to prevent fistulas. I just had to dissect a millimeter closer to the skin on the underside of the penis to access it. That soon became routine, which also made that step easier in boys to be circumcised.

Later, when a tempest arose from surgeons convinced that the price for this vanity was more complications, I searched through my database and wrote a paper showing the numbers of fistulas and glans dehiscences were the same whether the operation concluded with circumcision or a foreskin repair. When others speculated there had to be more skin problems when the foreskin was reconstructed, I replied that very few boys needed the skin revised whether they were circumcised or made to look natural.

When a few colleagues agreed on these points but worried the repaired foreskin did not always look natural, I adjusted the technique to make it look better. When some declared the repaired foreskin would not work properly when the boy matured during puberty, I showed examples of it working just fine in teenagers and challenged them to show their proof to the contrary.

I may have paid my dues that year in Seattle to join their society, but I remained very much an outsider. Few surgeons have their own data to bring to a debate, and some resented that I did—even though anyone could start their own database. For my part, I enjoyed the vigor of the exchange, hearing different perspectives and polishing my responses, all the while thinking innocently, and wrongly, that we debaters could laugh together over a beer afterward.

Meanwhile, I smiled at the irony that a urologist from the land of routine circumcision traveled to Europe and Latin America and Asia, where circumcision is much less common, encouraging surgeons to repair the foreskin in their patients. Because it is no laughing matter for those boys to have their hypospadias fixed and still look different from everyone else. I learned to do it and did not understand why others refused to. As it turned out, Sweden was one of the few countries in the world I visited where surgeons routinely reconstructed the foreskin. Most urologists in most other countries preferred to cut off that skin without a thought of the consequences that a naked glans might have in a locker room of boys with covered ones.

At the opposite end of my university career I planned another trip to learn something new, inviting myself to Japan to watch an operation I did not think should work: a graft repair done in one stage.

I frequently gave witness to the miracles of grafts, but done as plastic surgeons taught: first sewing them flat onto the penis, and then waiting until new blood vessels grew in before rolling them into a tube six months later.

In fact, during my year in Seattle, I read a 1940s account of a graft that was harvested and rolled into a tube in a one-stage repair. When Graham Humby, a pediatric surgeon working in London during the Blitz, removed the bandages, he saw that half the tube had died, while the part resting against the penis lived. Although he did not realize it, Humby's experiment proved that grafts should be placed flat to reliably gain the vascularity they need before they are tubularized.

But then I read a manuscript that described taking and rolling a graft during the same operation, successfully.

"I just want to see how you do it," I explained to my friend, Kaoru Yoshino. "Because it doesn't make sense to me."

"It works!" Yoshino insisted. "I showed you our data."

"Yes, you did, and that's why I need to see you do it!"

She looked down. "I don't think we can invite you to watch us operate."

I let the matter rest, sensing her refusal was a sign of respect.

But I would not be deterred.

"Kaoru, it will be an honor to visit your hospital and watch you operate. We can all learn from each other," I wrote her in what grew into a chain of emails back and forth over the following months, as I tried to nudge her, politely, until it was no longer polite for her to refuse.

Then I faced another hurdle.

"The university will not pay for this trip," Jimmy Loftin, the Urology Department Manager, declared when I submitted the routine paperwork.

"Why not?" I asked. "It's an academic visit."

Jimmy shook his head no.

Making no headway, I added, "I want to learn a new operation *to help patients here.*"

"I understand, and I'm sure it's worthwhile," Loftin replied. "But if you want it paid for, the Japanese will have to do that. Even then, with the new university rules, the chairman will still have to approve your time away."

And that struck a raw nerve.

"I've already told Claus[22] that reducing my travel is not going to make me work any harder," I complained, "given the fact that, despite my time away, I still earn more than double what I'm getting paid!"

Searching for an end to this conversation, the manager advised, "Really, the best way for you to do this is to use your vacation time."

I arrived a few minutes late to the operating theater, distracted by the Rube Goldberg handwash system whose doors opened and closed in a precise sequence to first deliver a pick to clean under my nails, then a hand brush followed by an exact portion of cleanser, a rinse for my soapy hands, a last coating of sanitizer, and finally, gusts of air just sufficient to dry. I was so amused that I washed my hands twice.

Yoshino already had the case underway, assisted by her mentor, Saboru Tanakazi, who returned from retirement for this event. When she realized I was watching, the lead surgeon's hands began to shake.

I sensed her embarrassment and leaned over to say, just loud enough for all the young surgeons gathered around the table to hear, "I have a tremor, too, in my left hand of all places. Mine annoys me enough to take Inderol[23] before I operate."

Her hands soon steadied.

They degloved the penis and Tanakazi injected saline to check for the downward curvature most boys with proximal hypospadias have. As expected, the penis bent as it grew firm. Yoshino cut across the urethral plate and then dissected it a short distance toward the scrotum. Tanikaze injected again, and I was surprised to see the penis spring upward, completely straight.

"Well, that's nice," I said in a whisper to no one.

The surgeons pushed on without comment, as though this was usual. They were nearing the part I had traveled to watch. But before stitching the foreskin into a tube, Yoshino prepared the glans to wrap around the new urethra. For a second time I shook my head in wonder. She dissected the sides of the glans apart as though laying a book open

---

22. Claus Roehrborn, the Urology Department Chairman after John McConnell.
23. *Inderol* is a blood pressure medicine which taken in small doses controls fine tremors.

in the middle, like I did, but then changed the angle to free the two wings farther upward in a maneuver I had never seen before.

Then the surgeons tubularized the foreskin graft and sewed one end to the hypospadias opening and the other to the tip of the glans. I noticed how the extra dissection they did minutes ago made it easier to bring the glans around the graft and stitch it together without tension.

"Kaoru, that was way more dissection on the glans than I've ever seen anyone do," I mentioned afterward, as we sipped green tea waiting for the next patient to be brought to the operating room.

"It was how we always do it," she explained. "The glans is smaller in our boys, and this dissection prevents dehiscence."

The second boy had similar hypospadias, the penis bent down to a meatus in the middle of the scrotum. I watched as the two surgeons began the repair, degloving the skin, performing an artificial erection, and finding the penis curved to what I guessed was at least fifty degrees. Yoshino and Tanakazi then cut across the urethral plate, just as I would, and dissected behind it down the shaft of the penis, as I would do, and then repeated the artificial erection. Once again, the penis grew firm and stood straight.

What are the odds of that? I asked myself, knowing that most of my patients would still have a bent penis at this point. But these surgeons clearly were not surprised as they continued their routine. Yoshino opened the glans like she did before, and I saw again that she began dissecting the same way I did, but then went much farther.

As they moved on to roll the foreskin graft and sew it into place, the very steps I came to watch, I sat on a stool with my back to the surgery scribbling notes, trying to capture in words the movements they used to open the glans so wide.

The next day brought two more operations for proximal hypospadias. Already I was less interested in their tubed grafts than I was curious to see if the penis would straighten again the same way, and if I had managed to describe their glans dissection accurately.

The three of us sat together that evening drinking Sapporo while the chef grilled thin strips of beef and placed them on the counter before us to share.

"This is my favorite steak house," Tanakazi declared as the first round of Kobe was plated. "But I don't think it is as good as your steakhouses in Texas."

I wrestled a slice with chopsticks. "Well, it's certainly *different* than a Texas steakhouse," I replied, glancing at the patrons lined down the counter as though sitting at a sushi bar, sipping cups of sake or glasses of beer rather than red wine from oversized goblets, and watching small slivers of meat rather than sixteen-ounce New York strips, sizzle on the grill. An older male host, rather than an attractive young woman, seated new arrivals. "Yeah," I explained, "the steak is delicious, but everything else is pretty much the opposite of home!

"Thanks again for arranging these cases," I said, returning our discussion to the operating room. "I learned a lot."

I struggled to take another bite with the chopsticks.

"And I was especially intrigued by two things: how cutting the urethral plate straightened the curvature in every one of those boys, and how much more you open the glans than I do. When we transect the plate, the penis almost always stays bent, so we have to do corporotomies to lengthen the underside."

I set my chopsticks down and made hand motions to illustrate those maneuvers.

"Yes, we know," Yoshino answered. "Sometimes we have to do that, too, but it is not common here."

"And I was impressed by that glans dissection. It looks like it really decreases tension on the closure. What's your rate of glans dehiscence?"

"Less than 5 percent," she told me. "I think we had just three in our last 150 patients."

"That's less than half of what I have after proximal repairs! It was worth coming here just to see how you do that."

I did not mention that those tubed grafts I almost begged to see and then traveled so far on my own dime to watch would not work for me, since they would not survive on top of corporotomies.

Tanikazi ordered a round of local whisky to end our meal in a toast to friendship.

"We are happy that you visited us," he said, raising his glass.

How ironic that the notion of academic freedom originally referred to the right of scholars to freely travel in the pursuit of knowledge. That I did for many years before the dean imposed restrictions, visiting nearly forty countries scattered throughout the world to lecture, operate, and to learn. It was only a bureaucratic annoyance that I left on my first visit before I worked at the university long enough to earn a day of vacation. But now, years later, travel had to be *justified* to the department chairman, who was pressured by his superiors to scrutinize every request.

Without that freedom I would not have returned from Sweden having learned to repair the foreskin in boys with hypospadias, and in the years that followed, families would not have traveled to the university specifically for me to provide that service when their local urologist refused. Without my trip to Japan, I would not have learned the better glansplasty method which soon reduced complications for my patients at the university. And if I could not demonstrate surgery outside the university, how many boys would be harmed in how many places because their surgeons could not come to Dallas to watch?

I met Bracka again on a darkened stage in the conference hall of the All India Institute of Medical Science, the preeminent teaching hospital in Delhi. I retreated there, ignoring signs forbidding food and drink, in urgent need of an air-conditioned respite after a fiery breakfast before the workshop began.

I opened the conference by telling the audience that I used TIP for every distal hypospadias. In fact, I had not used another operation for the last sixteen years, and if TIP worked for me in so many boys, it would also work for the surgeons listening. TIP could also repair proximal hypospadias, if the penis was no more than slightly curved and easily straightened with a single plication stitch on the topside. Otherwise, when the bend required cutting across the urethral plate, I tried Byars flaps, but every patient had complications afterward. *100% complications!* Now I relied on the two-stage graft repair I learned from Bracka, which had half as many complications, but still more than my proximal TIPs.

That was sufficient incentive to keep probing the boundaries of that operation. So, when I heard one of their colleagues, the Indian surgeon Emil Bhat, describe a different maneuver to straighten the penis without transecting the urethral plate, I was willing to give it a try.

"After all, it's not a new idea to mobilize the entire urethra," I reminded the audience. "Adult urologists have done it for years repairing strictures." Using that concept, I explained, "We can lift up the urethral plate, do corporotomies under it to get the penis straight, and still do a TIP," emphasizing that point with a dramatic picture of the plate raised high in the air off the penis it was still attached to on each end. A caption reported I had done that in six boys so far, and not one of them had a complication.

Bracka followed my lecture, still warning of the cat's arse that skin flaps made, and still advising two-stage grafts for proximal hypospadias. But now he had changed to the Snodgrass method to repair distal cases with a single operation.

A third surgeon completed the morning of lectures. Joao Pippi-Salle, a short Brazilian everyone knew as Pippi, could not restrain his abounding enthusiasm behind a lectern, and so he paced back and forth across the length of the stage as he described his struggle to perfect Duckett flaps, rather than discard them as Snodgrass and Bracka had done. But, having reached the pinnacle of his success, Pippi had to admit that the penises he repaired with flaps did not look normal like those made by TIPs and grafts.

"I tell you it was very frustrating to work so hard to be one of the best in the world with flaps and not be able to match these guys," he admitted in an excited accent as he turned toward Bracka and me with a big smile.

Then, looking back over his shoulder, he added with a wink and a grin to the crowd, "So I became one of them!"

After lectures, the three of us were led from the auditorium straight into a mob of surgeons anxious to ask just one more question, or show us pictures from a difficult case for advice, or snap a photo standing with the renowned visitors. And the first snap unleashed a frenzy, like a school of feeding fish, drawing in others also wanting a photo who handed their cameras back and forth and squeezed into each other's shots as the celebrities smiled into lenses aimed from left and right, unable to take another step through the swarm of admirers.

Finally, we were pulled away and hurried through corridors back to a time and place where nurses still sharpened IV needles to reuse and powdered the surgeons' gloves in little cubbyholes beside the operating theaters, like my mother did in the early 1950s before I was born. We changed into aged cloth scrubs, mine so large they could accommodate both me and a friend, and exchanged our shoes for plastic flip flops.

Then we were each shown to a different operating room, where cameras stood on tripods rising high over the foot of the tables and assistants stood nearby with microphones in hand waiting for the show to begin. A tangle of cables snaked back and forth from a control desk jammed into a side hallway where a director sat waiting to beam the operations down to an eager audience.

Bracka's patient was ready first. He adjusted the height of his stool and did a microphone check before starting a proximal repair. I took a few pictures of him sitting to operate, without a mask, in the British tradition.

Both Pippi and I stood to do our operations, fully masked, each beginning with a distal TIP. All three surgeries played simultaneously on a large screen in the auditorium, the moderators calling attention to a key maneuver and the director activating the microphone in that room for that surgeon to comment.

Meanwhile, as one visiting professor described what he was seeing or doing, the other two might have to pause for a few moments waiting their turn to show something important that they were seeing or doing. So the operations lurched forward in fits and starts, and the surgeons watching saw jumbled bits and pieces they had to piece together like jigsaw puzzles into three coherent pictures.

From operating in workshops several times a year, I had learned to describe the important steps clearly and succinctly before the audience's attention wandered to another room. And it was easy when Bracka or Pippi was in the other room, since the three of us did the same operations in much the same way. But because we were working simultaneously, I heard the comments but rarely witnessed their surgeries.

In the future I would end the confusion of multiple operations done at the same time and organize a workshop in Dallas beamed around the world by webinar to teach surgeons everywhere one operation at a time.

Until then, I did the best I could to model for the delegates how I operated back home, despite the foreign surroundings, despite assistants who struggled to help the way I wanted to be helped, and nurses challenged to load my tiny needles ready for my left hand to use. Despite cameras that encroached on the operating field to send images to the audience that were sometimes blurred, and microphones that might screech and crackle more clearly than they transmitted my words.

It was raw, unrehearsed, unpredictable performance art. Rock bands might play twenty different cities on a tour, but the songs, the instruments, the stage, the lights, the microphones, and the speakers were always the same. Like them, I did the same operations over and over in different locations carrying my own instruments and sutures, but I constantly worried that the operating theaters, the supporting cast, the audio, and the video might disrupt the show and confuse my message.

On this trip, I finally tired of the nurse never handing me anything ready to use, so I stopped and laid my instruments and sutures out on the Mayo stand so that I could help myself. That worked better but took longer. But there was nothing I could do to remedy the cautery; a disposable being used for the nth time that shocked me every time I pushed the button to stop something from bleeding.

Later that evening I stood in line with Bracka and Pippi for a buffet dinner served outside to the delegates on the hospital grounds. Fortunately, most of the attendees' energy was spent after the earlier photo frenzy and a day overflowing with lectures and surgeries, so the three of us managed to eat in a relative calm interrupted by only a few final questions and a last quick snap of a photo.

I flew home exhausted, as I usually did after a workshop, feeling my very soul had been sucked from me by surgeons desperate to learn as much as they could in so little time. Could they see the operations well enough to realize how deeply I incised the urethral plate? Did they hear me explain when to do a proximal TIP and when to do a two-stage graft? Were the words and pictures on my slides convincing enough to persuade anyone to give up the flap repairs their mentors taught? How would I ever know?

I thought it curious that my first invitation to Latin America did not come from next-door Mexico, but instead from faraway Chile. I did not know what to expect after flying more than ten hours to land only one time zone away from Dallas in Santiago. But I looked forward to sampling their version of Mexican food, imagining a similar cuisine spiced, I supposed, with different peppers than the jalapenos and habaneros that fired the Tex-Mex I knew. So, it was a surprising disappointment to be served basic meat and potatoes, with dinner rolls rather than tortillas. In fact, the only tortillas I saw on this trip were hanging on a rack inside a convenience store and labeled Made In New York City!

The lectures I gave were, however, a new experience. Few surgeons at the conference spoke English, so interpreters sat in a booth at the rear of the auditorium listening to me speak while simultaneously translating my words into Spanish transmitted to headphones worn by most in the audience. I was amazed the translators could listen in one language while speaking in another, especially when I took questions afterward and was immediately confused when I left on my headphones and heard Spanish as I spoke English.

The audience had to be confused, too, listening to the lecture in their language while looking at my slides written in English.

"You have to help me translate them before my next trip," I told our fellow, Juan Prieto, a Columbian, when I returned home.

It happened that I was scheduled to travel to his country a few months later and I wanted that audience to both hear and read my words in their native tongue.

But when Prieto completed that task and I looked through the presentations, I could not read my own slides or recall what they said. How would I give a lecture without the usual prompts on the slides? I asked him to sit with me and review his translations, but soon decided it would be more efficient if I used Google to translate the specific words I had to recognize to remember what to say. Soon I acquired a repertory of hypospadias nouns, along with a few verbs to link them together into descriptions of my operations.

On this second trip I thought I understood some questions, or at least bits of questions, though I still relied on the interpreters to be certain and to translate my responses. Then, after hearing the concerns of surgeons in the audience, I returned to the hotel that evening and made some new slides to add to the next day's lectures, translating them myself with Google's help.

The occasional grins of the surgeons told me when the computer chose a word they would not have used. Still, I was satisfied that my lessons were easier to understand when the audience read and heard Spanish, even if my version was not always precise.

Later that year I was invited back to Chile for a different conference. This time I made all my own slides in Spanish and asked Prieto to proofread them. That process finally stirred long dormant memories of the basic Spanish I learned in college and never used afterwards. I decided to try giving one of my lectures in Spanish, surprising those in the audience who recalled I could hardly speak a word in their language six months earlier.

After that, I gave all my lectures in Spanish when I visited Spain, and again when I was finally invited to Mexico. Most surgeons complimented my new proficiency, although one host sitting across from me at lunch in Puerta Vallarta laughed saying my Spanish was *horrible*, trilling the Rs exuberantly in a way my tongue would never mimic. Nevertheless, like other lessons these visiting professorships taught the teacher, the Spanish I learned soon helped me better explain hypospadias to parents at Children's, where many spoke little English and interpreters were not quickly available. Soon I was speaking in Spanish before and after surgery, and through much of the day in the clinic.

I am sure no one wanted to hurt me, but there were some close calls in these many travels. When the driver veered off the main road into a small village near the pyramids and a horde of farmers wielding hoes and sickles immediately surrounded the car, peering suspiciously through the windows at the foreigner inside.

Or when I walked along the shore outside the hotel in Rio de Janeiro at dusk and was captured by a gang of teens who held my arms tight as they rifled through my clothes looking for money. I was relieved that none of them brandished a knife.

There was an all-day adventure in Bosnia floating down a river in a scorching heat with nothing to slack my thirst except the water flowing past or a local moonshine packed onboard. My dehydration finally reached the point that IV fluids were needed. Even worse was the extreme bout of Delhi belly incited by the smallest possible taste of an Indian relish my hosts insisted I compare to Mexican salsa back home.

Sometimes I returned from these trips discouraged. Like the time I was asked to start a proximal repair late in the afternoon and discovered the camera turned off and the delegates shooed out before I was even halfway through the case. And when I learned that despite several visits to a well-known center nothing there had changed, because the chief was less interested in what I had to say than in using my reputation to fill seats in the auditorium with paying customers. Or the time the host curried favor with another visiting professor by asking him to do a complex reoperation, and that surgeon repeatedly asked me what he should do next.

What was the point of taking time off from my practice, flying away from my wife and kids, traveling twenty-four hours in economy so cramped I could barely open my laptop, operating with a nurse who not once in two days loaded a needle right for my left hand, or teaching in a workshop where the video quality was so poor the audience could barely discern what I was doing?

What about the time in Aleppo where the operating theater had no standing stool to level me with an assistant who stood a good foot taller, and there was a long delay while someone hammered together a wooden box for me to stand on? Which worked until the operating table hydraulics failed and it kept sinking down and having to be pumped back up by foot, over and over, until I resembled a Texas pumpjack until the surgery was done.

Or when there was an AV delay starting a workshop in Athens and the chief of anesthesia declared she would not do the second operation, despite an auditorium filled with surgeons waiting to see it, because she was not paid extra for working overtime. I replied I would not be paid for doing that case either.

But most discouraging were those surgeons who smiled when they met me and took seats near the front of the auditorium where they would be seen by others, who nodded in agreement with what I was saying whenever our eyes met, yet resisted my message, refusing to rethink their practice despite a mountain of evidence proving they should.

Surgeons like the moderator who heard me introduce TIP in Galveston and declared, "I'm not convinced to change what I've been doing," and still was not convinced to change years later despite all the data reported from around the world that proved TIP was better than a Mathieu.

Occasionally someone would stand up in a meeting to challenge my testimony, but more revealed their true beliefs through a snide remark or a comment tinged with skepticism. I never seemed to find a good response to those provocations, if there was one. After all, I made changes in my own practice to do better and could not understand why others would not.

One day after returning from a workshop in Russia, I told a trainee that the host surgeon hesitated to let me repair a boy with a graft after several flaps had failed.

The anesthesiologist overheard our conversation and looked over the drapes to explain, "Warren, don't you know that the first time you hear something new it's a bad idea?"

I nodded.

He continued, "Then the second time you hear something new you remember that you've heard it before. And by the third time you hear something new, you answer that you've been doing it that way for a long time. You just haven't gone there often enough!"

In 2009 I flew from Dallas to Dubai and then on to Dhaka, half a world and another universe away. In a decade of travels, I had never seen children lying head to toe down long corridors with only thin mats to cushion them from the floor because all the beds in the hospital were always full. I had never seen such desperate looks from parents who huddled on the ground with them, hung their laundry in the window to dry, and watched over small cooking pots to feed them while they stayed in those hallways. And I had never seen such a wealth of patients brought into ORs more scarcely provisioned—the Mayo stand set for my hypospadias surgery with one adult-sized scalpel, one forcep, one pair of scissors, one needle driver, and one package of a suture much too large to use in a child.

"Where are the other sutures?" I asked.

"This is all the hospital provides," my host explained. "The family has to buy the rest on the streets and bring them here, if they can afford to."

I wondered how surgeons could possibly do a repair with only one suture even if they tied knots until there was literally nothing left to tie. I needed a minimum of five, and often several more.

I was never more relieved that I brought my own instruments and sutures, and never so despairing of what I could teach surgeons who would never know my abundance of supplies. In fact, I had to question if boys born into families so hopelessly poor even needed to have their distal hypospadias repaired. Should a country so overwhelmed with the poverty I saw on the streets, and in the hallways and operating rooms of its largest teaching hospital, spend scarce resources for surgery that might fix the penis but not improve the boy's life?

But I had prepared lectures and brought supplies, and there were surgeons who came great distances to learn, and parents thrilled to have a foreign doctor repair their son's hypospadias. So, I lectured and operated as best I could, struggling to meet my personal commitment to always do in other countries the same operation in the same way that I would do at home.

Eager surgeons surrounded me in the conference room after my lecture, and I answered one last question from twenty more questioners who followed me down the hall when I finally walked away. I was corralled in the OR by surgeons pressing close around the operating table, straining for a glimpse of the surgery and holding their cellphones high overhead to take pictures. And when one of them asked to snap a photo with me afterward, a hoard of others soon joined the fray wanting a photo too.

After surgery my host and I were invited for tea in the office of the senior hospital administrator. We sat in black cushioned chairs around a gleaming mahogany table and were served from a brightly polished silver tea service by an aide wearing dark slacks and a crisp white shirt. We sipped tea with milk and sugar refreshed by the chill of air conditioning, a luxury not shared anywhere else in the hospital. Only the blind would not see the contrast between the shining white walls and sparkling tile floors where the administrator worked, and the gloomy wards with stained walls and dirty floors where the doctors worked, and where the fortunate children lay in beds whose rails were chipped and rusting while the rest slept on mats out in the hall.

As we chatted, I asked the administrator who chose which sutures to buy for the surgeons.

"Those decisions are made over my head, at the Health Ministry," came the immediate reply.

That night the conference faculty all went to dinner in the outdoor courtyard of a western hotel. I happened to be seated at a round table across from the Assistant Minister of Health and next to the surgical chief I met before in AIIMS, who tried to start a conversation.

"Minister, what percent of GNP is health care in Bangladesh?" Devendra Gupta asked, tossing a softball question.

The official looked back at him, uninterested. "I don't know, actually," he replied, without a hint of embarrassment.

Everyone else at the table was embarrassed, though, that the Assistant Minister of Health did not know, and apparently did not care that he did not know, what piece of the pie his government devoted to health care for its people.

I seized an opportunity in the awkward silence. "Minister, why doesn't your office ask these pediatric surgeons seated here what sutures and instruments they need," I said with a wave of my hand toward them, "instead of giving them adult sutures and instruments? After all, that would decrease complications, and save your ministry the money you're spending for redo operations *on children*."

All eyes turned to the minister, waiting for him to respond. But in that exact moment a band suddenly started playing on a stage right behind our table, and when everyone looked toward the sound, the minister slithered away and did not return.

Two years later I again flew all day from Dallas to Dhaka, this time greeted by a different surgeon who invited me into her minivan for a drive of countless hours down congested roads that belched dust the entire way to Chittagong, the second-largest city in Bangladesh. Along the journey, we stopped so that I could sample five varieties of bananas, admire roosters thrust toward me by hopeful street vendors, and to see if the man casting his net into the murky green waters of a roadside pond hauled in any fish for dinner.

I was soon exhausted by the people everywhere, squatting on the ground, carrying huge bundles on their heads, clinging to the outsides of buses overfilled on the inside, steering bicycles and pedicabs stacked impossibly high with bamboo sticks or sacks of onions, driving little green taxis and huge motorized trucks and even the occasional Mercedes, all in a back-and-forth weave making a Gordian knot of traffic that slowed progress wherever we went.

After a rest, little Tahmina Banu took me to the hospital to wade through a sea of boys waiting in a large ward so dimly lit that a trainee held a flashlight while I examined their hypospadias. I selected the few to be operated and explained to an entourage of surgeons how I would repair the others, had there been more time. A nurse trailed behind, squirting my hands with antiseptic.

Then it was on to the operating theater where every square inch of space was filled with surgeons anxious to see me work in person, rather than watch the screen in a conference room. I struggled to find room in that squeeze just to move my arms.

When the surgeries were done it was time for lectures. I was the only visiting professor at this workshop, so my message was not lost in an endless splitting of hairs by guest surgeons determined to account for every possible contingency at the risk of confusing everyone else listening. In that moment I recognized the genius of Bracka's teaching for many years that all hypospadias could be repaired using just one operation. One operation that doctors trained as urologists or general surgeons or plastic surgeons working anywhere from the finest US operating rooms to the most impoverished operating theaters in Bangladesh, could focus on getting right.

My lesson was nearly the same, that all hypospadias could be re-paired by TIP or a two-stage graft. Two operations that were versions of the same idea: to make a urethra from the urethral plate that should have made it in the first place, or from a substitute plate formed from a graft when the penis was bent.

Again a teeming mob engulfed me afterward in a photo frenzy of surgeons passing their cameras back and forth to get a "snap" with Pro-fessor Snodgrass. When the crowd finally drifted away, three young surgeons lingered behind.

"We saw you in Delhi a few years ago," one of them told me as the others smiled and nodded enthusiastically.

A second added, "Yes, and we have to admit that when we heard you describe your TIP, we all thought it was a bad idea. We worried that incision into the urethral plate must surely scar, like strictures do if you cut them the same way."

I smiled back at them. "Well, many surgeons had that concern in the beginning, but now there are a lot of data from many different insti-tutions showing that it does not."

"Yes, professor, we know that. Thank you. When we saw you were coming to Dhaka, we went to hear you again. We took a picture with you then too," one of them said, grinning even larger as he held up his phone for me to see.

"And after your lecture and surgeries we talked and decided we should give your operation a try," another one explained.

Their happiness predicted where the story would end.

"This time we came to Chittagong to tell you we are doing your op-eration all the time!"

"We are all very pleased with the results."

"Thank you very much."

I looked at them smiling from ear to ear and realized that even a visit to the most desperate place served a purpose.

"Thanks for telling me. I'm glad to hear your results are good," I told them.

But as they walked away a weary sigh escaped my lips. "I just can't visit everywhere three times."

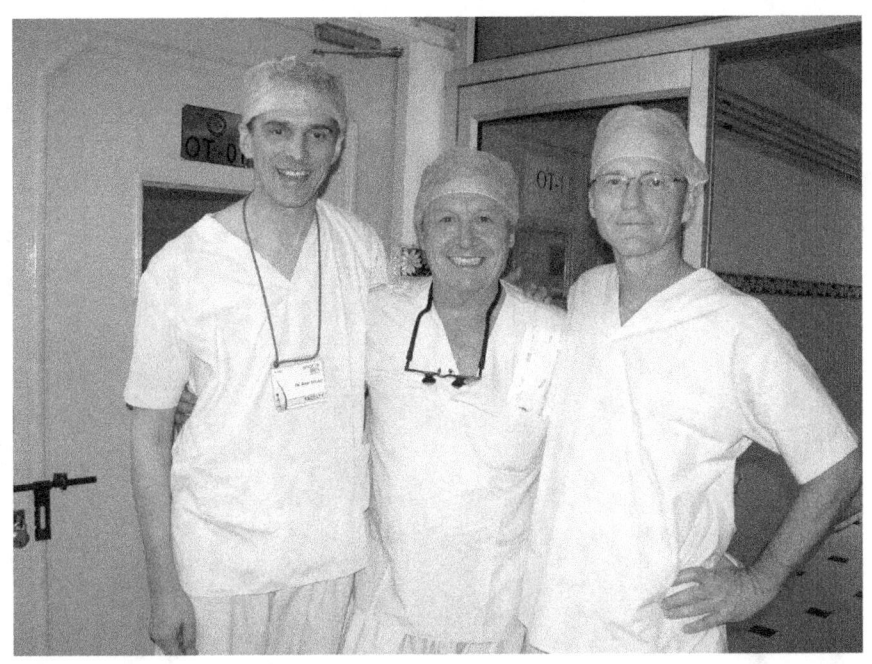

Bracka, Pippi-Salle, and me in India

◀ CHAPTER 7 ▶

Turned Away in My Own Country

Although I flew to the far corners of the world to lecture and operate, there were far fewer invitations for visits within my own country. The first came in 2001 when Tony Caldamone, one of the early converts to TIP, asked me to explain the operation to the urology residents at Brown and then spend the weekend at his house on Cape Cod. Four years later, Pippi-Salle invited me to Toronto for a steak cookout before a hypospadias symposium began the next morning at Sick Kid's Hospital. Though not in the US, that urology program was integrated into our professional societies.

There were not many others. Once a senior department chief bumped into me at the airport and remarked his group would have to get me up for a visit that never came to pass. Another mentioned his trainees were hoping I would come lecture, but that invite never arrived either. Over the years I have been a visiting professor eight times in the US, and eighty-one times in forty other countries.

I wondered about this and imagined several explanations. Maybe my colleagues thought TIP easy enough that they did not need to hear Snodgrass describe the key steps, its nuances, and intricacies. Probably some hesitated to have me lecture their trainees knowing the data I would cite taught lessons different from the dogma they quoted. Undoubtedly, at least a few were jealous that an operation was named for me, even though I did not give it that name.

It could be that the encyclopedic knowledge of hypospadias I gained reading all those articles during that year in Seattle came across as arrogance. Or some were irritated I did not stay in one lane but developed expertise in other conditions besides hypospadias. Maybe I once made a comment standing at a microphone on the floor of a convention that hurt someone's feelings. A friend mentioned that my neutral look, when I was neither happy nor mad, came across stern and could be unsettling.

It was impossible to know. But I was the same person teaching the same lessons and making the same comments with the same expressions on my face who was enthusiastically invited all over the world, and usually for more than one visit. I finally accepted the truth of the ancient maxim that a prophet can be welcomed everywhere and yet be turned away in his own country.

So it was an unexpected honor when I was asked to organize the 2005 Society for Pediatric Urology program, scheduled in San Antonio. I had a year to consider the topics and speakers and wasted no time planning a meeting filled with fresh ideas.

Naturally, the day had to begin with hypospadias. But, in an unexpected twist, I chose a panel of surgeons to discuss options when TIP could *not* be done, specifically after failed surgery when the urethral plate had been removed or was too scarred to use. I knew that nearly everyone in the audience would choose some variation of a skin flap, and Doug Canning agreed to describe those the way that Duckett taught him. That set the stage to show the alternative I learned from Bracka, when multiple flaps done by multiple surgeons failed that boy I struggled to help when I first arrived in Dallas.

I was not going to give this or any other lecture. If anyone could persuade Americans to rethink the dogma of flaps, it was Bracka, the world's most experienced surgeon using grafts. And just in case a few in the audience missed that point, slipping out for coffee or standing in the back of the room chatting with a friend, I scheduled Bracka to follow up with a second lecture presenting his "Alternative Views on Hypospadias."

As expected, Bracka riveted the audience with his contrarian thoughts on grafts and flaps, delivered in that British voice which makes the words sound all the more intelligent. I was pleased, though Bracka wondered afterward how anyone survived the broiling heat of summer in San Antonio.

A note arrived in the mail a few weeks later from one of the Americans who attended the conference. "I consider the meeting a success if I hear one new idea for my practice," the short message began, repeating an adage my father often said. "I wanted to tell you that I brought back several from yours!"

That one day as program director earned me a three-year term on the Society for Pediatric Urology executive committee, which entailed arriving to the annual meeting a day early to hear reports and vote on several items of business. There was nothing more required from me, or most others on the committee, since the bulk of the work was done and most decisions had been made beforehand by the secretary. What I found most interesting was this peek behind the scenes at the politics of our profession.

But I forgot an important lesson I learned while president of my college fraternity: to never make a proposal unless you already have the votes for it in your pocket. I had known for years that different places taught different lessons to their fellows, resulting in a "Boston way," and a "CHOP way," and many assorted other ways to do the same things.

"Maybe the SPU should have a curriculum committee to help standardize training," I suggested with an innocent shrug when discussion turned to that topic, not realizing the strong defenses jealously guarding each of those fiefdoms.

I think that is what vetoed a nomination to make me the next SPU secretary. Or maybe it was the lecture I was invited to give that lampooned a popular surgery on the bladders of children with spina bifida.

Earl Cheng beamed a huge smile as he pumped my hand afterward, exclaiming, "That was *great*! Exactly what I hoped you'd say!"

But my nurse told me someone sitting behind her sneered, "He's not even a real pediatric urologist," and a division chief pulled me aside to chide, "We don't need another Duckett," which was clearly not meant as a compliment.

Regardless, I admit to feeling ambivalent when my dapper, bow-tied friend Marc Cendron called to discuss me taking the job of secretary when his term ended.

"We're busy organizing the first-ever joint congress with the Europeans for 2010," Cendron explained of his brainchild, "and it's going to take a lot more work coordinating the program with them."

Despite the honor of being asked, I immediately envisioned all the meetings that this would require, and sensed all the agendas that would have to be weighed and balanced, and imagined all the egos that would have to be smoothed in the process.

And here was likely the key reason I was not given that political office or invited by my peers as a visiting professor very often. Rather than stroke egos, I challenged complacency.

It proved a blessing to not spend time coordinating an American/European congress when I needed to reorganize our group at Children's. Strand eventually left the university after I was made chief, and I interviewed several candidates for a faculty position before convincing a Brit who was interested in moving that he could survive summers in Texas. In fact, I still laugh how the gentle Duncan Wilcox *insisted* on visiting during the Fourth of July specifically to sample the heat, and how a cloud providentially covered the sun just as he landed and then kept Dallas in an unseasonably pleasant shade until the moment he flew off again a few days later.

"It seems the rumors of your summers are exaggerated," Duncan pronounced as he left.

Wilcox quickly built a practice from our surplus of patients, but then abruptly left a short time later, chasing the offer to become his own chief in Denver. That left me the only full-time faculty since Baker spent half her time in the lab, and Harrison spent half his time anywhere else than in the hospital.

Now I had to absorb Wilcox's patients into my own bustling practice. Rather than see forty patients in a day of clinic, I somehow managed to rush through seventy and then dictate all their notes and letters to the referring physicians. Even then the managers at Children's pressed me to work faster when the wait for nonurgent problems stretched more than three months out.

Simple math proved it was impossible to provide the best care to patients allotted less than ten minutes of my time in the clinic. Surprisingly, I never did that calculation, but instead found company in the boasts of other chiefs that their days were just as busy. Nevertheless, our group clearly needed more faculty, which meant I had to start another search for candidates to interview and court.

Meanwhile, I found other opportunities to teach and to learn from colleagues. John Duckett launched the Pediatric Urology Winter Forum to give an excuse to his university, and a tax write-off to the IRS, for a week of skiing every year in the Rockies—choosing that awkward name to convince both it was a legitimate academic conference. Which it was, albeit a rather small one that never gathered more than twenty-five surgeons to give lectures in the early morning and late afternoon while spending the rest of the day on the slopes. Nevertheless, this was the meeting where I met Mitchell and Lackgren, Caldamone, Cendron, and Canning, and sat bubbling in a hot tub in Telluride as I discussed my future with Jeff Waxman.

Duckett also began a course during the American Urologic Association congress, the one where he showed pictures of hypospadias and asked panelists how they would repair them. After he died, Mike Mitchell revamped the course and its faculty, adding me the same year I moved to Seattle. In that era before PowerPoint and laptops, I used Kodachrome slides that are long since misplaced. I probably spent most of my allotted time discussing distal TIP and how deep and long that key incision had to be.

The AUA course had to be renewed every year, and over time both the faculty and their messages evolved. Mike Carr was the first to drop out, leaving Mitchell, former Duckett fellow Larry Baskin, and me. At some point, Mitchell handed the program over to Doug Canning, and then both he and Baskin stepped away, taking with them the legacy of Duckett and his flap repairs. I invited Pippi-Salle to join me as I refocused the program on TIP and the staged grafts we both used.

This new version consistently attracted around sixty surgeons, which was enough to please the AUA. As I did with all other lectures, I revised my presentation year after year even though the program always received the highest possible marks. It was a once-a-year chance to bring others the latest news on hypospadias, and I was an obvious choice for the messenger since my work made most of that news.

Still, most of those who attended were foreigners, and I could not help but nurse a frustration that few Americans, and none of the most influential leaders, came to listen. I had to remind myself each year not to focus on those who were not there, but to instead sow seeds that would bear fruit in those who were.

When I was invited as a visiting professor, I divided the time between lectures on hypospadias and other topics in pediatric urology which intrigued me at the moment. The same curiosity and drive for perfection that powered my research on hypospadias inevitably spilled over into nearly every other facet of the specialty.

For example, I shared my vision for "Hypospadias Without Flaps" with the pediatric urology group at Vanderbilt, but also discussed the "Management of Slings Without Augment for Neurogenic Incontinence" and "Reflux: Shifting Paradigms." Despite my emphasis on hypospadias, those patients did not fill more than a tithe of my clinic slots or a third of my OR schedule. There were plenty of other patients with urine leakage from spina bifida, or infections due to bladder reflux, not to mention obstructed kidneys, undescended testicles, and a whole assortment of other conditions to occupy the remaining time.

In fact, my first fellow complimented the diverse practice I built after he finished his training in 2005. "I expected you to do a lot of hypospadias, which you do, but I am impressed by all the other surgeries you do too," Selcuk Yucel told his mentor. "I hope my practice will be the same."

His mentor took pride in that practice, not fully realizing how much those other interests distracted from my primary focus.

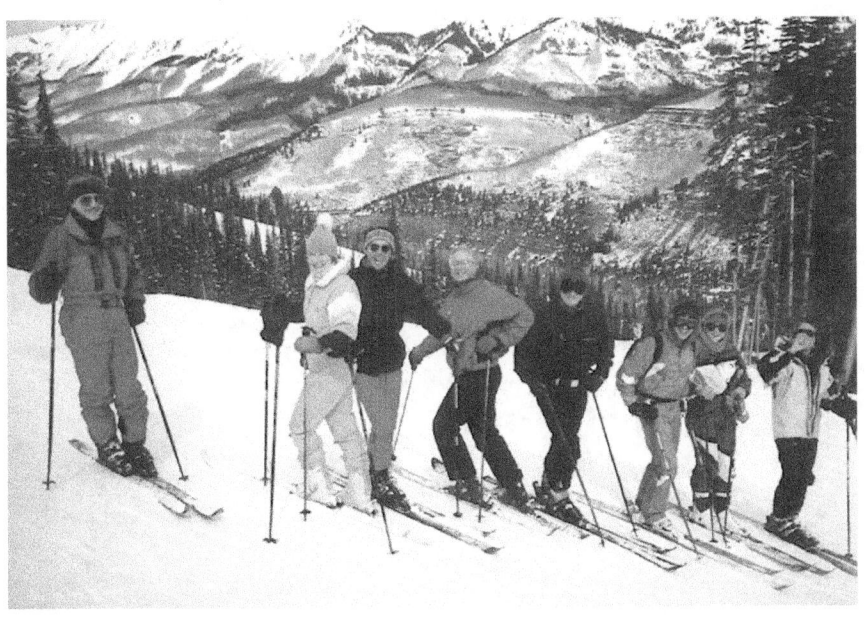

Me (far left) and Duckett (4th from left) at the PUWF in Telluride.

◄ CHAPTER 8 ►

I Need to Dummy Code Your Databases

She sat down in one of those wooden chairs stamped with the seal of the university that residents are given when they graduate.

"I would like to talk about my future," she announced, beginning our negotiation. "I want to stay in Dallas, but I know that you don't keep the people you train."

I sunk back into a leather chair on the opposite side of my desk, elbows resting on the arms, fingers meeting just below my nose, eyes narrowed, as I listened carefully to her opening statement. *Because they don't bring anything new to the group*, I added silently, finishing her sentence. I sometimes commented to trainees how some institutions train people and then keep them forever, making their programs increasingly insular over time. "Despite what we know about inbreeding . . ." I would sometimes conclude.

"So, I've done some homework and learned that the university has a master's program in Clinical Studies."

I raised my eyebrows into a question, signaling I did not know about this degree.

She read my expression and explained, "It's like an MPH,[24] but without all the math. And so far, they've not had almost any surgeons do the training, so I'll probably get accepted."

Then she returned to her rehearsed proposal.

---

24. An *MPH* is a Masters in Public Health degree.

"Anyway, you would have to hire me to the faculty and give me 50 percent protected time[25] while I do this program."

I remained quiet as a sphinx.

She buttressed her argument. "We both know that you want someone in your group with this training." Then she advanced to close the deal. "This way I get the job I want in Dallas, and you get someone to organize your clinical studies."

And just like that, my fellow Nicol Bush bargained her way into a career at the university.

Having witnessed the power of my hypospadias database, I created new spreadsheets for other interests in my practice. One to hold information on the bladder neck repair I devised for children with spina bifida, and another to store results of my Deflux injections to stop reflux.[26] When I questioned the best way to locate a testicle that could not be felt, I made a database to organize the findings. And after Bush and I considered various projects for her master's studies, we made another database to record how many children developed scars in their kidneys following urinary infections.

One day I carried my laptop to the operating room to enter data after a Deflux treatment. A resident happened to see me sitting in the corner typing and recognized an Excel spreadsheet open on the screen.

"Can I look at that?" Amit Gupta asked.

"Sure," I replied, pushing the computer toward him. "It's my Deflux database."

Gupta studied it a few minutes and then asked for a copy.

"No problem, we just have to add you to the IRB[27] first."

When the paperwork was official, I handed Gupta a thumb drive with the database. Two weeks later he handed back the results from 259 injections organized into seven tables, with univariate and multivariate statistical analysis identifying factors that predicted success or failure. I

---

25. *Protected time* was given to Bush to do her studies, reducing her obligation to see patients in the clinic and do surgeries.

26. *Reflux* is a condition in which urine flows backward from the bladder up the ureters to the kidneys. *Deflux* is a substance injected through a scope into the opening of the ureter to prevent this.

27. The *IRB*, or Institutional Review Board, reviews all research involving humans to be certain it is done according to ethical standards.

understood the columns listing how many patients had which grades of reflux, and the tables that showed the varying anatomy of the orifice and how many injections of how much Deflux I used to change it. I even understood the analysis of grade and anatomy versus the volume of Deflux I injected to see if any or all of those predicted results. But Gupta had to explain the final table reporting odds ratios and confidence intervals that determined which of these observations were the most reliable.

And then all I had to do to finish a manuscript ready for publication was write an Introduction and a Discussion to bookend these Results, highlighting the key findings and summarizing the take-home messages that could help other surgeons. It was the easiest, and one of the best, papers I had written.

There was one analysis that stood out because it was different from what the hospital statistician calculated from the same information.

"That's because he didn't really understand the question you wanted answered," Gupta explained. "It's better when doctors can do their own statistics, since they know what they want to know."

I needed no more convincing. But there were few urologists like Gupta who understood not only how to do surgery, but also how to study the surgery to see if it could be done better. After all, he was exceptional, a graduate from AIIMS, in Delhi, who somehow worked his way into the Master of Public Health program at UT Southwestern, and then persuaded the Urology Department to give him one of its few residency positions. Gupta would later graduate to fellowship training at Sloan Kettering, a preeminent cancer center, recruited there by one of my mentors to reorganize their urology cancer databases.

I had already reorganized my first hypospadias database. Distal TIPs had different results than proximal TIPs, so I divided them onto separate sheets to make them easier to review. A first look at TIP used for redo surgeries showed those outcomes were different, too, needing a new database to house them. Then, as I gathered more patients with severe hypospadias, and more with complex problems after failed operations done by others, I created yet another database to record the two-stage graft repairs I learned from Bracka.

It took only a few minutes after surgery to enter the details I thought were important, and even less time in the evening after clinic to record follow up. Most patients had no problems after their repairs, and those complications that happened were easy to list into separate columns of fistulas, glans dehiscence, meatal stenosis, and urethral stricture.

When abstract deadlines approached for a national congress, I would look through these databases for ideas to analyze and results to present. They became the proverbial gifts that keep on giving, kept fresh by adding new columns as I thought of new questions to answer.

I also reviewed these data for the most up-to-date information to share with audiences before leaving on visiting professor trips. Or, if I read an abstract that someone would present at an upcoming congress that warranted comment, I would first check my own data on that subject. When I suspected I was seeing a complication more often than I should, I tallied my data to learn if it was true and then considered how to adjust the operation to make it better.

Sometimes I told trainees about Brantley Scott, the visionary who developed the inflatable penile prosthesis, and, somehow, in the days before Excel, found a way to store his results in one of the first Apple computers. Before attending a congress, Scott updated his information and then downloaded it onto a floppy disc that he carried into a local shop in whatever city the meeting was held to transfer onto Kodachrome slides.

How much easier it was to do all this now with laptops and Excel and PowerPoint! But I was limited by the way I set up my databases, typing words into the little boxes on the spreadsheet. I could count the number of patients who had a TIP or a two-stage graft repair, see how long they were followed after surgery, tally the number of fistulas and glans dehiscences or other problems, and then calculate the overall rate of complications. But I could not do a more sophisticated evaluation of my data to learn what factors predicted if these problems would occur—the sort of analysis that produced odds ratios and confidence intervals.

"I have to dummy code your databases," Bush explained to me one afternoon during a break in her master's classes.

She completed the required reams of IRB paperwork and then I gave her access, but this time more than a couple of weeks would pass before that task was done. The 259 Deflux injections that Gupta re-coded were in just 168 patients with a few columns of data. Bush faced well over a thousand patients with more than thirty columns of entries apiece spread among four different databases, all to be translated from words to the ones and zeros of computer language. It was a mammoth undertaking piled on top of her master's studies, patients in the clinic, the operations they needed, and an infant son who kept her awake most nights.

The fruits of her efforts were a harvest of papers updating both distal and proximal TIPs and describing a new algorithm to guide decisions in reoperations. Next came the first, and only, publication focused entirely on glans dehiscence. And then there was a fifth paper that used complex statistics to learn that the age when a patient has surgery does not affect the results, countering conventional wisdom that younger boys have better outcomes. Which eased the guilt parents feel when they, for one reason or another, could not schedule repair at the time the surgeon thought best.

Bush and I established a pattern writing those first manuscripts together. Once the new master database was ready, I entered the information after operations and follow-up clinic visits to keep it current. When we had a question to study, Bush formatted the statistical program and ran the analysis. Then we reviewed the results and what they meant. Next, I wrote a draft of the scientific article introducing our question, explaining how we studied our patients, reporting the results of our research, and then discussing how others could use what we learned. She described our statistical analysis, and read through the manuscript suggesting changes, which I then made.

Weeks after we submitted a manuscript to a journal, the editor emailed back reviews. Requests for a clarification, comments on how our work could have been better analyzed or reported, disagreements with our conclusions. I took the reviewer comments and broke them down into questions and statements that required a response, forwarding those regarding statistics to her to answer. Then I revised the manuscript in bold type to highlight changes for the editor when we sent it back. Bush reviewed those revisions to finalize them.

Sometimes reviewers noticed something we had overlooked or

gave an alternative explanation for our results. Other times I joked a reviewer must have imbibed a few too many adult beverages before reading our paper. She wondered if some reviewers were qualified to judge our statistics. We were both occasionally exasperated to have to answer questions from reviewers that were already answered in the manuscript. But I had learned to let an initial wave of irritation wash over, knowing that if a reviewer asked something or argued some point, there would be readers who were going to have the same question or disagreement. It was time-consuming and sometimes annoying, but the process made our papers better.

Before our collaboration began, I had to parry a challenge to TIP using my original database. The first article, published in 1994, concluded it could be used for "distal hypospadias with minimal chordee." The next one, co-written with Koyle and the other surgeons two years later, went a step further to declare the operation "widely applicable" to the many variations in anatomy that these boys have.

I had not used a different operation to fix distal hypospadias after my first TIP repair. And it appeared many others had not either, at least judging by the headlines of their articles calling TIP "A Near Ideal Way To Correct Distal Hypospadias," or "The Perfect Repair For Virgin Cases Of Hypospadias."

But in 2000 the *Journal of Urology* published a report from Australia that claimed there were more complications if TIP was done when the urethral plate is narrow. Those surgeons wrote that they did the operation exactly as I described it, and so they had to conclude that boys whose plates were less than eight millimeters at the widest point—nearly a quarter of their patients—needed a different repair.

The editor of the *Journal* did not ask me to review this manuscript before deciding to publish it. The most immediate remedy afterward was to write a letter to the editor suspecting the Australians did not, in fact, do the operation exactly like me. More likely, they did not incise those "narrow" urethral plates deep enough. But that letter was not published for a full year, and then was mixed in with other letters to the editor on a variety of subjects where it was easy to overlook.

So I combed through my database and found that I had measured the urethral plate in enough of my own patients to write a rebuttal article. Two-thirds had a plate measuring less than eight millimeters before I did the TIP incision, but only one of those developed a complication afterward. That 2004 article repeated the main point of my letter, that the complications those authors reported were not the fault of their patients' anatomy, or from using TIP, but rather occurred because the surgeons made a technical error in the most important step of the operation.

That should have ended the discussion. But surgeons had heard exaggerations about other operations enough in the past to now eye TIP with some suspicion. Like me, they also recalled how Duckett wrote that MAGPI could be used for all distal hypospadias, as long as the penis was straight, until Gibbons and Gonzales sorted through boys to learn that some had anatomy that resisted it. Which implied that complications after surgery happened because the wrong repair was chosen, not because the surgeon did a key step of the right operation wrong. And that conclusion led to the first version of the AUA hypospadias course, where Duckett showed slide after slide of distal hypospadias for two other surgeons to argue over which operation was best.

But the 159 patients I reported in 2004 were *consecutive* boys with distal hypospadias who *all* had TIP repair. That many patients likely had all the anatomic variations a surgeon would encounter, yet most of the operations were a success.

Still, the matter was not resolved. In 2009 the *Journal of Urology* published another article written by different surgeons repeating the charge that there were more complications if TIP was done when the urethral plate was narrow.

This time I asked the editor, "Why didn't you send me this paper to review?"

"Warren, you can't review all the papers on TIP," he replied, dismissively.

"Of course not," I agreed. "But I should have been asked about this one, especially since they wrote that *half* their patients shouldn't have had a TIP because of a narrow plate. I published, in this journal, that I haven't used another operation for distal hypospadias in years, so, obviously, a narrow plate is not a contraindication."

"Well, you can write a letter to the editor."

"That no one will see for a year. In the meantime, boys are going to be hurt if surgeons go back to doing operations that are not as good as TIP because of this paper."

Instead of writing another letter I wrote another article, the one with Bush after she reconfigured my database. This time we analyzed results in 426 consecutive distal hypospadias repairs all done using TIP, emphasizing again that we could find no anatomy that the operation could not fix. Proving that surgeons did not have to go back to the days when the anatomy of each boy had to be scrutinized, and the surgical drapes covered with hieroglyphics, trying to choose the right repair. And this time we chose to publish in a competing journal, the *Journal of Pediatric Urology*, which introduced the article in 2010 with an editorial declaring TIP the *gold standard* for repairing distal hypospadias.

Meanwhile, centers around the world were reporting similar results as mine, without warning there were some patients with distal hypospadias who needed a different operation. As best I could tell from discussions at meetings and during my travels, most surgeons were doing TIP most of the time, though some still clung to the operations they learned from their mentors, while others were persuaded by these articles in the *Journal of Urology* to return to the operations they did before TIP.

I told the story of proximal TIP as it stood in 2010 to my fellow skiers gathered again in the mountains of Telluride for the PUWF. But before speaking, I took an Inderol to control the anxiety of a pounding heart standing before them, even though they were friends.

I began by describing the first patient to have that operation, the one who my nurse suggested needed a TIP incision.

"He healed great. His penis looked totally normal and there were no complications. Naturally, I decided to do it again."

But then I had to wait more than a year for the next opportunity and told my colleagues that the painfully slow drip of boys with proximal hypospadias into my practice was the main reason I moved to Dallas.

"I used the same stitches and suturing that I was taught in residency for Duckett flaps in those first proximal TIPs. So, I was shocked to see the complication rate was 54 percent, including 33 percent fistulas!" I confessed. "I changed the stitches and changed from sewing the urethra in one layer to two layers. And, since it's hard to keep even tension on a long running suture line, I started interrupting the first layer."

I went to the next slide. "These modifications helped. As you can see, the next time I looked at my results, the overall number of complications had decreased to 25 percent, with only 10 percent fistulas. That was encouraging," I said, watching the small group of surgeons as they looked at my numbers, "but it was still a lot of fistulas." I advanced the slide again.

"All the boys in those first two series had their neourethras covered by dartos. I made another technical change and started using tunica vaginalis in a third series." A slide showed a picture of that dissection. "Dr. Bush and I recently reviewed those results. Only 13 percent had any complication, and *none* of those were fistulas. So, through technical improvements, the number of complications decreased from 54 percent to 13 percent and the number of fistulas went down from 33 percent to zero."

I looked at my friends again. "Meanwhile, I was also searching for the best answer when the penis was so bent that TIP couldn't be used. I tried Byars flaps, since they seemed popular, but *every one* of my patients had a complication. Then I changed to variations on Bracka's operation, and my complications decreased to 50 percent, which was better, but still a lot more compared to proximal TIPs."

The next slide showed that dramatic photo of the urethral plate held high in the air above the penis it was still connected to. "When I heard Bhat talk about elevating the plate off the corpora to straighten the penis, I started using that maneuver so I could do more proximal TIPs. And that seemed to work . . . at first," I continued, showing the early data. Then I clicked the mouse for the next slide. "Until some of those boys returned with febrile urinary infections or urine retention due to strictures.

"Most of them didn't stricture, but nearly one of every five did." I clicked the mouse again and a text box appeared with the admonition to stop doing proximal TIPs when there was more than a slight bend, that I designated as thirty degrees. "So now I don't elevate the plate anymore or try to do a proximal TIP when the penis is bent that much. Those have a Bracka repair."

Then I summarized. "I moved to Dallas to define the limits of TIP.

Now I can say it is the best choice for all distal hypospadias, and for proximal hypospadias when the penis is straight, or nearly straight. The main contraindication to TIP is ventral curvature of thirty degrees or more, when it's better to transect the urethral plate and do a two-stage graft repair."

Afterward, one of the participants commended me, "If every pediatric urologist chose just one topic and then studied it as methodically as you do, we would have the answers to most of the problems we see in no time."

But then I overheard another one sneer, "We're going to need a wide-angle lens for our group photo to fit in his big head."

◄ CHAPTER 9 ►

Now I Had to Teach Fellows

"That means we'll have to start a fellowship program," I told John Mc-Connell, moments after he named me the new chief of pediatric urology.

"Warren, that's absolutely *not* going to happen!" he replied emphatically. "Our department takes great pride in its residency training, and bringing in fellows complicates everything."

"That may be, John, but you just charged me to create an *elite* division and elite in pediatric urology is a fellowship training center."

I did not know McConnell well enough to realize the chairman would categorically state that something I asked was not possible, only to inform me the next day that the matter was resolved. But there was no problem and no urgency. The new division was nowhere near ready to begin training fellows, who would be capping their five or six years of general urology residency with another two devoted exclusively to pediatric urology.

A checklist of requirements had to be met to receive national accreditation for a fellowship. Our group already had a funded research lab where the fellow could work the first year, but Baker needed to add infrastructure for their education in basic sciences. Similarly, although we had a clinical research program and regular conferences to discuss patient care, those had to be built larger and modified to incorporate fellows. Bringing in fellows also meant adjusting clinic and OR assignments for the urology residents, so that all the trainees could participate in patient assessments and surgeries. And, since everything costs money, someone had to pay the salaries for the new fellows.

"Of course, we won't be ready to start a fellowship anytime soon, John, but we should build the division with that goal in mind and then decide when the time comes."

I was writing our application to the ACGME[28] two years later when the first email from a Turkish urologist, Selcuk Yucel, arrived.

> Dr. Snodgrass, I would like to do a pediatric urology fellowship with you and learn hypospadias. I have already spent a year in the basic science lab of Dr. Larry Baskin. What do you think?

I had to respond that Yucel was applying a year too early, and then I heard nothing more for the next several months until I opened a second email from him.

> I have been offered a fellowship in Australia. What do you think? Do I accept this offer?

I typed back:

> Selcuk, Congratulations. Maybe a bird in the hand is best for you, since we are just now submitting our application for accreditation. It will still be some time before we can offer a position.

That paperwork was completed, and our application sent to the ACGME in time for its review in December 2004. But, somehow, the packet was left on a secretary's desk while the committee met, so no action was taken and would not be taken for another six months, which was well after the fellowship match had passed. There was no appeal for their oversight, and no way we could interview applicants even though our program was certain to be approved at the next committee meeting. We would have to wait another year to begin.

Then a third email arrived from the Turkish urologist.

> Dr. Snodgrass, I turned down the position. Now what do you say?

---

28. *ACGME* is the Accreditation Council for Graduate Medical Education, which sets the standards for training after medical school, including fellowships.

I answered he was welcome to start in July.

Yucel was the first of nine fellows to train with me. Although our program offered several attractions, no doubt the opportunity to study hypospadias surgery with me encouraged applicants to rank Dallas Children's higher than more established programs with larger reputations. Certainly, that motivated Yucel to hold out for a position while we finished credentialing.

It was also the reason our second fellow, Ali Ziada, decided to train in Dallas, planning to take back home to Cairo lessons to decrease their complications.

"We do TIPs," he explained, "but we don't do them right."

Another applicant told me how confused she was struggling to understand which operation among many to do for hypospadias, since the chief where she was completing urology residency still analyzed the anatomy in each case to decide.

"I looked too, of course," Candace Granberg told me, "but I was never sure I would reach the same conclusions he did, so I worried I might do the wrong operation instead."

Which recalled my own residency and the lingering uncertainty from Gibbon's sketches on the drapes when we started a repair. Her decision was made when I explained I only used two methods to repair all hypospadias.

I was excited to teach fellows in a way I never felt training residents, who would use little of what I taught in their futures. The last place a doctor trains is the most important, and my lessons would help lay the foundation that these fellows would build their careers on. Unlike residents, they would arrive to the OR determined to learn all the key steps, nuances and intricacies I could teach them about hypospadias.

But I also knew those would change as time went by, as the operations I did continued to evolve. So the most important lesson to teach them was self-assessment, to review their work to be certain the results were good and the complications low—the 3Ps they watched me practice. I had to show them the best way to do those operations, but they had to realize that the best way might not have been found yet.

There would be no "Dallas way." Instead, my parting word to each one when they graduated was not to cling to what Snodgrass did when they were here, because Snodgrass might not be doing whatever that was the same way anymore.

It happened during a clinic day in June that every other one of my patients returning for follow- up after a hypospadias repair had a complication. That made for a long and difficult day, informing several parents that their sons were among the few who develop those problems after my surgery. The 5 percent after a distal, or the 15 percent after proximal repairs that I tell them is the risk beforehand, which every parent hears and assumes will not include their boy.

"We do everything we know during surgery to avoid a complication," I promise, "but someone's boy is going to have one anyway."

Now I had to slow down my hurry from one patient to the next because this discussion cannot be rushed. I had to tell the parents what I saw. Then I had to pause to let the news sink in. "I'm very sorry this has happened," I always said next, because I was. And frustrated that neither I nor anyone else had managed to drive those percentages lower. "No, I'm not sure why," I answered their question. "We've decreased how often it happens, but it still does." They wanted to know what I was going to do about it. "Nothing right now, except wait until everything's all healed. Then, in six months or so we can do an operation to fix it, which usually works," I reassured them.

What I did not learn at the university is that parents listening to this explanation really wanted to know if *they* somehow caused the complication to happen. Because they feel guilty that it happened to their son, and they worry they are responsible. But I would not hear those questions until my next career, when I made more time to listen.

They were also distressed that their son needed another operation when they hoped surgery was done. It is always discouraging to have this conversation, but I repaired a lot of hypospadias, which meant I saw a constant trickle of these complications afterward. What was unusual was that cluster of several on the same day.

I remember how my father, who did not do hypospadias surgery, was devastated when one of his patients had a complication after some other operation. How he stood in the office wondering why it had to happen to him despite his hard work to make everything right. I watched faculty during my training tell patients they almost never saw whatever complication occurred, which only made those patients worry even more. I heard surgeons who found a complication declare on the spot, "Well, I'm never going to do *that* again!" Even though *that* might still be the best operation since *all* operations have complications some of the time. I listened to discussions between colleagues during Morbidity and Mortality conferences and concluded there would be a more thorough search for the root cause of a complication if the names in the chart were blacked out and the records sent someplace else for other doctors to review.

It was the information in my databases that taught me to look past self-pity and self-serving excuses, and instead examine the operation that was done and the problem which occurred, and then ask myself if I made a mistake. But those answers came when we applied statistical analysis to groups of patients, while I had to face the boy and his parents one at a time. Did I make a wrong decision in all the many decisions taken during the course of his surgery? Or perhaps I made a technical error by stitching something too loose, or too tight? I usually could not find a reason, but it was always important to ask these questions.

The fellow happened to accompany me that day when so many boys returned with problems. Fellows came to my clinic in the first few months of their training, and then again during the last month for a refresher before leaving to start their own practice. This was Granberg's final day.

"Well, Candace," I said when the last patient left, "I hope you have the intestinal fortitude to do hypospadias surgery."

And without the slightest hesitation she looked at me and said, "You can do it because you know your numbers. You knew it was just a fluke that you saw several patients with complications on the same day."

Which proved the importance of teaching self-assessment. I was not taught to review my work in medical school, or during residency, or even in fellowship. The only faculty I knew who kept up-to-date data on his own results was Brantley Scott, using his Apple computer, and he was on sabbatical when I was scheduled to work with him. I suspect that to this day most surgeons who teach trainees do not know their own results, and so they cannot know if what they are teaching is best. I thought that collecting this information might be a redeeming benefit for all the troubles the Electronic Medical Record forced upon doctors when it came along several years later, so I tasked my last fellow to make that work in Epic[29] for hypospadias. But then I left the university before I could test the system Melise Keays devised.

When fellows arrived, I had to revisit how I taught hypospadias surgery. While it might be enough for residents to make and close incisions, fellows had to learn how to do entire operations that even experienced surgeons struggle to do right. And because they spent one year of their training in the lab, I had just one year with them in the operating room to accomplish that before sending them out to perform on their own. How much did they need to do to learn, and how could I allow them to do that and still get the same results with no more complications than when I did it all myself?

And just like when I became an academic surgeon at the university five years earlier, that task came with no instructions.

So, I looked back to my experiences as a trainee. I tried to remember how Edmond Gonzales taught his fellows hypospadias while I, a resident, watched. But those were memories from twenty years past, and all I could see was my mentor holding the penis while they incised the skin, picking up dartos tissues they cut to deglove the penis, and then . . . how he did the key steps blurred, probably because as the resident, I never did them. I invited Gonzales to Dallas as a visiting professor looking forward to the déjà vu of seeing him operate on a hypospadias again, but I was disappointed to see nothing that looked familiar.

I also thought back to that year in Seattle, but Mitchell rarely did a hypospadias repair and all I recalled was watching Mark Burns, a private urologist, do nearly the entire operation himself. That, and then chuckling as he finished, "And that's how I do the Snodgrass better than Snodgrass!"

After joining the UT Southwestern urology department, I went over to the adult hospital several times to observe one of my new col-

---

29. *Epic* is the name of one of the largest EMRs, used by many hospitals, including Children's when I was there.

leagues operate. More than once I saw the faculty talking a resident step by step through an operation they had obviously never seen before, and thought to myself it was better to *show* how to do it right than to *say* what to do next. And I undoubtedly cringed at all the attaboys the teachers dispensed.

The Gene Carlton I knew during residency was a man of few words, carefully chosen. There was no fawning praise to residents doing the job they were expected to do, but ample criticism when they arrived unprepared. I realized my chairman thought I was ready for the world one day in the last year of my residency when we were standing together in the surgery lounge waiting to begin an operation. The circulating nurse came in to ask Carlton how he wanted the patient positioned, and he looked at her and suggested, "Why don't you ask the surgeon?" nodding his head toward me.

I recall few other compliments during my four years there.

Coming from private practice I knew there was no more instruction after graduation, and no one watching who could tell if the surgeon was doing something right, much less doing it the best that he could. A compliment then meant little.

"You have to judge yourself," I told the fellows, "because you're the only one in the room who can. The nurse just knows if you're pleasant, and the anesthesiologist just cares if you're efficient, and don't lose much blood."

My first three fellows probably knew that truth already, since Yucel and Ziada followed a similar path as me to do their final training after being in practice a few years. Then Juan Prieto came to Dallas having already done a fellowship in Miami, because that one was not yet accredited and, therefore, did not officially count. In many ways these three were similar to the practicing surgeons who came to Children's to observe me operating, looking for the mistakes they were making and the subtle moves that could make good, better. My first fellows were more concerned to watch than to do.

So, by the time Nicol Bush started as the fourth fellow, my pattern was established. Neither she, nor any other fellow, would ever do any operation from beginning to end while I watched and assisted. Rather, I did most of the operation with them assisting, allowing them to do some important step in this patient, and a different one in the next. And I admit there were a few of those key steps that I rarely, if ever, allowed them to do, especially after the chief of another program told me, "Our results would be better, if we weren't always having to scramble out of some problem the fellow got us into."

My guiding principle was that the fellows could learn how to do hypospadias repairs by watching me do them, seeing the same steps applied to different anatomy over and over, day in and day out, week after week for their one year of clinical training. It was my responsibility to teach them two operations, and then they could go out and practice them on their own patients.

Nevertheless, I immediately recognized that Bush had unique skills. It was even clear to observers who saw us operating together, like the foreign visitor who came to Dallas just weeks after her clinical year started, and at the end of a day of hypospadias surgery commented to me, "You have a very nice setup here, and you are so lucky to work with an assistant who knows your every move!"

But not all the faculty shared my views on training.

"Warren, we need to set up a fellow's clinic where they can see their own patients and then do the surgery," Linda Baker told me several times, reminiscing about how her fellowship at Johns Hopkins was organized.

I could not imagine how this would work. Which patients with what problems would we schedule into that clinic? Who would review the fellow's decisions afterward? How would the faculty supervise their operations and what would we do if the fellow did not know how to do the operation they scheduled, or wanted to do something the faculty would not do themselves?

"Linda, maybe their time is better spent with us than doing things on their own," I responded each time.

When she persisted, I finally said, "OK, please go ahead and sketch out that plan so we can all review it."

Which never happened.

Meanwhile, I heard from the fellows how Baker might sit at a desk in the OR working on a research grant that was due by midnight, her back turned while they practiced what little they knew on a child assisted by a resident. I realized this teaching style was not unique to her, and I knew she was just as critical that I never relinquished control to see how much the fellows could do on their own. But the "see one, do one, teach one" model placed training above caring, and I was determined to keep the welfare of patients the central focus.

While I was confident the fellows graduated able to repair hypospadias, there was no *proof* that either my or Linda's style for teaching them worked. I thought I could tell from what they were allowed to do if they had the technical skills needed to cut and sew and make a penis normal, and I showed them how to hold something different or cut something at a different angle to improve those skills. I also proved they had the knowledge to manage patients with hypospadias before and after surgery by testing them constantly. For example, a fellow might hear conflicting views regarding the best age to repair hypospadias and ask my thoughts.

I would always answer, "That's a really important question. What *is* the best age?" and if they could not recite to me the available data on that subject today, I was certain they would be able to tomorrow. Whatever their skills, whatever their knowledge, it was my job to push them to a higher level of skill and knowledge. Everyone can improve.

All doctors remember that the orders they wrote as medical students had to be countersigned by an intern, a resident, or a faculty physician, someone with those initials MD after their name. And then, in the twinkling of an eye, they had those initials after their name and were suddenly responsible for what was done to a patient.

All surgeons recall how they watched several faculty do the same operation differently, thinking during the case, *I like that move, I'm going to do it that way too,* or, *Wow, I'm never going to do that when I'm in charge!* It was easy to judge when their judgment did not count, but the very first day after graduation their decisions were final. A young surgeon can ask advice from his new partners, but those new partners expect him to already know what to do.

Only the few who choose academic surgery face the added challenge of going from trainee to teacher in that twinkling of an eye. One day they are fellows, and the next they are faculty, with residents and fellows looking to them for guidance. I had twelve years in private practice to develop as a surgeon before I instructed others. Bush found trainees standing opposite her in the OR expecting her to teach before she proved to herself that she could do what she had learned.

So Bush started her career worried. Could she teach residents and fellows how to do things right? Did the bits and pieces I allowed her to do come together to make the same operations I did with the same results? I thought they did, but I did not know.

Bush decided to prove the value of her protected time and devised a study to find out. She contacted Ziada and Prieto who preceded her, and the two fellows who followed her, Ted Barber and Dan DaJusta, asking them to send their results from repairing distal hypospadias when they began their own practices. She then compared those, combined with her own, to my outcomes during the same time.

"Look at this," she told me when the data were all organized. "All five of us had the same results, and there was no difference in ours versus yours!"

No statistical difference in the complications that ranged from the low of 3 percent that she achieved to a high of 13 percent that another of the former fellows reported.

Despite whatever opinions others might have about the best way to teach, here was proof that my method accomplished its goal. But there was a bigger truth in these numbers that Bush immediately recognized.

"This means there doesn't have to be a learning curve for distal hypospadias."

If they were taught right and learned what they were taught, then even young surgeons could perform at the highest levels from the beginning. Of course, the converse of that was also true.

Which meant it was less important how mentors teach than what they teach. My comment to the SPU executive committee may not have been politically correct, but the idea that fellows should all be taught an evidence-based curriculum was professionally correct.

◄ CHAPTER 10 ►

You Sure Know How to Run a Group

I was surprised to learn that Duncan Wilcox operated on more boys with proximal hypospadias while he was at Children's than I did. Because he had more open slots in his clinic for the schedulers to fill when patients called for an appointment. Although Wilcox was an experienced surgeon, it would have been the same had new faculty arrived fresh from their fellowship training.

I did not give the scheduling process much thought during my first years as chief. The primary goals then were to get the phones answered promptly and the patients in to be seen without the long delays so common in academic centers, and in the other departments at Children's. There were no guidelines issued for the schedulers to direct boys with severe hypospadias to me, or for that matter, girls born without a vagina to Linda Baker, who watched me take grafts from the mouth and decided those could work to make her patients new ones.

As a result, my number of first-time operations for proximal hypospadias actually decreased after Wilcox arrived, to no more than a handful at the midpoint of my university career in 2007. When he left, I counted how many he did and realized those would have easily doubled my tally had they been scheduled with me. Furthermore, his patients had more complications than did mine, although his results were the same as would be reported a decade later by surgeons at Boston Children's and CHOP and Texas Children's.[30]

30. Those three papers published between 2015 and 2017 reported complications in 50 percent or more of proximal repairs.

Bush made her pitch to join the group the same year that Wilcox moved away, and I also recruited Patricio Gargollo, who was completing his fellowship training and wanted to establish a robotic surgery program. They say a crisis is a terrible thing to waste, and the urgent need to hire both these faculty and support their aspirations presented the opportunity to follow the lead of adult urology and subspecialize our reorganizing group.

"Patricio, tell me the cases you can do on the robot, and I'll refer them to you," I offered Gargollo to entice him to take the job.

Then I promised Baker all the girls with genital problems to speed along her research. Like me, Bush wanted to repair hypospadias, but her master studies left little time, and in any event, she would have to wait into the future for the proximal cases and redo surgeries that I intended to make my specialty. I gave her a few extra distal cases in the meantime. When I hired Micah Jacobs a few years later, I sent him all my new patients born with spina bifida.

And so, having first built a diverse practice in pediatric urology, I divested myself of major parts of it. I looked up at the picture of Gene Carlton looking down at me from the wall behind my desk, and recalled how he pioneered urology subspecialization twenty years earlier by similarly giving away pieces of his own practice to younger faculty, like Edmond Gonzales, so they could gain expertise and build their academic reputations.

It just made sense. If hypospadias happens in only one-half of one percent of boys, and proximal hypospadias in just one-tenth of those, there was no way that every pediatric urologist could do this surgery and expect to provide the best care. Not to mention other conditions the group treated that were even less common.

As expected, soon my number of proximal repairs increased to twelve a year. There was no way to know then that this was *six times more* than most other pediatric urologists in the US, whose average of only two a year would not be reported from the Board of Urology until 2011.

Of course, more surgeries also meant more patients returning with complications. After I managed to reduce fistulas in proximal TIPs, the most common problem was glans dehiscence, which seemed to happen more often than after distal TIPs. That was easy enough to verify, and a simple calculation from the database verified my suspicion.

Why did the glans come back open in only a few of my distal repairs, but over three times more often after the proximal ones? The same surgeon did the same repair using the same suture to sew the glans, yet the results were significantly different. Maybe, I thought, the smaller glans that some boys with proximal hypospadias have made it more tenuous to close over the new urinary channel.

Once again, Bush organized a study to test my theory, recruiting Dan DaJusta, our fellow that year, to measure the width of the glans in infants with proximal and distal hypospadias. They soon confirmed that the average size of the glans in proximal cases was, in fact, a few millimeters smaller.

And that seemed an easy fix. It is well-known that male hormone grows the penis, and many urologists use testosterone before surgery to enlarge a glans they deem to be small. That treatment dates back to a patient who went to the Mayo Clinic in the 1950s after several attempts to repair his proximal hypospadias failed. A surgeon there took one look at his penis and declared that no operation was going to succeed until testosterone grew it larger. After that, a few papers reported measurements documenting that growth, but no one ever showed that making the penis bigger improved the results of the repair that followed.

I decided to give testosterone before surgery to those boys with smaller glans until it grew to the average size of those with distal hypospadias since they had much less dehiscence. Bush and I then devised a protocol using measurements to decide who to treat and when to stop treating them.

At first, I gave the standard dose found in every textbook. But when I remeasured the glans a month later, most had not grown. So, I doubled the dose of testosterone and measured again, and then doubled it another time if there was still no response until the glans reached the targeted size. Then surgery was scheduled. Other boys with proximal hypospadias whose glans already measured the desired size were not treated. I added all these patients to the database, along with a new column indicating whether or not they received testosterone beforehand. No one had ever done a study like this before.

One Friday evening I was grilling a steak at my beach house in Galveston when my cell phone rang.

"Warren, are you sitting down?" Bush began the call.

"As a matter of fact, I am," I replied, swirling my glass before taking a sip of cabernet.

"Good. Because I just spoke with Carlos, who ran the numbers . . . and testosterone *doesn't* work!" she informed me, her voice infused with the excitement of discovery.

"Seriously?" I asked, drawing out the syllables.

"For sure. I've looked at it every which way and the answer keeps coming back the same. Testosterone grows the glans bigger, but complications stay the same."

"Well, you'll have to hold that thought," I told her, cradling the phone on my shoulder as I set down my glass of wine and reached to turn over the steak. "I'm not going to burn my dinner listening to you describe the stats! We can talk later."

Bush was right. No matter how she and Carlos Villanueva, the fellow, set up the statistical analysis, the message remained that testosterone, given in sufficient doses, managed to enlarge the small glans, but the boys who needed it still had more complications than the boys who did not. In fact, her modeling said that testosterone became a new risk factor for complications. Since the goal was to decrease glans dehiscence, and not just to enlarge the head of the penis, testosterone treatment failed.

The following Monday I stopped using testosterone. I had no idea what to do next to solve this problem, but chance favors the prepared mind. A few months later, the glansplasty I watched Yoshino and Tanikaze do gave the answer.

It was not just my practice that improved with specialization. Soon Gargollo learned that he did more operations on the robot than any other pediatric urologist in the US. Baker's list of vaginoplasties grew to the point that she could say her method worked better than the other ways surgeons tried to make a vagina. Jacobs began rapidly gathering the patients he would need to study bladder problems in children with spina bifida. And Bush was making a name for herself reporting clinical studies like these on glans size and complications.

The faculty all knew I expected them to set up their own databases. Now, when the time came to write abstracts summarizing their research for national meetings, those spreadsheets gave them fresh material to analyze. In a few years our group consistently had as many or more presentations as any other center in the country, including larger programs with more faculty longer established in academic circles.

A senior colleague remarked at one convention, "Your group always has the most interesting talks."

All this made them better teachers too. I frequently reminded everyone that the fellows would pass on the mistakes we taught to the children they operated in their future practices. As they focused attention on more patients and fewer conditions, it was easier for the faculty to review their results. That helped Gargollo recognize that one operation he was doing with the robot had too many complications, which led him and the fellows back to doing it in the traditional way, because not everything new is better. As word of this evidence-based teaching spread, the number of applicants wanting to do their fellowship training with our group exploded.

Specialization also improved efficiency. We could see more patients and do more surgery when we moved through clinics and surgeries with less uncertainty and hesitation. That brought in more revenue, and soon our group was one of the most productive at Children's—not because we focused on making money, but because we focused on taking better care of children.

It is no accident that the best and most successful medical centers in the world—the Mayo Clinics, the Sloan Ketterings, and the Texas Heart Institutes—are all filled with specialists doing the few things they do best day in and day out.

After a discussion in his office one day, the Urology Department Manager told me, "You sure know how to run a group!"

But specialization in pediatric urology was something new. And knowing the natural response to a new idea, the murmurings from some in the group were no surprise. The faculty who did not see the example of adult colleagues specialized to treat only cancer or stones, but only saw our difference from other pediatric urology programs. Who grumbled that some operations paid more than others, even though everyone was salaried and bonused under the same university regulations. Who were not satisfied with their own pie, but wanted bites from everyone else's too. But everyone had to give up something to get what they wanted most, and no one gave up more than I did, since my pie was the largest.

Despite these quibbles, I considered specialization my greatest achievement as division chief. It was also one of the first things my successor would dismantle. It was astonishing how quickly the clock ran backward to fewer national presentations, fewer fellow applicants, and less revenue. And fewer faculty, when the experts in hypospadias and robotics left for new practices where their expertise was recognized.

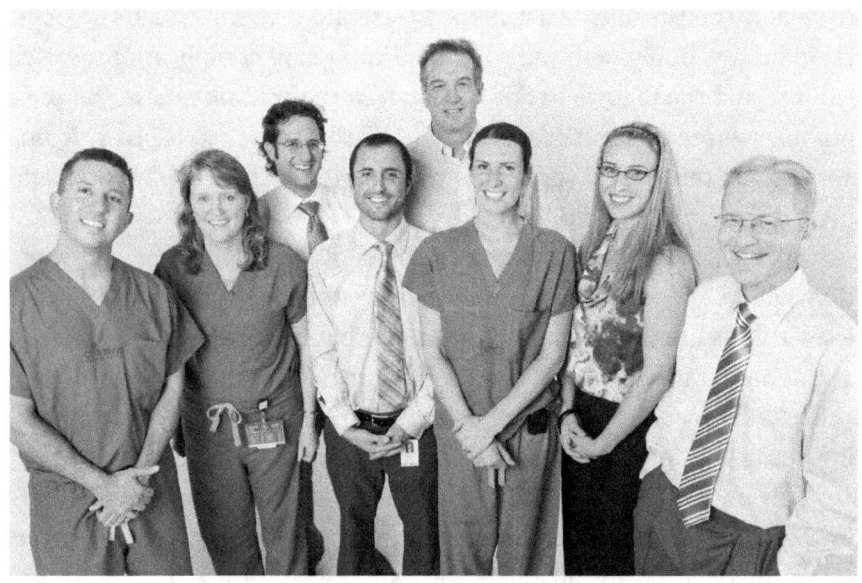

The Dallas Children's Urology Group in 2012. Gargollo, Baker, Jacobs, Villaneuva (fellow), Harrison, Granberg (fellow), Bush, and me.

◄ CHAPTER 11 ►

We Bring In Specialists to Do the Rare Cases

As the plane descended, I looked through my briefcase for the itinerary. The papers Janet Parker, my secretary, always prepared before I left Dallas that listed arrival and departure times, the hotel reservation, the schedule of lectures and surgeries, and my contact person. I did not recall seeing it, and now I could not find it despite looking through each compartment twice.

A young woman waited just beyond the jetway holding a sign with my name and steered me away from the other deplaning passengers to an elevator that took us to the ground floor. A car pulled near as soon as I exited. She opened the back door for me and then sat in the front next to the driver.

We drove a short distance around the terminal to another entrance, where the guide led me to a booth to present my passport. I glanced to the right and saw other passengers queued in long lines waiting to be processed. The officer returned my passport and the escort walked with me to claim my luggage. As soon as the carousel started turning and I saw my bag emerge, she spoke briefly into a walkie-talkie clipped to her collar, then loaded my suitcase onto a cart and walked me through customs and out the door. A different car pulled up. The woman shook my hand and left, and then the driver took off without asking where I was going.

Forty minutes later he pulled into the Hilton, where a bellman took my suitcase while I registered.

"Dr. Snodgrass, we have you on an executive floor for one week."

"Do you have any messages for me?" I asked the receptionist.

"No, sir," she replied as she handed me the room card.

I took the elevator to the eleventh floor. My bag arrived as I stood on the balcony of my room admiring the view of the sea to the right and the sprawling city of Tel Aviv on the left. I unpacked and sat on the bed, wondering what the plans were for the week. There was no envelope on the desk with instructions, and I had no number to call.

With nothing else to do, I changed into swim trunks, rode the elevator back to the ground floor, collected a towel, and went down to the beach for a swim. The sea was a pleasant cool, and the beach was filled with Israelis escaping the July heat.

An hour later I returned to the room to watch the sunset from the balcony. Still no message. My arrival resembled a scene from *Mission Impossible*, and now I could only wait for instructions.

Normally, the host would meet me at the airport, and then review the schedule of events enroute to the hotel. Sometimes, a trainee was dispatched to collect me, or a driver stood waiting holding a card with my name, and the meeting organizer would give me the final plans over dinner. But this time I landed without an itinerary, and still had no idea who my host was, what I was supposed to do, or when I was supposed to do it.

The phone finally rang. "Professor Snodgrass. This is Rabbi Firer. Welcome to Israel!"

I strained to understand the accented mumbling.

"We have arranged a visit for you to Jerusalem tomorrow morning."

Well, that's a nice surprise, I thought, wondering how far away Jerusalem is from Tel Aviv.

"A guide will pick you up from the hotel at 8:00 a.m., so you have time for breakfast," the rabbi continued. "You will see some patients Tuesday morning and operate on three boys Thursday. I look forward to having dinner with you Wednesday."

During the drive the next morning the guide recounted the history of their state, pointing out, for example, the ruins of battles along the roadway preserved as memorials on the ascent to the Holy City. Then he told of celebrities he had toured around the country, most recently Rahm Emanuel, President Obama's Chief of Staff, who brought his family a few weeks earlier to celebrate his son's bar mitzvah at the Wailing Wall.

"And how are you special?" he asked, glancing toward me.

"I'm not, really," I answered, as I watched the landscape flying by.

The next day Rabbi Firer came unannounced to the clinic where a local pediatric urologist and I were examining a few boys with hypospadias. The rabbi walked in dressed in Hasidic garb, wearing a black yarmulke with an open-collared white shirt, black trousers tucked into shin-high socks, and tassels from his tzitzit undershirt hanging out over either hip. I noticed we were about the same age and height, although the rabbi had a distinguishing long grey beard, and curls of hair tucked behind his ears.

"It is nice to meet you, professor. Thank you for sharing your expertise with us."

I replied it was an honor to be invited. Then I resumed clinic under the interested eye of the rabbi, who stood just off to the side where he could watch without interfering. When the last boy was examined and sent away, the rabbi reminded me of our dinner the following evening, and then asked my plans for the afternoon. Hearing there were none, he promised to send a driver to the hotel at five o'clock for a trip to Caesarea, north of Tel Aviv.

After my visit to Jerusalem, I was excited to see the ruins of a city built by Herod the Great and named in honor of Caesar Augustus. I already knew the city was built overlooking the sea, centered around a harbor created in the open waters by a massive artificial jetty considered a wonder of the ancient world.

"You want to go to Caesarea? Right now? That will take an hour in this traffic, and the park will be closed!" the driver protested as I clicked my seatbelt. "I will take you on a tour of Tel Aviv instead," he declared as we sped away from the Hilton.

Before I could respond, the phone in the car rang. After a brief discussion shouted in Hebrew, the driver made a U-turn, and looked at me suspiciously from the corner of his eye.

"He said not to worry about the time. They will keep the park open for you."

And so it was. We arrived as the site was closing and walked in like fish swimming upstream against the current of people flowing out from the gates.

"Take as much time as you want!" the guard called out as we passed by.

The next evening I dressed for our dinner in a tie and jacket, to show respect to the rabbi whose work, Google explained, had been honored with the State of Israel's highest award. Rabbi Firer sat at the head of an oval table hidden under a white paper cloth, wearing the same traditional clothes as he had at clinic the day before. He took two cell phones from his pockets and rested them nearby. Then he introduced me to his colleagues seated to the left, as a waiter silently brought in the first course of our meal. While the others started eating, the rabbi took off his glasses to wipe them clean and turned to his visitor.

"Tell me how you fix hypospadias."

I took stock of him and the others, gathered in this small room on the fifth floor of a box-shaped building nestled in the orthodox Jewish community of Bnei Brak, bordering Tel Aviv, and considered how to explain the complex surgery to men whose only formal education was in the Old Testament and related religious writings. Then I held up my finger and pointed to a spot below the tip.

"Most boys with hypospadias have a distal opening, with the tissues that should have made the urinary channel, the 'urethral plate,' running from there to where the opening should be," I began, as I would to a family in the clinic. "To correct that, we make incisions—"

The Rabbi cut me off with a dismissive wave of his hand. "*Anyone* can fix distal hypospadias. We want to know how you do *proximal* hypospadias."

My face betrayed an instant of surprise, as I looked again at this bespectacled middle-aged man fingering his tassels.

"Well, I use the same technique if I can, making a longer urine tube from the urethral plate."

"So, you don't need to use a skin flap in your urethral repair?" the Rabbi asked. "This is why we brought you here," he added, nodding toward his associates.

Now I recalled the letter I received months ago, connecting the name Ezra Le'marpeh to this building and Rabbi Firer to this man. A letter that asked me to help a boy with proximal hypospadias who had been circumcised on the eighth day, in the Orthodox Jewish tradition, which meant he did not have foreskin to make a flap. The letter mentioned sending the boy to Dallas for surgery, but now I realized they had flown me to Israel to do that repair.

"Flaps are the most popular way to fix proximal hypospadias," I explained, "but I decided years ago to see what surgery looked like without them. I never use flaps."

The Rabbi resumed his questioning. "What is the complication rate using your technique? How many fistulas and meatal stenoses or strictures do you have?"

I marveled at this inquisitor. Not many parents knew these words. Even some of the young residents beginning their urology training did not know the "urethral plate" and could not define "meatal stenosis" after surgery.

"Rabbi, I keep a database with all my results. When I first started doing proximal repairs, my complication rate was 54 percent after TIP and 100 percent with flaps, which is why I stopped doing flaps. I made some technical changes to the TIP operation and now the complication rate is 15 percent, which was recently published. Those are fistulas and glans dehiscence."

"How many strictures do you have?" the Rabbi asked again.

"Almost none," I answered. "Meatal stenosis and strictures are more common with flaps than with either TIP or the grafts I do."

I told how plastic surgeons consider the blood supply to the ends of foreskin flaps to be unreliable, which meant they had a greater chance to scar into those complications. I saw Firer glance over to Rabbi Wolfe, one of his assistants, as though confirming a hunch.

Our conversation continued back and forth through the main courses. As dessert was served the Rabbi reminded me that I would do three operations the next day, including the circumcised boy they had written to me about, plus two others with complications after earlier surgeries.

"I'm looking forward to watching your operations tomorrow," he said, ending our discussion with another surprise.

Then Firer changed the subject. "Professor, what do you do besides hypospadias?"

I thought a moment, and then said, "Some of everything, really, but mostly surgery for neurogenic bladders."

The Rabbi smiled. "That's very interesting," he replied. "Tell me about the Zhou procedure."

Maybe it was not such a wonder that the Rabbi knew so much about hypospadias, I thought during the ride back to the hotel. After all, they brought me here to operate on boys with hypospadias, so he might have spent some time reading up on it. But Firer had no idea I would mention neurogenic bladder, yet he had heard of a new treatment from China just beginning tests in the US.

"All evening the rabbi talked to me with the knowledge of a fellow," I told Freddy Rosenberg, the insurance executive who sat across from me at dinner and was now driving me back to the hotel.

"Trust me," Freddy answered, "it's not just hypospadias or urology. He knows this much about *everything* medical. All the doctors are surprised the first time they meet him."

Nearly a year passed before another letter arrived from Ezra Le'marpeh, the Rabbi's nonprofit organization, inviting me for another "vacation" in Israel. I laughed at this formality. *No one sends letters anymore*, I thought, as I typed my acceptance to the email address listed in the letter and clicked SEND.

This time I was less amazed by the guided shortcut through the airport, and the spy movie pickup from the terminal and delivery to the hotel. This time I did not worry about the schedule, knowing I would get a call detailing it sometime that evening. When the car left a half-hour late the next morning, I was not surprised that the phone rang, and the guide eyed me curiously after a conversation with an unknown person in Hebrew. I almost anticipated he would then whisper a password that opened a gate to a small parking lot where, I was told, even Benjamin Netanyahu, the Israeli Prime Minister, could not park. It seemed natural that just as the car rolled to a stop my door was opened and I was hurried away for a tour of the tunnels that run alongside the Western Wall of the Temple, which was another triumph of Herod the Great. And, of course, my entire journey through this passageway was recorded by a photographer into an album the rabbi presented to me at dinner the next evening.

But this time I was worked harder, the vacation cut shorter to make more time in the operating room. This time there was another patient or two waiting to have their proximal hypospadias repaired, plus several more suffering from complications the rabbi wanted me to fix. Most of these looked like that boy who first opened my mind to Bracka's repair, and by now, I had many years' experience removing scarred tissues and replacing them with healthy grafts taken from inside the mouth.

This time Yoram Mor, a pediatric urologist trained in London, arranged the OR schedule and assisted during the operations. There was nothing I had not seen before, or was unsure how to correct, but the back-to-back-to-back difficult cases were a fatiguing challenge. I would have never scheduled my day like this at home. And, despite Mor's training, he did not know these operations that I was doing and so he could not know how I wanted help.

It was late every evening when I returned to the hotel exhausted, so late that one night even the executive dining area was closed, and I had to order room service before collapsing to sleep.

Freddy drove me to the airport at the end of the week.

"I guess we will be seeing you again in six months," he said, referring to the second operations that would be needed to finish the two-stage repairs I had started.

"I'm sure the rabbi will find plenty to keep you busy," he chuckled as he said good-bye.

By the next trip, a routine was developing. I would begin with a day of sightseeing while recovering from jet lag, followed by several days confined in the hospital operating. There would be dinner one night with the rabbi and his colleagues around the same oval table in the same square building, and another dinner with Freddy in an upscale restaurant somewhere in Tel Aviv.

The operations were reliably difficult, a concentrated dose of severe hypospadias mixed among failed surgeries to be redone. It resembled my practice back home, but only if you took away all the distal operations, and the much easier hernias and undescended testicles and surgeries for reflux that dispersed the strain of these most demanding hypospadias repairs.

"I think you should come and help me do these cases," I told Bush when I returned from my fourth adventure at the end of 2012. "It will be good for you to see so many difficult cases all at once. Besides, you'll enjoy meeting the rabbi. He's like a matchmaker who connects patients with the doctors they need."

Even with her help, the days operating ran into the night. But, as I predicted, the cases were less fatiguing, and the decisions were more certain, working together. Although we had rarely operated together since her fellowship, Bush and I quickly found a rhythm again. We complemented each other, advising when a stitch seemed out of place or an oblique incision into the skin needed to be made, and shared the steps in long operations like a relay team passing the baton to a fresh runner.

"Wow, those were amazing cases," she declared, as we waited for Freddy to collect us for dinner. "It was like a year's worth of the hardest operations packed into one week! I'm so glad you invited me."

We arrived a few minutes ahead of Smadar Wieler, Freddy's assistant, and found a table. Freddy, dressed as always in a sport coat and tie, ordered a bottle of wine, always Israeli, and always red even though we would be eating fish in this popular restaurant on the beach. Then Smadar walked up, and she and Bush looked over the mezza of appetizers, choosing several for us to share.

As we settled into the meal, Freddy politely asked Bush how she came to be a urologist, a woman in a field best known for treating men. She certainly did not resemble a typical urologist, given our society was filled with short, balding, bespectacled men. In contrast, Bush stood tall with a dancer's lean body and straight blonde hair, kept long once she realized there was no hiding her Dallas Cowboy Cheerleader past. I laughed silently at the answer I knew was coming.

"Who better than a woman to be a penis expert?" she replied, with a coy smile.

As Freddy blushed and Smadar laughed out loud, Bush asked what his connection was to Rabbi Firer.

"He is a special man, as you have seen," Freddy answered. "Somehow, with no medical training, he knows more than most doctors, at least more in many fields from urology to cardiology to neurosurgery to cancer treatments . . . everything, it seems."

He sipped his wine and poured another glass.

"Many people contact him every day to ask his advice, and he connects them with the best doctors to get the best treatments."

Bush remembered how I described the rabbi as a medical matchmaker.

"Yes, that's it," Smadar agreed. "There's no one else quite like him."

"Sometimes a patient has a problem that is uncommon, or more complicated than usual, and the rabbi knows it will be difficult for them to get good treatment in Israel," Freddy continued. "We are a small country, so we bring in specialists to do the rare cases."

"Like us," I added.

"Yes, like you. Everyone knows the name Snodgrass for hypospadias, so we bring you here to do the hardest operations."

"But the first letter I got from the rabbi asked if he could send a patient to me in Dallas. Then I ended up here instead," I replied, puzzled at the question I had never before thought to ask.

"In Israel, everyone has insurance, and they can pay a little extra for treatments abroad. But that can be very expensive, especially in the US," Freddy explained.

Smadar continued the thought. "After the bill for one cancer patient we sent to Colorado nearly broke our whole budget, Freddy started a program to fly specialists here, where at least we can control the costs!"

"Your company will pay for people to go outside Israel?" I asked. "I've never heard of insurance anywhere doing that."

"In Israel every life is sacred," Freddy answered, recalling his own family's experiences during the Second World War. "And we think insurance should help them, not fight with them about the care they need," the insurance executive continued, implying the contrast to US companies. "Unlike in your country, the major insurances here are all nonprofits. I work with the rabbi to get people that care."

"Since we don't have a fee agreement with your hospital in Dallas to fix the costs, we bring you here," Smadar said, finishing the story.

Not long after returning home, I arranged a meeting with the Chief Financial Officer at Children's.

"I want to discuss a fixed price that we can offer international patients to come here for hypospadias surgery," I opened the bargaining.

"We already have something like that," he replied.

I studied the small man who seemed the caricature of a bean counter, trusting numbers over reason.

"What I hear is that the hospital charges way more than its best contracts pay if people don't have insurance," I countered.

"Well, we offer a steep discount if they pay in full at the time of service," the accountant parried.

"But if you charge $100,000," I argued, using figures rumored to be true, "and then discount that 50 percent, the overall fee is still way more than what Blue Cross, or any other company for that matter, would pay you."

The administrator stared at me, impassively. I searched for any other argument that might penetrate his stone heart.

"Remember, these families also have to pay for flights and hotels. If we price surgery too high, they won't be able to afford to come here, and then the hospital will make nothing!"

"We have to cover our costs."

"Yes, you do," I agreed. "And those costs will be the same as they are for insured patients."

"But if we fix the price and someone needs emergency care after surgery we could lose money," the accountant insisted, holding his ground.

"And that has never happened after a hypospadias repair in the ten years I've worked here," I almost sneered.

Several more meetings with the CFO yielded no progress, and this debate remained at an impasse until I cornered Doug Hock, the Chief Operating Officer, in the hallway. I made the hospital's second-in-command a simple proposal.

"Why don't we set the hospital fees somewhere above Medicaid and somewhere below whatever the top-paying private insurance con-

tract is?" I asked, using my hands to indicate the range available between these extremes.

I could see the gears turning.

"Doug, y'all make money off of Medicaid," *and a good thing too*, I
thought, considering that over 90 percent of the patients coming to
Children's were insured through that government program.

"So, for sure you'll make more money from these patients, and you
won't even have to spend a dime authorizing[31] them. They'll just pay
you cash up front, in full."

There was no hesitation.

"Sure, we can do that. Give me a week to get some figures together
and we can agree on the fee."

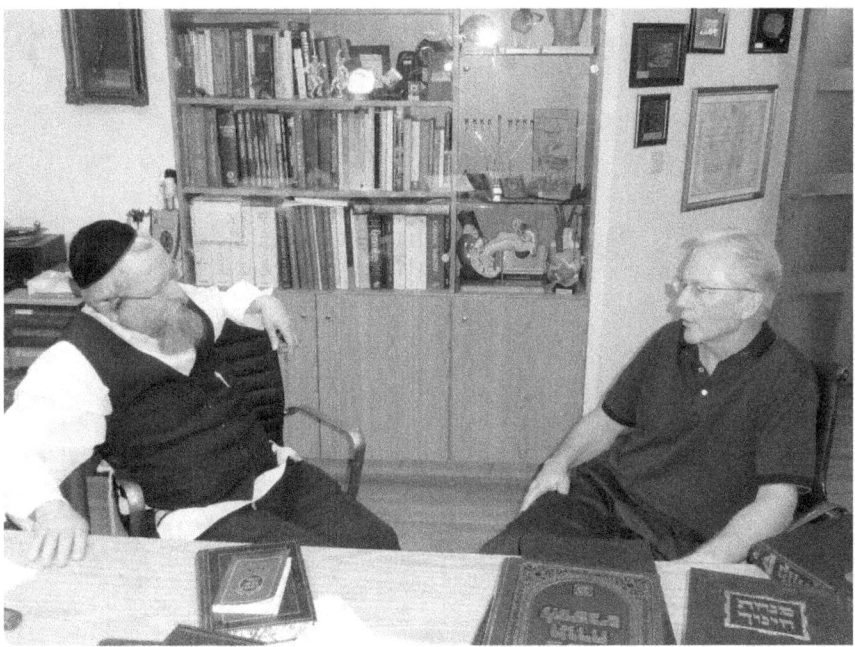

Rabbi Firer and me in his office.

---

31. *Authorization* is the approval required by insurance companies in advance of an operation or
other treatment.

◀ CHAPTER 12 ▶

I Only Heard He Was Innocent

It was a never-ending frustration that half the pediatricians in Dallas trained at Children's, but only a few referred their patients to the academic specialists there. The majority supported the town pediatric urologists, who, like them, were in private practice. When I arrived, I drove around the city introducing myself to these community pediatricians, emphasizing my private practice roots in the hopes they would see me as a kindred spirit. The hospital supplemented these efforts, highlighting my worldwide reputation in its magazine and newsletters, and promoting me as a speaker in its educational programs.

"None of this is working," I complained one day to Chris Dougherty, the vice president overseeing community outreach. "It's so irritating that patients with hypospadias are sent to our competitors, who then do the 'Snodgrass repair' without anyone ever telling them they could have it done by Snodgrass himself!"

Knowing that information on the internet is available all day every day, in contrast to quarterly magazines and sporadic lectures, I proposed some sort of website that would let parents know what Children's and I had to offer them.

"That would be a pay-per-click campaign," Dougherty replied, and then explained the mechanics. "It's a great idea," he admitted, "but Children's has never done it, and it will be a challenge to convince the bosses to spend the money."

"What if I pay to get it started, and then they can see the results?" I proposed, already annoyed at another example of the administration's shortsightedness.

And so I spent $1,000 from my own pocket for Children's to start a pay-per-click ad in the Dallas-Fort Worth region. That proved such a good investment that a few months later the hospital paid out of its pocket to expand the campaign nationally, which I learned when two colleagues at the AUA complained they saw it every time they googled hypospadias. That was exactly what I hoped parents would find.

Soon a dribble of new patients followed those ads into Children's to see me, enough for my nurse, Kate Walden, to need a white board to keep track of them. Never very many, but enough that she and I both noticed when the stream would, from time to time, dry up.

"They must have turned off the ad again," Walden told me several times when weeks passed without any new contacts.

Dougherty would explain that the budget had been adjusted, meaning decreased, and the ad ran out of clicks, or that there was turnover in the department running the campaign and something must have fallen between the cracks. Soon the ad would resume, and patients would find their way here again.

Then Dougherty left Children's. I was assured the campaign would continue; the administration buoyed by the quarterly reviews of its performance. In fact, the statistics were so encouraging that the hospital decided to expand the program to include other services in addition to my hypospadias repairs.

But every one of those new initiatives soon floundered.

Then, during yet another round of belt-tightening in the hospital, driven by rumors that Medicaid funding was about to be cut, the entire pay-per-click program was abruptly closed. Once again, my nurse and I discovered this when no new patients contacted us, and I was only able to salvage my campaign by convincing the bean counters that, unlike the others, it paid for itself.

"It's so crazy," I confided to Walden when the ad was renewed, again. "This is the most effective way we have to attract patients from the community, and the hospital keeps turning it off, without even telling me!"

Meanwhile, I continued journeys to foreign lands, teaching others what I was learning about hypospadias in live-surgery workshops. Although I did all the usual academic activities: presenting my work to congresses, writing peer-reviewed articles, filming teaching videos of operations, I also knew that five-minute PowerPoint presentations, paragraphs of words describing operations, and videos editing two hours of surgery into eight minutes, could not convey essential messages as clearly as an actual operation viewed live.

All operations are a series of steps fused together to make a repair. Each of those steps might be done in different ways. For example, some surgeons make the TIP incision using scissors, like I do, while others prefer a knife, and a few, a needle-tip cautery. Or they might tubularize the urethral plate in one layer or two, with stitches penetrating the lumen or staying beneath it. And the order of the steps can make a difference.

I sometimes told an audience, "I'm standing here because I did the TIP incision under direct vision, and so I could see how the plate widened and that I didn't need a flap. Duckett hinged the plate *after* he sewed on a flap by just sticking a knife down the meatus and cutting blindly. So, he couldn't see what I did."

I explained over and over, year after year, how to do each key step in a TIP repair. Still, live-surgery workshops were scheduled year after year around the world and attended by scores of surgeons, many of whom were having complications from doing the operation wrong, despite thinking they were doing it right.

How many times did a surgeon watch me incise the urethral plate and then say, "Now I see my problem! You're cutting much deeper than I am."

But unlike many visiting professors, I did not relish these performances. It did not stroke my ego to operate in front of peers. In fact, I was careful not to promote myself as a gifted surgeon, but instead emphasized to the others watching that they could achieve the same results as mine, if they did the key steps of the operation the same way that I did. Still, the invitations to workshops kept coming; a testament to the struggles surgeons have repairing hypospadias all over the world.

A 2007 workshop brought Pippi-Salle, Bracka, and me back together, this time in Kosovo, for the usual lectures and live-surgery demonstrations we were now well accustomed to doing. But first the three of us found time for a beer in a café the afternoon before the meeting began. Soon, we were reminiscing about other adventures when our paths converged, and the many places we had each visited but at different times.

But not in the US, where live surgery is rarely demonstrated. In fact, I had never heard of a workshop devoted to hypospadias that showed operations in my home country. Even the other surgeries that were commonly done by visiting professors when I was a resident had mostly come to an end.

Maybe hospital attorneys discouraged live surgery, citing the theoretic liability of a visiting surgeon. Perhaps meeting organizers were reluctant to wade through the stacks of paperwork required to credential a renown surgeon to do a single operation. Or maybe local surgeons did not think there was enough to learn from a visitor to justify confronting the attorneys and filing reams of documents to make it happen.

But that stream of patients drawn to Dallas by pay-per-click suggested otherwise. At least half of them wanted help when surgery by other pediatric urologists had failed, and as their numbers slowly but steadily increased, I decided something had to change. So I met with the hospital internet technicians, the Continuing Medical Education staff, and the head nurse of the OR to set into motion planning for a live surgery workshop at Children's geared for US surgeons.

Naturally, I wanted to duplicate the most successful workshops I had participated in.

"We'll need a split screen so we can show two surgeons operating on different cases at the same time," I told IT. "And we'll want microphones to transmit comments and questions back and forth between the auditorium and the operating rooms."

Then, to avoid confusion and call attention to key maneuvers being shown, I informed CME, "We have to invite a moderator," since they handled those arrangements.

Finally, I met with the head OR nurse to say, "We're going to need the two best circulators and techs who normally work with us to make sure the cases run smooth and the rooms turn over fast."

But I wanted to extend the reach beyond the usual workshop. While the emphasis would be on live surgery before a live audience in the hospital conference center, there would be some US colleagues who could not attend because they had to cover call, some fellows who would not be given time off to come, and some foreign surgeons who could not afford the travel or obtain the necessary visas. Consequently, I decided to also broadcast the show live by webinar, and I asked IT to make that happen too.

I chose the rather cumbersome name *Data-Driven Decision-Making in Hypospadias Surgery* to emphasize this course was not going to be a typical debate between surgeons arguing their opinions.

"The visiting surgeon and the moderator will both give lectures," I told Bush as we discussed details, "but I want to speak first on evidence-based practice to set the tone for the meeting."

To further ensure a clear message to the participants, I wrote two syllabuses to accompany the operations. One described each key step they would see, with photos and illustrations to supplement the live images on the big screen, and space for them to write notes. The other reviewed published data regarding preoperative, intraoperative, and postoperative decisions: the age to do surgery, whether to give testosterone, the sutures, catheters, and bandages to use, assessments afterward to check for complications, and many other questions that were asked again and again at other workshops I attended.

Every detail had to be right. I calculated we would need two ORs running two full days to demonstrate first-time distal and proximal hypospadias repairs, a fistula closure, and both easier and harder reoperations. To simplify local arrangements and transportation to and from the conference, I asked the hospital to reserve a block of rooms at a nearby hotel that provided shuttle service. The hospital agreed and also promised to cater lunches in the auditorium on both days so the surgeries could continue without interruption.

The most important decisions were also the easiest: who to invite to operate and to moderate? I confirmed my choices with Bush.

"We'll get Pippi to operate, since he does surgery pretty much like we do, and he's also perfect to lecture. He can tell other surgeons that he was once a flap guy, but now he's converted to TIPs and grafts."

"He'll be great," Bush agreed, "and it'll be good to have someone besides us talking about two-stage grafts to an audience who mostly still does flaps."

"That's why we need Aivar to moderate," I continued. "No one else in the world has his experience with grafts. In fact, this'll be the second time for Americans to hear him talk about them," I reminded her. "I invited him to the SPU in 2005, and you know the story about hearing something new; this time at least some people will remember they've heard about grafts before."

"OK, but didn't you tell me he doesn't keep up with his results? How'll that go over in a data-driven workshop?" she asked.

"The audience probably won't notice, since they don't either!" I laughed. "But at least Aivar can answer basic questions about grafts to get them thinking, and he's probably the best moderator I've seen at a hypospadias course."

Once the program was finalized, the CME department issued the official invitations to Pippi-Salle and Bracka, secured Pippi-Salle's operating privileges, and arranged their travel to Dallas. Meanwhile, the PR department helped advertise the event, and dietary drew up the lunch menus. I was left to complete the course materials and select the patients for surgery. Finally, after more than two years of preparation, the first US surgical workshop on hypospadias was ready.

I sat down for a quick breakfast Friday morning, an hour before the workshop began, and read emails while I ate. There was a message from the department chairman.

> Warren,
>
> I have some questions about Bracka. The residents found some disturbing things on the internet about him. Does Children's know about that? You should have told me. What if word gets out and I didn't know about him?"

I thought back to a breakfast in Kosovo, when Bracka said he was arrested early one morning after a former patient filed a complaint against him with the police for inappropriate behavior. In the ensuing publicity, another two or three patients made similar accusations. Bracka's credentials to work were suspended while he awaited trial.

I hammered a fast reply:

Claus,

I knew he was accused, but a British court found him innocent. His credentials were restored, and he resumed seeing patients until he retired months ago. I invited him over a year after the case closed. Children's managed all the arrangements for both visiting professors. They didn't say anything to me about any concerns.

I invited Bracka because he knows more about grafts than anyone else in the world. I learned a lot from him, and I wanted him to teach others too.

I paused, reflecting for a moment how the chairman never showed much interest in the affairs of his pediatric division . . . telling me every time I asked for advice, or needed his assistance, or simply wanted to update him on some matter, "Warren, you are in charge of pediatrics."

Still, it seemed prudent to add:

Sorry I didn't discuss this with you.

Then I hit SEND, and wondered if I had crossed some ethical boundary. I invited a renowned surgeon, one of the best in the world, to help other surgeons needing help for their patients, after Bracka was accused but declared innocent by a court of law.

I read through Claus's email again and saw that my boss did not tell me to remove Bracka from the program. In fact, I thought Claus must not have been too concerned since he did not call me but sent an email that I might not have seen until the course was over. And with that thought, I rushed out the door to arrive to the course on time.

Over one hundred pediatric urologists attended that 2011 workshop in person; mostly US specialists, with a sprinkling of foreign surgeons traveling from as near as Canada to as far away as Japan. Another untold number watched on computer monitors in over forty countries and most of the twenty-four time zones worldwide. I was relieved the surgeries flowed smoothly, and together with the lectures, clearly conveyed the core message that TIP is the best operation for distal hypospadias, and staged grafts are superior to flaps for proximal repairs. These were new concepts for many of those watching, especially hearing the benefits of grafts after being taught that flaps are inherently better.

As expected, Bracka helped keep it all straight, calling attention to key maneuvers as Pippi-Salle and I operated, while sprinkling in anecdotes from his own experience. His signature cat's arse dismissal of flaps seemed a perfect contrast to the normal appearance of the meatus our operations showed.

This workshop also debuted Bush on the international stage. The live-surgery program opened with her demonstrating a distal TIP ending with a circumcision; the most common hypospadias operation done by everyone watching, and therefore, the most important one to show. I was impressed, and a little jealous, that neither her voice nor her hands betrayed any sign of nervousness performing before such a large audience.

After Bush's operation was underway, I started a distal repair and reconstructed the foreskin in the other room. Few, if any, of the US surgeons attending had ever seen the foreskin repaired to look natural.

Then the workshop moved on to more complex operations: Bush assisting Pippi-Salle while I continued operating in the other room with the fellow, DaJusta. Surgeons in the auditorium and around the world saw how TIP and two-stage grafts should be done to repair proximal hypospadias and operations that had previously failed.

When the show ended, Children's collected standardized evaluation forms from the attendees as they filed out of the auditorium. A week or so later, the CME department emailed a summary of their responses to me. Bush and I read through them and then forwarded the report to hospital administrators involved in the workshop. Doug Hock, the COO, emailed back.

Warren, Evaluations are never all "Excellent" and "Very good," but you didn't have a single negative comment. Congratulations!

Many participants also sent me separate messages.

Great course, glad I came.

Thanks for organizing this. I learned so much!

This was the best meeting I've ever attended.

I specifically remember that David Ewalt, the private pediatric urologist who declined to join our academic group, wrote:

Warren, Good job. You should repeat this course in a few years.

I had one final duty after the workshop: to host some sightseeing for the guest faculty, which was an expectation at every workshop I attended. Bracka had already seen the highlights of Dallas on the way to the meeting in San Antonio, satisfying a long-standing ambition to visit the set of the TV series where JR Ewing once roamed.[32] So, the next morning, Bracka, Pippi-Salle, and I loaded into my car for a drive down the interstate from Dallas through Houston and over the bridge into Galveston.

"Two years ago I was operating on a Friday morning when my medical school roommate called," I began the background story. "He shouted over the phone, 'Warren, where the hell are you!' I said, 'In surgery, like every Friday . . . why?' *'Because it's our thirty-year class reunion!* You need to get your butt down here. Everyone else is already here.'"

"So I Googled and found out there are flights literally every hour between Dallas and Houston. I flew down Saturday morning, rented a car, and drove to the island to find everyone still asleep from a party the night before!"

I glanced over at Bracka sitting next to me and smiled in the rearview mirror at Pippi-Salle in the backseat before continuing.

"Since I had a car, I drove around visiting old haunts. This was two years after Hurricane Ike, and I noticed that property was selling cheap. So a few months later, I ended up buying a house on the beach to retire to! One of those built up on stilts. It had some damage from the storm,

---

32. *JR Ewing* was the fictional star of the TV series *Dallas*.

and the contractor literally just finished working on it, so this is my first chance to see it all fixed up."

We arrived in the afternoon, climbed the stairs to the front door, and stood in the main room admiring the view of the sea through the new windows. Bracka congratulated me.

"Well, I must say I can understand why you would want to retire here."

"Are you planning to quit soon?" Pippi-Salle wondered.

"I want to work full time another three years," I replied. "That gives me time to finish training a successor, probably Gargollo, or maybe Bush, although I don't think she wants it, to take over the division. Then I'll go to a three-day workweek and spend four-day weekends here!"

But that dream was not to be.

The next day morning, Pippi-Salle and I were drinking coffee and checking our emails before Bracka was awake. I saw a message from Marty Koyle, who had recently moved to Seattle.

Warren,

I need to ask you about Aivar. He's supposed to come here next week, but I don't think we can let him visit. How did you get your university to allow him in your course?

I typed back.

Marty,

The course was run by Children's. Are you referring to his trial? You know he was found innocent.

Minutes later there was another email.

"Warren, have you seen the Medical Council report? A resident here found it on the internet. Look it up and then let me know what you think."

I thought for a moment and then remembered a British plastic surgeon mentioning a rumor that some disciplinary committee might launch its own investigation after the trial. "They are under pressure to take action against doctors, and now that Bracka is retiring he would be an easy target." But I heard nothing more, except a request from Bracka's attorney to reference a statement I wrote before the trial summarizing Bracka's contributions to hypospadiology, if there was another inquiry.

I moved to the sofa and googled Bracka, seeing the same news articles I had read before; the earlier ones reporting the accusations, and the later ones announcing the Royal Court's verdict declaring him innocent. But now I saw new headlines saying that Bracka was "struck off" by the General Medical Council following their own investigation.

"Pippi, did you know that Aivar had his license revoked in England?" I asked, as I kept reading.

"No," he shook his head, "I only heard he was innocent."

"That's what I heard too. But here's an article saying there was a second investigation that found him guilty and took away his license."

I looked up from the computer confused how he could be found both innocent and guilty of the same charges.

But Koyle mentioned the actual General Medical Council report, so I changed the search terms multiple times and finally found what the resident in Seattle must have seen. A wave of nausea surged through me as I read that Bracka admitted he had exposed himself "to a small number of patients, to show how they should look and function after surgery."

I carried my computer back to the breakfast table and pushed the screen over to Pippi-Salle to read, wondering if this was what the urology residents at our program also found and showed to Claus. But that was not possible, I decided, or Claus would have called immediately to remove Bracka from the course.

Then I closed the search and wrote another email.

Marty, you have to cancel Aivar.

That evening over dinner, I told Bracka I had heard there were more developments in his case.

"Yes," he replied, without hesitation. "The GMC struck me off, which does not really matter since I am retired."

"But how could it happen that they took away your license after the court found you innocent?" I persisted, studying his expression while keeping my face blank.

"It was all political correctness," he answered. "They could show the public they are disciplining doctors by taking away the license I no longer use."

"Does that affect your pension?" Pippi-Salle asked.

"Not at all," Bracka replied, shrugging his shoulders. "As I said, it was perfect for them."

I probed deeper. "But Aivar, they say you admitted to having inappropriate conduct with patients."

"Actually, I denied that," Bracka corrected, looking first at me, and then to Pippi-Salle. "My attorneys encouraged me to fight that conclusion and told me I would win that case too," he explained, confidently, without the slightest hint of guilt. "But I'm tired of this. Besides, the Royal College of Surgeons paid the attorney fees for the trial, but any additional costs would come from my pocket. I did not think it was worth spending my pension to defend a license I don't use anymore."

I sat a moment processing all this. "I guess I can understand that?" I finally replied, raising the last word into a question as the conversation ran its course to an unconvincing conclusion. "But you should have told me when they took away your license."

Bracka and Pippi-Salle flew out the next day from Houston. I drove back home, still unable to reconcile what I read in the computer with what I heard Bracka say. Was he guilty or innocent? And if he was guilty, did the good he did for so many in any way mitigate the wrong he did to others?

I thought about the many times he had spoken to urologists and decided that those of us who heard his message and converted to grafts could carry on that teaching ourselves. And with that conclusion, I vowed never to participate in another workshop with Bracka.

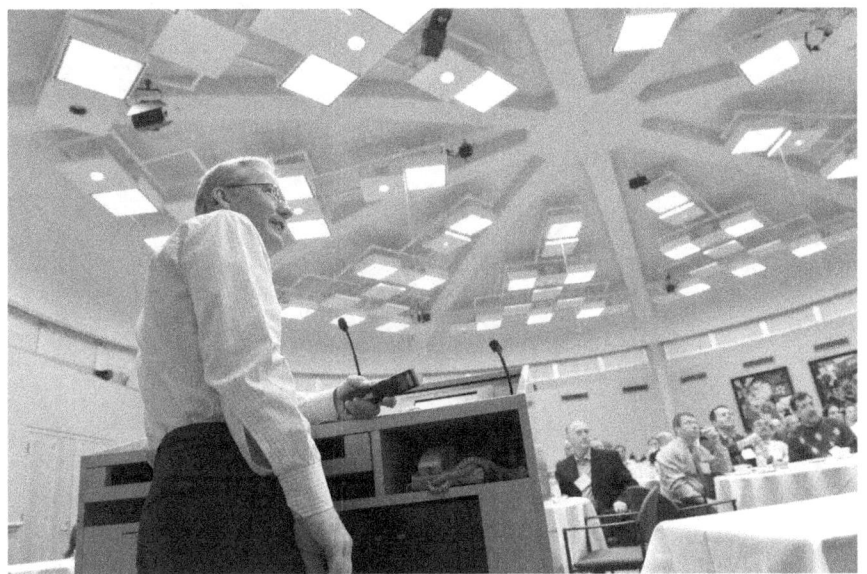

First Children's Hypospadias Workshop, 2011. I am introducing the program.

◀ CHAPTER 13 ▶

It Took an Atomic Bomb to
Get You Out of There!

The job of division chief carried a burden of meetings. Meetings to discuss which calls to the clinic to answer live and which to roll over to the phone tree. Meetings to review the current waiting time for a new patient appointment, and when we specialized, meetings to decide how the schedulers should guide patients to the correct surgeons. Meetings to analyze the group's billing and collecting, to make certain we did not charge too much or too little according to ever-changing, often confusing, and sometimes contradictory rules and regulations. Meetings to plan new satellite offices and meetings to renegotiate contracts with the current satellites. Meetings with the other surgical chiefs about the goings-on in the OR, and meetings with hospital administrators when our group wanted new equipment, like a robot for the OR. Meetings with the adult urology faculty. Meetings with the pediatric urology faculty. Meetings with the residents and fellows, and meetings with the nurses and secretaries. Meetings with the department chairman, like the one who made me chief, and the other who granted the pediatric group autonomy.

Of all these hundreds and hundreds of meetings over my fourteen years as chief of pediatric urology, one stands out as unique. A gathering of all the chiefs of the various surgical and medical divisions, the heads of nursing, and the top hospital administrators that I recall only happened once during my tenure. Mixed among several agenda items was an announcement of a change in nursing policy, explained by the chief of nursing. She stood up and turned to face the group, holding a microphone.

"In the past, incident reports were sometimes used to identify nurses for possible disciplinary action. This seemed to *discourage* reporting of important events, and so, effective immediately, nurses throughout the hospital will be *encouraged* to report anything that appears out of the ordinary without fear of punishment so that we can identify areas for improvement."

As she sat back down, Ann Roberts, the administrator running Medical Staff Affairs, took the microphone.

"And when an incident report mentions a *physician*, it will still be routed to my office and reviewed according to the policies and procedures outlined in the hospital bylaws."

As this news sunk into the audience, one physician raised his hand. "So, to be clear, do I understand that *nurses* are being encouraged to write more incident reports and not worry about being punished? But if they mention a *doctor*, he or she will be investigated and possibly disciplined?"

"Yes, that's correct," Roberts responded, quite matter-of-factly.

A murmur of hushed voices grew louder around the room like the rising hum of cicadas early in a summer evening. As it reached its crescendo, Doug Hock suddenly jumped to his feet and commandeered the mike. His face visibly red, he scowled at the medical leaders of the hospital and declared, "We're doing this because all over the country physicians are out of control! We intend to change that here at Children's!"

The seeds of this fruit were planted several years earlier, when the hospital flunked a routine accreditation update, and the new CEO was rumored to decree that any nurse involved in a mistake found during the next review would be fired. In a classic example of unintended consequences, reports against physicians skyrocketed as nurses reasoned they could blame the doctors for an incident since the hospital could not fire them.

As it happened, I was one of those early victims. On a day when a foreign surgeon was visiting to observe several hypospadias operations, the OR nursing educator coincidentally decided she would refresh her skills and circulate my room, meaning she would locate and open supplies as they were needed. And on that same day a brand-new surgical tech was assigned to my room for the first time, on the presumption that her history of once having done adult urology cases at another hospital made her sufficiently qualified to pass special instruments and load tiny sutures during a pediatric hypospadias repair.

It was a recipe for the disaster that followed. The tech did not know what instruments and sutures were needed, and when I asked for something she did not have, the nurse educator had no idea where to find it. Over and over through the first case, I waited for supplies I always used to be found and opened, and then had to show the tech which was a Gerald forcep and what was a caliper while reloading every needle she passed right-handed for my left hand. These delays meant increased swelling in the tissues I was operating, more anesthesia for the child, growing anxiety for the parents waiting longer than expected for the surgery to end, and frustration for the next family whose son became increasingly irritable because he was not allowed to eat.

On top of all that was the effect this confusion had on the visitor who traveled halfway around the world to improve his hypospadias surgery but could not help but be distracted by these miscues and delays, and his embarrassment that my team appeared so incompetent.

Between cases, I happened into the charge nurse in the hall. I explained the situation and mentioned the foreign surgeon trying to learn.

"It's not their fault that they don't know my routine," I said in defense of the nurse and tech. "But it's also not fair to my patients, or to my visitor, to have to wait for everything that should already be open and ready in the first place."

Realizing the delicate circumstances, I asked the charge nurse, "Is there a way you can fix this without hurting anyone's feelings?"

When the next case began, there was a familiar circulator and scrub nurse, and the remaining surgeries ran smoothly.

Two days later a hand-delivered letter stamped PERSONAL AND CONFIDENTIAL arrived from Medical Staff Affairs, demanding my presence at a peer-review committee meeting Monday at 8:00 a.m. to respond to credible complaints that I created such a "hostile work environment" that both the nurse and the tech asked to be reassigned to another room.

I called the committee chairman and insisted they first interview the nurse's aide, the anesthesiologist, his fellow, and the urology resident and fellow who were all eyewitnesses, and then let me know if the committee still needed to question me.

He did, and they did not. But the committee's initial reaction to the complaint had been to assume the physician was at fault. Why else would a nurse, a tech, or other hospital employee accuse a doctor, unless that doctor had done something wrong? I had to demand they fact-check the complaint, which found the nurse educator had taught for so long that she forgot how to do, and the new scrub tech had exaggerated her urology experience. Both embarrassed, they conspired to blame the surgeon.

This change in hospital incident reports added still more meetings to my list. Soon I had to discuss a time-out complaint with one of our faculty. A newborn arrived for a circumcision in the office, and while the nurse took Mom to the waiting room, Harrison began the procedure. When the nurse returned moments later, she asked if he had done a formal time-out, declaring out loud the name and birthdate of the patient, the procedure he was about to do, and that all needed supplies were available. He innocently replied no, since he was the only person in the room, had just confirmed with both Mom and the nurse that this baby was there to be circumcised, and could see all the instruments were open and ready to use. Following the new hospital policy, she wrote an incident report, and the physician named had to be investigated by the chief of his division—me.

Another time Bush was doing surgery on a testicle, and when she handed back a partly used suture, the small needle bounced off the Mayo stand. Both the surgeon and the tech saw it fall away from the operative field toward the floor, but a diligent search by the circulating nurse did not find it. Giving up, the circulator looked online at the hospital policy and read that no further measures, such as an X-ray of the patient, were needed when such a tiny needle was lost.

But the policy did require an incident report, and since a surgeon was involved, a copy was routed to Ann Roberts and into the machinery of physician discipline. Once again, the chief of urology had to hold a meeting and then write a report to declare there was no physician mis-behavior to report.

In this toxic atmosphere, it was inevitable that some incidents mentioned me, who, as division chief, could not investigate myself. In that circumstance the policy called for review by the chief of surgery. That happened when I was about to do elective surgery on a girl with spina bifida to repair the drainage tube from her kidney. She had just been anesthetized when my fellow happened upon a report in the computer that her urine was infected with yeast. I canceled the operation until that could be treated.

"So the child had unnecessary anesthesia," the chief of surgery began the meeting.

"She had anesthesia for a couple of minutes," I clarified.

"Well, it was your responsibility to review all pertinent data on the patient before taking her back to the operating room," Bob Foglia countered, as though reading from a manual.

"That test was ordered by the nephrology service, which, for some reason, didn't treat the yeast even though they knew she was scheduled for surgery," I tried to explain. "The last culture we knew about from a couple of days earlier was negative. Since we didn't know anyone ordered another test, we weren't looking for those results."

"But you found them, and that should have happened before starting the case," Foglia persisted.

"The fellow happened to see that report while checking on something else after the child was already in the room," I responded. "Regardless, we did the right thing by delaying the surgery. It wouldn't have been safe to continue."

This back and forth continued several more minutes, Foglia grinning the whole time like a cat swatting at a cornered mouse. Finally, he rendered his verdict. The report had "minor merit."

Minor merit was also the conclusion when I asked for the foot pedal to operate fluoroscopy during an examination of a baby with complex birth defects.

"We need to keep an eye on the amount of X-ray the baby is getting," I reminded the junior faculty I was assisting.

The radiology tech reported I yelled at her and accused her of not following directions, which prompted an investigation by the head OR nurse.

Afterward, the nurse told me, "This tech files incident reports all the time. I spoke to everyone in the room, and they all said nothing happened. I've passed that along to Dr. Foglia."

But Dr. Foglia was not satisfied. "Why would she say that if you didn't yell at her?"

"Apparently because she wants to control the fluoro," I answered. "I think that's all in the report from the head nurse."

"Yes, I read that. But I still think you didn't handle this the best way. I'm going to rate it as having minor merit."

And there was that smile again as he said it.

I began to wonder what "minor merit" actually meant, and how many "minor" merits added up to something major.

An envelope stamped PERSONAL AND CONFIDENTIAL from the Medical Staff Affairs Office enclosed the answer.

"According to the bylaws of the hospital, a physician who is named in three incident reports determined to have merit during a two-year period will undergo peer review by a committee comprised of medical staff officers."

I read those words angry at myself for not protesting above Foglia when he insisted on finding merit in every incident report when others found none. Angry that Foglia labeled an incident "minor" so as not to arouse a stronger reaction from me, or scrutiny of his judgement from others, all the while knowing that the key word was "merit." There were no grades of guilt. And that realization made me all the angrier knowing that now it was too late to stop the wheels of bureaucracy from grinding over me.

The head of the peer review committee explained their mission, telling me they would not rehash complaints, but determine if they established a pattern of misbehavior. He made clear that it would be thorough, warning, "Our investigation will go wherever it goes, and will take as long as it takes."

They planned to interview nurses, aides, techs, and secretaries in the operating room, hospital wards, and my clinic. It was not my business who they chose to interview, but for the appearance of fairness, I could suggest some names for the committee to add to their list, if they had time.

Then I did not hear anything more. Weeks passed by, and the only evidence of the investigation was an occasional remark from someone the committee had questioned. Then one morning I arrived at my office and found the Institutional Review Board combing through my research files. More time passed. Next, I was told to appear before a different committee.

"We want to know why you invited a visiting professor to Children's who had his license revoked."

"I invited an internationally renowned surgeon to teach in our hypospadias course. I knew there had been some accusations about him, but an English court found him innocent."

"But he lost his license."

"I didn't know that. It happened months after I asked him to moderate, and by then Children's had taken over all the paperwork for both the visiting professors. They obviously didn't find that out either."

Then the silence returned. I worked each day with the shadow of the investigation lurking at the edge of my thoughts. I moved though the poisoned air of the hospital worried that some remark, or some look on my face, in some unguarded moment would add to the suspicion against me. I knew I was innocent, but started to wonder if I was guilty.

Even my wife said I *must* have done *something* wrong to merit such a lengthy inquiry.

Then a mom filed a complaint that a medical student who accompanied me during a clinic visit leered at her son. The head investigator sneered, "Can't you behave when you know we are watching?"

I made an appointment with the department chairman, who told me he had already discussed the investigation with the University Vice President at Children's and was advised to let it run its course.

"That's not a surprise," I replied, "seeing how he and Foglia are best friends. Claus, they go hunting together and even take vacations together. He's protecting Foglia."

But Roehrborn said no more, looking away. He had already said enough, spending most of our scheduled time describing similar situations involving the adult faculty that he had taken care of. I walked away reminded that the chairman had long ago washed his hands of pediatric urology after granting it independence to run its own affairs.

There were times when I was overwhelmed by the unknown happening around me, anxiety churning my gut and pounding my heart into exhaustion with worry about my career and the future of our group. I drove alone to the coast one weekend and walked for hours on the beach, but the cool waters ebbing and flowing over my naked feet did not bring calm. I begged for peace, but those prayers can take time to answer.

I finally asked for some idea when all of this would end, admitting to the chief inquisitor that I could not sleep because of it.

"You're supposed to have trouble sleeping," came the curt reply.

At last I was summonsed before the investigators to hear their verdict. We gathered in a conference room of Medical Staff Affairs, where I was directed to a seat opposite the three of them. Ann Roberts sat nearby, beside someone taking notes of the proceedings, apparently to supplement the audio recorded by a tape player positioned in the middle of the table.

The chairman summarized the findings of their investigation. I had no IRB violations. While it was unfortunate that a surgeon who had his license revoked was invited to the hypospadias conference, they acknowledged that I was not aware of that.

"We spoke to people all over the hospital who work with you," the chairman said, coming to the point. "Eighty percent told us you are an excellent physician and surgeon, and that they enjoy working with you."

I thought how any politician would be ecstatic over those polling numbers.

Then the chairman screwed his face into a stern expression. "The other 20 percent said you set high expectations and they sometimes get intimidated."

The doctor seated to his left quickly added, "But they also told us that if their child needed surgery, they would want you to do it."

"So that sounds like a good report, overall," I suggested, feeling hopeful.

"What concerns us is if a nurse or a tech is intimidated by you, they might not do the right thing in some situation and a patient could get hurt," the chief inquisitor harshly rejoined.

I thought about that for a moment. Here was the crux of the matter, yet I knew that the reports that led to this investigation came because I insisted the right things be done for patients.

"Well, your committee has investigated me for nearly six months. You've looked through all my files and talked to nearly everyone in the hospital. Did you find a *single time* when that happened?"

The chairman cocked his head slightly to think, while the other two committee members turned to look at him. The one on his right finally asked, with maybe the slightest hint of sarcasm, "Yeah, Karl, did we find that ever happened?"

"No."

And this likely explained the protracted course of the witch hunt, as the committee searched high and low month after month to find some fire behind all the smoke that Foglia blew. Not that it mattered. The same university vice president who was a friend of the chief of surgery mandated that to keep my position as urology chief, I had to undergo evaluation by a psychiatrist, who promptly declared my mental health was sound.

Meanwhile, it appeared that other investigations into the other chiefs of surgical divisions were more fruitful. In this season of inquisitions, two chiefs of heart surgery were forced from Children's, leaving with the chiefs of ENT and plastic surgery, while the chief of neurosurgery stayed but was demoted from his position. About the only one who remained unscathed was the chief at the center of this maelstrom finding fault in everyone but himself. Then I heard a few years later that Foglia abruptly resigned and left Children's.

Each year the Urology Department hosted a symposium in honor of its first academic chairman, Paul Peters, that tightly wound chief who others warned before my residency interview could have a heart attack any moment. Roehrborn planned a reunion of sorts for this occasion in the spring of 2013, several months after the Children's investigation ended, and invited John McConnell and other luminaries from the past to return. He then asked various faculty to prepare lectures, and even suggested a title for me: *From Harry Spence to TIP: Progress in Hypospadias Surgery.*

I did not often lecture to adult urologists, but I always used the opportunity to tell them how the 3Ps I learned doing hypospadias repair showed the way to improving results of any surgery. For this occasion, I wrapped that message into the history of the department, recalling how ideas of Harry Spence, the first pediatric urologist in Dallas, and John Duckett, a former urology resident in Dallas, helped lay the foundation for TIP repair.

This lecture was also an opportunity to thank the chairmen who helped me build the pediatric urology division. First, I explained to the audience, "Dr. McConnell made me an offer I couldn't refuse, and then said, 'Now that you're the chief, go and create an *elite* program!'"

Next, I looked to the current chairman. "When Dr. Roehrborn took over the department he told me, 'Warren, manage your own program.' Of course, he did that at a time when it was easy to cut loose the pediatric group, since it was losing money!" I laughed.

"Well, I hope the division now meets y'all's expectations," I continued, looking at them both. "We have six faculty, up from four when I became chief. And two of them, Dr. Jacobs and Dr. Bush, have master's degrees to improve clinical studies. They help supervise *eight* prospective clinical trials we have in progress, which may be more than any other pediatric urology program.

"When I arrived, pediatric urology had one satellite office in Plano, which lost money. Today we have four satellite offices and are about to open a fifth, and our division is one of the few at Children's that makes a profit.

"We also started a fellowship training program, which defines 'elite' in our specialty. And I'm proud to say we have now graduated eight fellows who work in academic centers around the country and internationally."

But I was most proud that the pediatric group had specialized and used the final moments of my time to name each faculty, show their picture, and mention their area of expertise. Gargollo was likely the best and certainly the busiest, robotic surgeon among all pediatric urologists in the US. Baker was one of a few pediatric urologists with NIH funding for her lab and was recognized as an expert in vaginal reconstruction. Jacobs was working with Gargollo to treat children with spina bifida and planned to create one of the first programs in the world to help teens with that condition transition into adult life. Finally, Bush shared hypospadias surgery with me, and would eventually take over my practice.

Despite my reluctance to become a division chief, and the mistakes I made in that role, it was clear that our division stood among the elite pediatric urology programs.

A week later, Roehrborn informed me that it was inappropriate to forecast Bush as my successor for hypospadias.

"She has the best hands for hypospadias surgery of anyone I've worked with," I replied. "She also dummy-coded my whole database and has written a lot of papers on hypospadias with me. She's the natural choice."

"But it looks like favoritism," Roehrborn argued.

"Claus, I mentioned all the faculty and their area of expertise in that lecture. I've given all my surgery that Gargollo can do on the robot to him. I've given all my new spina bifida patients to Jacobs. I've given all my girls with genital problems to Linda. The one who has to wait the longest is Bush, since hypospadias is the one area I'm not giving up. That hardly seems like favoritism."

"Well, some might see it differently."

"What I see is that when John Duckett died, CHOP had no plans for who would continue his hypospadias program. When Mike Mitchell retired, there was no heir designated to care for children with bladder exstrophy."

I sensed I was not making my point.

"Claus, Doug Husmann told me about a meeting he had the day after he became the urology department chairman at the Mayo Clinic. The president shook his hand, and then asked the names of the two people he was going to prepare to take over his position *eight years* from now. That's how they maintain continuity!"

"Well, some people think hypospadias is not that special. I've heard it said that distal hypospadias to a pediatric urologist is like a TURP[33] to an adult urologist; it's something everyone can do."

"Except that a distal hypospadias done wrong can ruin a boy's penis for life."

I was appalled that someone in our group made this comparison, and that the department chairman believed it. I left our meeting wishing I had thought to say, "If distal hypospadias is so easy, then why do I get invited all over the world every year to help surgeons do it better?"

I found a sticky note on my loupes box when I finished surgery one Friday in late July.

"Meet Dr. Roehrborn at Dean Ginsburg's office at four today."

The nurse who took the message was gone, and it was already three-thirty. I signed some paperwork, spoke to the family of the last patient, and left Children's with just enough time to walk across campus to the Tower, the twelve-story box that overlooked the university. I rode the elevator to the eleventh floor, wondering what this meeting was about. I could not think of any business that I, or our group, had that concerned a dean.

Roehrborn was already seated at the far end of a long conference table. Dean Ginsburg invited me to sit opposite him in the middle of the table, several places away from the chairman.

"Warren, a matter has come to our attention that needs to be investigated," Ginsburg announced, casually, with a smile, as though we were about to leave to get a beer together. "The president has asked me to conduct an investigation. Meanwhile, effective immediately, you are relieved of your duties as the chief of pediatric urology."

I glanced toward Roehrborn, who stared resolutely at the table, trying desperately to shrink his large frame from view. Then I looked back at Ginsburg.

"OK, but what exactly are you going to investigate?"

Ginsburg leaned back in his chair and clasped his hands behind his head, still smiling broadly.

---

33. *TURP* refers to the transurethral resection of the prostate, a common operation done by adult urologists at that time.

"I actually don't know! Dr. Roehrborn is going to fill me in about that on Monday."

Roehrborn kept staring down, saying nothing.

"All I can say right now is that it has nothing to do with the investigation at Children's. We know you were found innocent in that."

I exited into the simmering heat of Texas July, unsure what had just happened. I was no longer division chief but did not know why. And what game was the dean playing to announce my demotion while saying he did not know why, either? The only memory I could possibly link to this turn of events was a request over a month ago from the legal office for all my email traffic related to Bracka and the hypospadias course, but the dean said there was something new.

Once again, I was under investigation, but this time I was not told the alleged high crimes and misdemeanors worthy of a dean's attention. Maybe because of that, or maybe because the last investigation looked everywhere and found nothing, I did not feel the doubt and would not have the restless nights that haunted me for six months at Children's. Rather, the greatest irritation arrived in an email that Baker sent the very next morning—Saturday—to the entire faculty and staff of pediatric urology. Announcing she would be making a list of changes to the practice on Monday, now that she was in charge. And that without even the courtesy of a phone call to me first. I noticed she had already updated her title to Interim Chief. I had always signed my emails with just my name.

Then Bush told me she heard that a reporter from the newspaper was snooping around.

"Whenever someone mentions anything about sex abuse, like with Bracka, a reporter's going to look into it," she said. "And you know how sensitive the university is right now about the *Dallas Morning News*, after all that bad publicity about residents operating unsupervised at Parkland," which led to a federal investigation that threatened to close the hospital.

Two weeks later, and with no further contact from the dean, the time arrived when each year every faculty at the university renewed their annual contract. Somehow, I never thought it odd that our jobs were guaranteed just one year at a time, unlike nearly all other jobs that continue indefinitely after a person is hired. But this year I glanced over the familiar boilerplate to see that the no-compete clause had been radically expanded from a limited zone around the medical center to a twenty-five-mile radius from *any location* where Children's had a clinic. Those four satellites I bragged about at the symposium now meant I was banished from practicing in Dallas and the surrounding suburbs if I left the university.

I recalled McConnell once saying, "Of course, you don't have to sign it . . . unless you still want this job," and knew the response from the university would be the same this year too.

The new contract went into effect on September 1, 2013, a Sunday. Monday was the Labor Day holiday. Tuesday, I was called to Roehrborn's office. The chairman introduced a slender man in a dark suit from the dean's office who sat silently through the proceedings that were about to unfold. Then Roehrborn looked down at the table, again, and informed me this would be my last contract with the university, sliding an envelope toward me as he spoke.

I took out a letter and read that the invitation to Bracka did not meet the "University's standards." Now I connected the dots and glared at the two men.

"So, this was all a sham. There was no investigation. The university's afraid the newspaper's going to run another story that'll make it look bad, so you're letting me go. Oh, but first you made me sign a new no-compete clause so I can't set up practice anywhere in Dallas." I paused, to no response. "Well, I guess this goes to lawyers next." Then I stood and walked out.

In mid-September the *Dallas Morning News* reported that I was demoted from chief of pediatric urology for inviting Bracka to our course. News behind the scenes made clear there was no interest at the paper in the story of a visiting professor who gave a lecture four years ago, until the university, desperate to avoid more publicity, instead ensured publicity by making it a current event. I was amused to read that I had made no comment on the matter, since the reporter never bothered to contact me for a comment.

The mystery of how this story came to a *Dallas Morning News* reporter so many years after the fact was explained by another rumor. Word circulated that the reporter's child was referred to a pediatric urologist in town, who, during that appointment, told him he knew a story that might be of interest . . .

I had one opportunity to reverse the gears of the university: a meeting with the head dean, and thirty minutes to plead for my job. I was told that another director found himself in the same chair in the same office and begged the dean for mercy. But I thought that a job I had to grovel to keep was not a job worth groveling for. Especially not to one of those officials who made this decision without troubling themselves to ask my defense. I wanted my position restored and time for our group to complete an orderly transition to a new chief.

The answer was clear when the dean glanced down at his watch after precisely thirty minutes and then stood to show me the door.

Now I had one year to find a new job. I sent a few letters of halfhearted interest to academic programs advertising a position, but never followed those up. Meanwhile, I looked for an expert in employment law, later telling friends I found one of the best by searching for an attorney with an office on the top floor of the tallest building in downtown Dallas! Keith Clouse made an appointment to chat with Leah Hurley, the lead attorney at UT Southwestern, about the no-compete clause. According to him, it was a short discussion.

The moment he was introduced, she replied, "I know your reputation." Then, with a dismissive wave of her hand, she added, "Don't worry, we don't intend to hold your client to his no-compete."

Meanwhile, Bush weighed her options. She condensed her decision to a single sentence.

"I can stay at the U and try to keep the hypospadias program you've built here going, or we can start a private practice together, and I'll have to live in your shadow until you retire."

We studied this question from all the angles we could imagine, but in the end, it was the interim chief who answered it. Bush and I returned from an international workshop in October to learn that the appointment schedulers were instructed during our absence to spread new patients with hypospadias evenly among all the faculty. There would be no specialized hypospadias program for Bush to inherit once I left. It was the first step taken to tear down specialization within the group, and the shove Bush needed to give up a guaranteed salary and a promising academic career.

That decided, we had nine months remaining to notify our patients we were leaving the university, and then to find and equip a new office, credential at new hospitals, hire new secretaries and nurses, sign new contracts with insurance companies, design and launch a new website announcing our practice, file legal paperwork for the new practice with the state, and finesse Bush's no-compete, which Hurley was not so quick to dismiss.

Adding to this press of deadlines, 2014 marked the twentieth anniversary of the article that introduced TIP to the world. I wanted to celebrate this milestone during the fourth, and final, Children's hypospadias workshop, and since it was the university, and not Children's, that was at odds with me, the show could go on. First, I planned to look back to the beginning, telling a younger generation of surgeons how TIP came to be. That history included those first five surgeons who publicly endorsed the operation, and I invited them to come and tell their own stories.

I also wanted to look forward. I would tell the audience that twenty years' experience, systematically recorded into databases and carefully analyzed many times, proved TIP can successfully repair any case of distal hypospadias. That alone was sufficient reason to celebrate the operation. But I had also learned that TIP was *not* the operation to use for proximal hypospadias when the penis was bent. I would use this opportunity to stress again to colleagues not to make the same mistake I did by trying to straighten more than the slightest bend while preserving the urethral plate.

Influenced by our experience operating together in Israel, Bush suggested we also adjust the surgical program.

"It's hard for the audience to follow when the camera goes back and forth between operations, even with a moderator." She continued, "Besides, we've seen how efficiently we work together, so you and I can demonstrate in one room all the cases that we did before in two." That meant no visiting surgeon this year.

I opened the workshop repeating my mantra: "We fix all hypospadias using only TIP and two-stage grafts." Then I explained, "In many ways, these are the same surgery—TIP tubularizes the urethral plate, while two-stage grafts make a substitute urethral plate that we then tubularize."

I showed a slide covered in diagrams and arrows to emphasize how complicated it had been when I was a resident to decide which operation to do.

"These two repairs free surgeons from having to develop expertise in many types of repairs, and from the worry they might choose the wrong one for a patient."

If only the surgeons listening would hear this message. But I had surveyed fellows training around the US and learned that nearly half were still being taught to study the patient's anatomy before deciding between TIP and several other techniques. Even worse, every single fellow who answered the questionnaire said they planned to practice what they were taught in training.

So, I paused, and then asked the camera, "What if you're taught wrong?"

Then I challenged the teachers. "A mistake we *make* hurts one patient, but a mistake we *teach* hurts countless patients."

Next, I contradicted Duckett. "Most complications don't happen because a surgeon chooses the wrong operation . . . most complications happen because a surgeon does the right operation the wrong way."

And there was the foundation for this final workshop. Bush and I would demonstrate the best way to do our two operations. We would encourage surgeons to use the 3Ps to learn their own results, and then improve them. We would call for our profession to specialize both proximal hypospadias and redo operations so that fewer surgeons would attempt these rare and complex procedures.

Our message beamed from Dallas around the world to surgeons watching alone or in groups. I still remember that more than sixty met in Istanbul, staying up late into their night to watch. Emails poured in from every continent, and many nations asking questions raised from the lectures or prompted by the live surgery that everyone saw clearly in HD. Nothing on this scale had ever been done in pediatric urology before.

On the final evening after the workshop ended, Bush and I hosted the original TIP surgeons to dinner at a nearby steakhouse. As we drank Syrah and relived the fun of the past three days, a jumble of emotions finally spilled out of me like blood from a deep cut—the pride in this international course reaching hundreds of our colleagues. The gratitude that Koyle, Caldamone, Hurwitz, and Manzoni[34] had the courage to try the new operation, and then to testify for it. The deceit by Bracka, who did not warn me when his license was taken away. The sadness that my academic career was ending. The frustration that so many worthwhile studies underway were doomed to collapse without my energy. The anger that the university so clearly and so deviously overreacted to fear of a news story. The stab in the back from the pediatric urologist who gossiped to the reporter. The weakness of the department chairman, and my certainty that McConnell, who hired me, would have managed things better.

I was embarrassed afterward, imagining the discomfort of my friends after they all flew away.

Bush listened, and then consoled, "They understood."

But I could not easily let go of the sadness and the need to mourn. Bush knew this was natural, and inevitable, but there was little time, and less each day to prepare for our future.

"It took an atomic bomb to get you out of there," Bush said at last. "Soon we will be thanking them!"

---

34. The fifth pediatric urologist who participated in the multicenter TIP report, Richard Ehrlich, was retired and did not attend the conference.

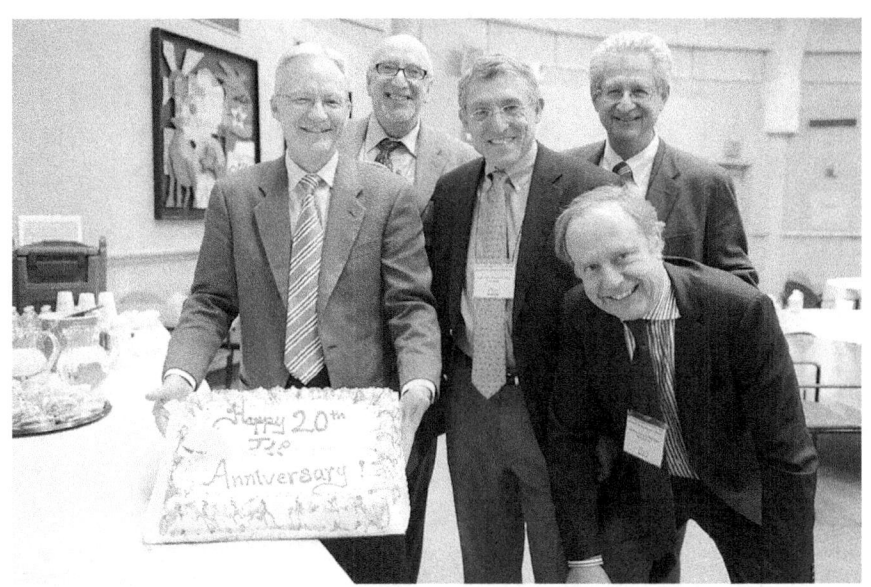

Me, Koyle, Caldamone, Hurwitz, Manzoni (front right)

STAG REPAIR

THREE CORPOROTOMIES

PARC Urology

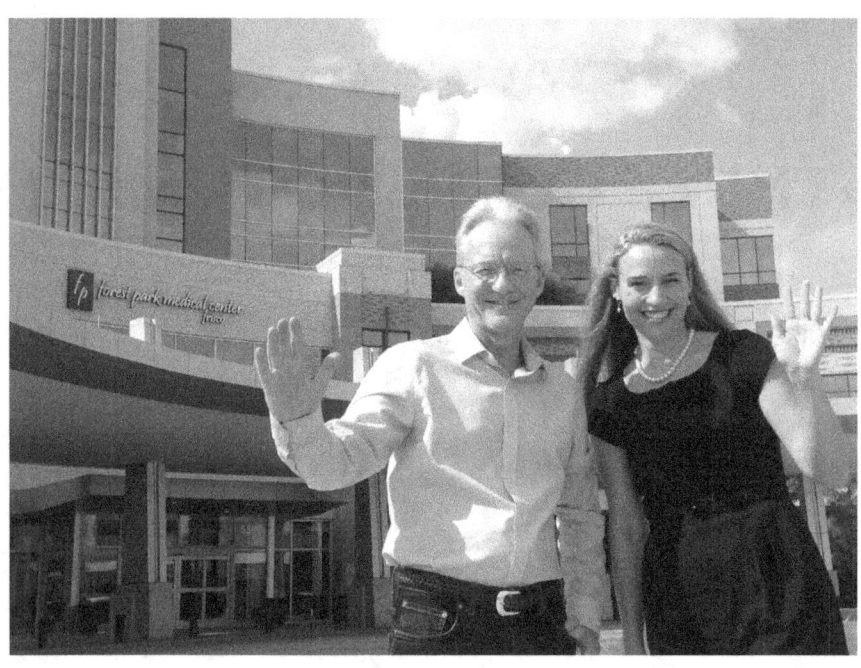

A photo from our first PARC Urology website showing Bush and me in front of Forest Park Medical Center

◀ CHAPTER 14 ▶

You Look So Happy!

"We need a pediatric urologist."

I ended the call not really sure what Forest Park was, and only vaguely aware that Frisco was a suburb growing up the tollway past my satellite office in Plano. The office that I now had to vacate, since the hospital had an agreement that only university faculty could hold clinics in Children's facilities. Somehow it seemed more than a coincidence that Kim Hines cold-called me just as Bush and I were growing desperate to find a new home.

I drove out to meet the physician liaison one afternoon for a tour.

"We're a boutique surgical facility, run by physicians," Hines told me as we walked through the hospital carefully designed to more closely resemble an upscale hotel. "Frisco is booming, and all the young families moving here want a place to take their kids if they need surgery. We have pedi ortho, ENT, and plastics already, and general surgeons on call," she explained. "But we need pediatric urology, and we can give you OR time right away."

The tour continued through the surgical suite, and I mentioned the supplies Bush and I would need: delicate needle holders and forceps, some small catheters, and the sutures with tiny needles we use for hypospadias repairs.

"Do you have any office space?" I asked next.

Hines led me across the parking garage into an office building. "There are several suites available," she said, "depending on how much space you need."

It was by far the most promising lead we had found, and I called Bush on my way back to Dallas to share the news.

She imagined the new practice in this state-of-the-art surgical hospital, and without seeing it herself, immediately declared, "My gut is saying this is where we belong."

The Texas Medical Board decrees that physicians changing practices must notify their patients where they can continue receiving care. The board also makes clear that when a doctor leaves a group, it is the responsibility of that doctor to give the notice. But the university, perhaps regretting its decision to let me out of the no-compete, sent its own letter to my patients which implied that I had moved away or died. Fortunately, the letter went on, they could make an appointment with any of their other pediatric urologists.

I learned this when several families called the office urgently, some of them distraught, asking what happened. I requested a copy of the letter and the mailing list the university used, to send out my own notification as required by the board. However, Hurley, the lead UT Southwestern attorney, refused. A lawyer sent a polite second request, which was also denied. So I told my attorney to inform Ms. Hurley that if she did not send over that list, I would report her and the university to the Medical Board. Being a native Texan, I added that we expected her to comply by high noon tomorrow.

But this was all just sparring for sport. I knew that when patients learned I was no longer available at Children's most would google me, and so what Bush and I really needed was a website announcing our new practice location and phone number. Stretching our shoestring budget, we hired a friend of my son, Phillip, to create the landing page.

Of course, the new practice also had to have a name to display on the website. Not long before we left the university, Bush and I sat outside on the patio of our favorite Tex-Mex restaurant sipping frozen margaritas while scrutinizing the possibilities.

"What do we want to be?" I asked, already knowing her response.

"A specialty center for hypospadias," she replied. "For all patients regardless of age."

"Then our name needs to say that."

Which led us to the challenge of naming something that, as far as we knew, never existed before. A practice devoted entirely to hypospadias repair.

"But we can't start out saying that," I reminded us. "Who knows how long it'll take to have enough patients to make that work?"

We snacked on chips and salsa, testing ideas on a napkin. Finally, after a second basket of chips and at least one refill of our margaritas, we settled on the cumbersome "Pediatric and Adult Reconstructive Center for Urology," which we immediately agreed would better be known by its acronym. And then we smiled that Forest Park would soon be home to PARC Urology.

Meanwhile, Bush spent countless hours studying paint chips, examining countertop samples, and comparing furniture swatches for the new office. Then she thumbed through catalogs looking for chairs to place in the exam rooms. Late one evening after work, she dragged me into Z Gallery at the mall to find paintings for the walls and knick-knacks for the waiting room.

She sent her choices to the contractor remodeling our office, deciding on a white color scheme for the cabinets and countertops to give the space a chic, modern feel. So we were surprised to walk through the dark, wood-grain décor that was installed by mistake when her preferences were lost under a stack of checklists on the contractor's desk. Bush could not restrain tears of frustration when she saw her vision of a youthful office rendered traditional and staid.

As the final weeks counted down to opening day, we still needed a manager to attend to all the administrative and financial concerns of the new practice. Our startup advisor reassured us several times that he had several qualified applicants, which turned out to be a total of two, only one of which seemed able to do the job. But Whitney Wells was not actually available when Bush and I interviewed her sitting around a table at a nearby Starbucks.

"He literally begged me to meet with y'all," she began the discussion. "I don't know him or how he got my contact information, and I told him I've already accepted another position." Then Whitney opened a briefcase and removed a stack of papers. "I read up on both of you, so I know y'all are pediatric urologists starting a new business. That means you'll need a company handbook with bylaws, policies, and procedures. Here are some samples I have that you could consider," she explained, sliding them across the table.

"Let me tell you my story," she continued without pausing to take a breath. "I was a waitress, and one day we were shorthanded, so I had to wait double the usual number of tables. It happened there was a doctor sitting at one of them who watched me hurrying back and forth and offered me a job on the spot! I started for him as a receptionist."

Bush and I exchanged glances indicating we were both impressed and a little amused by this quite young, yet thoroughly businesslike, applicant.

"I also opened the mail and happened to notice that payments from a few insurances for a couple of codes seemed off. So I made a list and tracked them, and confirmed they were less than the contracted rate. Next thing I knew I had gone from being a waitress to a billing specialist! Of course, now I'm an officially certified medical office manager."

I looked over at Bush again and saw her agreement.

Then I turned back to Whitney and asked, "What will it take to hire you?"

We also needed a program for our new computers to make appointments, schedule surgery, bill insurance, and track accounts—all the nuts and bolts the business side of a practice requires. That included creating patient records, which meant selecting an Electronic Medical Record system. Bush and I researched options, chose the least objectionable, and then devoted our entire first week, the first week of September, to customizing the program. All day every day we sat in the dark staring at a computer under the watchful eye of a technician flown in from the East Coast, enduring the mind-numbing torture of imagining all the problems our patients would have and then painstakingly building templates to speed data entry for each of those conditions.

I thought it would be less traumatic to poke needles in my eye. Bush constantly reminded me that we had no choice, if we did not want the EMR to dominate our lives past this one week. Demanding we look at a computer screen rather than at our patients, diverting attention from what patients were saying to what the computer insisted we record, consuming our time after clinic to finish the data entry we could not complete during clinic and stay anywhere near on time. And all that just for our patient notes. In a full week of doing nothing else, there was not enough time to finish the templates and also program the electronic billing the company promised would link to the patient records.

Then, only a few days after this torment, a routine system upgrade by the company erased every last vestige of all that work. No, it could not be recovered. It would have to be re-done. Yes, a technician could fly back to Dallas to help, but now on PARC Urology's dime since only the initial programming was included in their fees. No, they could not promise that future upgrades would not wipe away our templates all over again. Yes, Bush and I decided just three weeks into our practice that this contract was null and void.

Meanwhile, we had to eat, and the surgery we began the second week would not be paid by insurance for several more weeks, at the earliest. Fortunately, even though our jobs at the university ended the last day of August 2014, we were paid our final paychecks on September 1, providing enough to cover the first month of our new practice. Then a second check was mailed to each of us on October 1, reimbursing our unused sick time and accrued vacation.

There should have been one more of those final checks, our bonuses for earning way more than we were paid. But the university had changed the rules, declaring *bonuses* for last year's work were actually *incentive* payments for next year. And since we were leaving, there was nothing to incentivize. There was no appeal for this robbery, so Bush and I defied expectations and continued working as hard as usual right up to the very last day. Which meant we had no choice but to schedule surgeries after August 31 into our new practice when all our slots before then were filled and families wanted us, and not one of the other university urologists, to do it. That was so much surgery that we literally operated all day every day through the rest of September and well into October.

Having fired our EMR company, we had to find someone to bill all this work. With no other leads, we chose a local medical billing company highly recommended by a trusted colleague. Within days, our weeks of surgery were filed with the various insurances.

Payments started arriving a short time later. Bush and I reviewed them with our practice manager, and Whitney confirmed we were only getting paid around thirty cents on the dollar. She double-checked the numbers and then called the owner of the billing firm.

"What y'all have to realize is that private practice doesn't pay like it used to," Barbara lectured us during a meeting in Whitney's office in early December. She reached into her briefcase and then handed us both columns of figures and pages of brightly colored pie charts summarizing over two months of collections that clearly proved her point.

"This is no better than what Medicaid pays," Bush protested, expecting that payments from our Blue Cross, United Healthcare, Aetna, and Cigna contracts would be higher than payments from the state.

"How much money is outstanding right now from what you've billed?" I asked, hoping this was just a tithe of what we would eventually be paid.

"We've collected probably 80 percent of what you can realistically expect," Barbara replied, matter-of-factly, oblivious to the crushing weight her news delivered as she stood to leave.

"This means we can't afford to stay in business!" Bush exclaimed, unable to hold back tears of frustration that seeped out the moment the door closed behind Barbara.

We studied those many-colored charts again before she added, "We can't work any harder than we've been working, and these payments don't even begin to cover the cost of rent and our employees, much less leave any salary for us."

Certain there had to be a mistake, Whitney investigated and found dozens. Only the primary surgical code was listed on some claims, leaving off other codes for the additional work we did. Or, when several codes were filed, they were not listed in the correct order to ensure the maximum payment we were entitled to. Some claims did not include our provider numbers required to process the bill, while others gave a wrong bank account to receive the payment.

Confronted with these costly errors, Barbara reassured Whitney, "We know what we're doing. *We are billing professionals.*"

As the mistakes piled higher and our revenue fell lower, we saw no other choice but to declare another contract null and void. Whitney decided she could assume the role of professional biller, and almost immediately payments increased.

Temporarily. Even though collections improved, the money in our account still hovered just above bankruptcy. Searching deeper in the weeds, Whitney started adding the columns of numbers that accompanied payments and discovered that one major insurance consistently underpaid by 7 percent. Another declared it overpaid our bills and then "recouped" the excess directly from our bank account. When calls led to countless hours on hold and certified letters achieved nothing, Whitney tediously submitted complaints, one by one, to the Texas Insurance Board, which finally convinced those carriers to pay what they owed.

Yet these existential threats to my new life did not weigh on me like the last years at Children's and the university. I had no idea those burdens were so obvious until I realized that every single one of my old patients coming to the new office made the exact same comment.

"I love your new office! And, wow, you look so *happy*!"

Of course, problems with the EMR and struggles to force insurances to pay what they contracted to pay were not unique to us. Rather, the challenges facing private practice during this time drove many surgeons into large groups subsequently bought out by private equity firms, while others sold themselves to hospitals to manage their business. Bush and I were unicorns deciding to create and operate a small independent practice, but our recent experiences at both the university and Children's made us leery of new entanglements with larger entities.

Which exposed us to another crisis, when the anesthesiologist scheduled for the next day called Whitney to cancel. Everywhere I worked before moving to Dallas, a surgeon simply called the operating room to schedule a patient for surgery and then an anesthesiologist on the hospital staff would be assigned to that case. But there was a different system here. Surgeons had to first arrange for an anesthesiologist before an operation could be scheduled.

"I'm sorry, Whitney," the anesthesiologist apologized, "but I'm not going to be able to do those cases for Dr. Snodgrass tomorrow after all."

"Why not?" she asked, already thinking ahead to who she might find on short notice to replace him.

"Well, I just can't. In fact, no one in my group will be available," he added, closing the door to the most obvious solution.

"That's going to make it really hard to find someone," she pressed. "There has to be a reason why you, and your entire group, are suddenly not available to do cases you agreed to do weeks ago!"

The line went silent. Then he confessed in a sigh, "We can't do it because Dr. __ saw the schedule and told me that if I, or anyone in my group, did y'all's anesthesia, his group would cut us off." There was another pause. "I don't like this at all, but his practice keeps us busy . . ."

Now finding a new anesthesiologist was yet another task on our startup to-do list.

As was launching another hypospadias pay-per-click campaign. Whitney researched costs and we soon learned that the price for listing "hypospadias" had increased from that first ad at Children's to well beyond our budget. To gain exposure we could afford, Bush and I started writing detailed descriptions of how we treat hypospadias to attach onto our website, hoping Search Engine Optimization would bring our new practice attention. However, all these pages and pages of state-of-the-art content, with all the keywords and all the photos that programmers recommended, could not divert Google's attention away from generic descriptions of hypospadias posted by such behemoths as the Mayo Clinic, Johns Hopkins, and Boston Children's Hospital. After all that work, our webpage still languished in obscurity many pages off the first page of an internet search.

What did reliably appear on the first page whenever someone searched "Snodgrass" was that year-old *Dallas Morning News* article—a smear on my reputation that would continue year after year, indefinitely.

CHAPTER 15

A Goniometer to Settle This

One reason I was so happy despite all these difficulties getting the new practice started was our good fortune to find Forest Park. I could not help but smile every morning when I walked into the OR to greet the nurse and the tech assigned to me and Bush that day from a small pool of nurses and techs who all quickly learned our operations and how we did them. And then after surgery passed through the recovery room on my way to the pre-op area to meet the next family, walking by PACU[35] nurses who were learning how we wanted parents instructed to take care of their sons at home.

Bush and I had already handed the PACU detailed instruction sheets for those families. Answering the usual questions parents asked, both to reassure them, and to decrease the number of phone calls to us after hours when Mom changed a diaper and saw a few drops of blood, or a boy's cheeks turned red after a dose of Ditropan.[36] Then, to be certain everyone was on the same page, the head nurse asked us to also give a lecture to the staff explaining what hypospadias is, how we repair it, and what the nurses should expect in the PACU and tell the parents to watch for at home.

Those nurses were already impressed that the boys arrived in recovery awake, yet comfortable. One might expect that surgery on the

---

35. *PACU* is the post-anesthesia care unit where patients are taken directly from the operating room until they recover from the anesthetic.
36. *Ditropan* is the common name for oxybutynin, a medication given after hypospadias repair to reduce painful bladder spasms caused by the catheter, which can also make cheeks flush red.

penis would be quite painful afterward, but our patients rarely cried, and then usually because they were thirsty.

"I did a pediatric pain fellowship at Harvard," Matt Miller explained to them as they stood by the bedside. "They should never come out of the operating room hurting."

He and I worked together for years at Children's, Miller the anesthesiologist usually assigned to my room. As I was packing to leave, I told my friend that Bush and I would still be operating with him out at Legacy, the Children's branch in Plano, but we also hoped he could do our cases at Forest Park. It was not a difficult sale to the chief of anesthesia to allow Miller excursions into the private world, where higher reimbursements meant more money for their department, and once that was agreed, we no longer had to rely on sometimes unreliable private anesthesiologists to cover our cases.

Within a short time, Bush and I created an environment at Forest Park that resembled the one we left at Children's. Except that it was totally different. The staff at Forest Park *smiled* when we walked by. Pre-op *welcomed* our patients as though they were all VIPs. The nurses *wanted* to reinforce the post-op care instructions exactly as Bush and I explained them to the parents.

When someone at the next national meeting asked about the new hospital where we worked, I replied it was exactly the opposite of Children's, where staff rarely looked up when I entered, pre-op nurses interrogated patients searching for violations of their preoperative instructions, and the administration insisted the PACU give everyone generic post-operative instructions they purchased from some vendor, even if they conflicted with ours and ensured confusion and after-hours phone calls.

An obsession with rules rather than care seeped into every nook and cranny of Children's. I thought we would simply move our patients from the main campus near downtown to Legacy in the northern suburbs when we relocated, but that proved impossible. Only three weeks into this transition, I wasted forty-five minutes doing what should have taken five trying to give admission orders for a child preparing for surgery the next day. Epic, the hospital EMR, refused to accept them, so I finally picked up the phone to call the instructions to a nurse.

"I'm sorry, Dr. Snodgrass, but we can't take verbal orders," the nurse replied curtly.

"Well, I've been trying to enter them in Epic for almost an hour, but it's not working for some reason that even IT can't figure out," I explained. "My patient needs to get started on her pre-op antibiotics."

"I understand, but that's our policy."

I asked to speak to the head nurse only to hear the same refrain, even though the routine medications I was struggling to order were needed to make the operation safe, and verbal orders were allowed at the main hospital.

Finally, I asked, "If you *never* take verbal orders, what happens if there is some urgency and I'm in surgery somewhere else, or in traffic on the freeway, and can't type orders into the computer?

"Then you'll have to take a break from the operation or pull over to the side of the road. There are *no* exceptions." After a pause she added, "The other private doctors have the hospitalists admit their patients for them and they enter in the orders."

So, I contacted the hospitalist and explained the situation.

"I'd like to help," she told me, "but I already have three new patient admissions today and can't possibly add on another."

In contrast, at Forest Park I could call in orders, write them on paper, or enter them into the computer, whichever I preferred. And though there must have been some policy about incident reports, I never heard that anyone filed one. While the Children's administration threatened to fire nurses and discipline physicians, the CEO at Forest Park established an *esprit de corps* so strong that in the coming months when shenanigans at a sister facility strained its finances, the OR still managed to keep supplies on hand and employees showed up for work despite delayed paychecks.

Once we got started, our clinic and OR schedules were much the same as they had been during the last years at the university. But freed from the distractions of meetings and conferences, without residents and fellows asking questions, relocated far from all the policies and politics at Children's, and working with the same anesthesiologist and OR crew every day, our attention was better focused.

Maybe that helped connect the dots between three patients I saw scattered through that first year at PARC Urology. One returned with a second fistula after a proximal TIP, which signaled there was likely some underlying problem pulling the leak open again. Reviewing my notes, I read how I dissected the urethral plate high off the penis to help straighten more than thirty degrees of curvature, before I stopped doing that maneuver. Now, as I examined the boy in the office, I worried that his penis might be bent again. Which was exactly what Bush and I found when we reoperated.

A second boy had a recurrent glans dehiscence, and his penis, too, was bent. The third had no apparent complications but his penis looked hunched over, and when I tried to lift it upward, I felt tension and saw the scrotum rise with it. Both these boys also had proximal TIPs but without any special straightening maneuvers, which meant I thought at the time the bending was less than thirty degrees. Now we confirmed at surgery they both had recurrent curvature, which measured forty degrees in one and forty-five degrees in the other.

"I would do a plication again for this curvature," I admitted to Bush during surgery on the one bent forty degrees. "It doesn't look like very much."

"That's the whole problem with eyeballing it," she agreed. "That's why it's so important to actually measure it."

I injected saline into the penis again to create an artificial erection. Bush aligned a goniometer[37] along the penile shaft, placing the fulcrum at the point where the penis bent and adjusting the moving arm to the proper location of the meatus.

"Yes, it's definitely forty degrees."

"So, when I told people I only did proximal TIPs when the curvature was less than thirty degrees, I was actually doing it in some who had more than that because I didn't measure it," I confessed.

No one I knew measured curvature. Everyone just guesstimated how bent a penis was; some, like me, recorded their impression in degrees, while others described the curvature as "mild" or "severe" or "extraordinary." While it was easy to see if a penis was straight or

---

37. A *goniometer* is a type of protractor used to measure angles.

bent ninety degrees, when we started using the goniometer Bush and I quickly learned that eyeballing was not accurate between those extremes, especially curvature that our instrument measured from twenty-five to forty-five degrees.

In retrospect, I cannot believe that I never thought to measure it. An article published in the late 1990s reporting how surgeons straightened penile curvature criticized those subjective descriptions of mild and severe chordee,[38] but somehow its picture showing a clear plastic protractor pressed against a bent penis escaped my attention when I was collecting important publications on hypospadias and filing them away that year in Seattle.

Now I laugh at the memory of why I started measuring various aspects of hypospadias. It was my turn to lecture one morning at the PUWF, and almost the moment my first slide appeared showing a distal hypospadias, John Duckett leaped from his seat too filled with energy to simply raise his hand and comment.

"Warren, how do you decide where you're going to make your incisions beside the urethral plate?"

And before I could answer that, he pointed at the picture on the screen and demanded to know, "How wide is that plate?"

I raised a finger for him to hold that thought, and Duckett reluctantly sat back down while I advanced the slide to show the surgical marks. But before I could explain them, he jumped back to his feet demanding to know if I always drew those lines in the same place or adjusted them somehow to the circumstances.

My mouth opened, but his mind was speeding along faster, and he peppered me with more questions before I could speak. Finally his young associate, Doug Canning, tugged at his sleeve and suggested he let me continue so we could all go ski.

Then I showed a slide of the urethral plate before and after the TIP incision, and Duckett rocketed out of his chair again.

"How do you know how wide that little incision of yours makes it?" And without waiting for me to answer, shouted, "I WANT SCIENCE! WE NEED MEASUREMENTS!"

---

38. "Chordee: Varied Opinions and Treatments," published in 1999.

It was those measurements of the urethral plate that Duckett demanded which gave scientific proof that TIP incision made a narrow plate sufficiently wide when the Australians raised concern it did not. And then it was Duckett's lingering influence that led me to measure the glans and prove the smaller ones were more prone to complications. But I did not think to measure how bent a penis was, until one day at Forest Park when Bush and I argued about how bent it was.

Then she remembered an instrument she once read that hand surgeons use to measure finger joint angles and declared, "We can use a goniometer to settle this."

But the one the circulator found in the orthopedic set was too long to fit the penis.

"I can get it cut down for you," the scrub tech offered, and, in another sign of providence, the improved version he brought back just happened to have the correct arm shortened to fit our needs.

Soon we developed a routine. I injected saline to keep the penis firm while Bush manipulated the goniometer and read the degree of curvature it measured. I added a column to the database to record our findings. We quickly learned that most patients with proximal hypospadias are bent more than thirty degrees, in fact averaging seventy degrees, which meant I subsequently did even fewer proximal TIPs and more two-stage grafts.

And more ventral lengthenings to make the bent penis straight. I watched Bracka remove the urethral plate and simply declare the penis straight many times, but I do not recall seeing him confirm that with an artificial erection or hearing him explain what he did next if it was still bent. Rather, several times I held my index finger up bent to seventy degrees and asked Bracka how he fixed that. But he only mumbled something unintelligible before walking away.

The first boy I remember with that much curvature was the patient at the workshop in Istanbul who kept me awake imagining the steps I would take the next morning to lengthen the short side of his penis, before a rash canceled the operation. In subsequent patients I did traditional ventral lengthening, making a single incision across the bend and then patching the defect that created with a graft of tissue taken from a separate incision under the skin in the groin.[39]

Then I met Bracka and was convinced to change from skin flaps to grafts to make the new urethra. But that presented a dilemma. I could not place a urethral graft on top of the other graft used to straighten the penis and expect them both to develop the new blood vessels they needed to survive.

I was not sure what to do. I remembered hearing of "fairy cuts" done in the 1970s by the urology/plastic surgery team of Devine and Horton[40] to straighten the penis but could not find a description or an illustration of their method. I decided to incise across the corpora where they were most bent, in the traditional way, but then added a second and third incision a little above and below the first. Those three cuts released the tension on the underside of the penis to make it straight and healed without needing to be patched with grafts.

I published that these three corporotomies done without patches worked just as good as the traditional single incision that was patched. I eventually learned that my method worked better, although it would take another twenty years to convince a smattering of urologists around the world to use it.

The typical reaction of those who converted was always the same: "Those three incisions really do make the penis straight, and longer!"

---

39. Surgeons refer to this tissue as "dermis" and these grafts as "dermal grafts."
40. Charles Devine Jr. was a urologist, and Charles Horton, a plastic surgeon, in Norfolk, Virginia who performed hypospadias surgery as a team during the 1960s and 1970s.

◀ CHAPTER 16 ▶

Let's Call It Operation Happenis

We certainly had more pressing matters in those first months getting PARC Urology off the ground, but I was nevertheless determined to create the charity even if it had to then lay fallow for a year or two.

"No one at either Children's or the university would even talk to me about an endowment," I explained to Bush. "So now it's a priority for me to set something up right off the bat."

Even after paying our own salaries, and the salaries of our secretaries and nurse practitioners, plus fees to use Children's clinic space and their nurses, medical assistants, and schedulers at both the main campus and our several satellite offices, as well as the costs of flights, hotels, registration, and meals for meetings, membership fees in professional societies, the dean's tax,[41] and undoubtedly other expenses I no longer remember, the pediatric division I led at the university still had profits left over even though only three of the six faculty ever made more than they were paid. I simply wanted to set aside a portion of that surplus in an endowment.

John McConnell challenged me to create an elite division of pediatric urology, and this was another brick to build that foundation. I heard that Boston Children's Urology had three million dollars in their endowment. When John Duckett died, CHOP began raising money in his honor for a similar cash reserve. Seattle tried to bank on Mike Mitchell's reputation to establish a pediatric urology fund after he announced

---

41. The *dean's tax* is an assessment taken from the revenue earned by the faculty to help provide discretionary funds to the university administration.

his retirement. I did not want to wait until I retired, or died, to start an endowment for our division.

I had seen firsthand the value of having discretionary funds. When McConnell recruited Baker, he convinced Ross Perot to send her on a shopping spree for the test tubes and pipettes, the scales and micro-scopes she needed to set up a lab. McConnell also found a second do-nor to buy the new group X-ray and urodynamic equipment to assess bladder function that we needed to run a state-of-the-art clinic.

I floated several trial balloons to start a fund, such as capping our dean's tax and investing the remainder in an endowment. Or, convincing the dean to match our excess earnings and set that aside in the endow-ment. Or Children's could provide those matching funds with money it raised from donors. But I could never get so much as a hearing with any-one in power, not even when pediatric urology was the highest ranked *US News & World Report* program, adult or pediatric, at the University.[42] Roehrborn just shrugged his shoulders at the walls I kept running into.

Now Bush and I had only expenses and no profits. It was an act of defiance, and a show of confidence in our future, that made me insist on paying lawyers to file the paperwork establishing a nonprofit almost as soon as we named PARC Urology.

And, like PARC Urology, the new charity needed a name. Resigned to the fact that we would spend time and energy we did not have on this project, Bush first tried to envision what it would do. Visits to several websites of well-established nonprofits made clear the main goal was to raise money.

"So let's assume it's up and running and people are making dona-tions. What will we spend that money on?" she asked.

"I think one thing would be supplies for the operations we do at foreign workshops," I replied. "That's going to run us between $500 and a couple of thousand dollars depending on how many surgeries we do, since we don't have Children's to provide them anymore."

"OK," Bush agreed. "Along those same lines, I guess we could also raise funds to pay for a few boys to come here each year to have surgery

---

42. The orthopedic department at Texas Scottish Rite hospital ranked higher but was only loosely affiliated with UT Southwestern.

they can't get done otherwise." She thought another moment and then added, "Or, maybe we bring a boy and his urologist here so we can also teach the surgeon."

Which made us both think of Operation Smile, the charity for children born with cleft lip.

"We need a name like that," Bush declared, but neither of us could imagine anything suitable. "Operation Penis, Operation Hypospadias . . ."

Yeah, those won't work," I smirked. "Operation . . . what?"

A visit to her brother in Houston, and maybe the bottle of wine they shared one evening, filled in the blank for a name.

"Operation Hap-penis," Bush announced when she returned. "What do you think? I think it's brilliant! Clever, and just edgy enough to make people pause and then laugh."

I thought about it for a moment, and then laughed. "Yeah, that's perfect."

Legally established and wittily named, the next step was to appoint someone outside of PARC Urology to a Board of Directors. Someone to provide a different perspective, and to make clear the nonprofit had greater aspirations than being an arm of our practice. Our first choice was Tony Caldamone, one of the original TIP surgeons, and a pediatric urologist widely respected for his calm and reasoned demeanor.

"I'm not so sure about the name," he responded to our invitation. "I can imagine that being a problem." Then, in a follow-up call, he asked, "How much are we each donating to get it started?"

Neither Bush nor I had thought of seed money.

"Well, then, what if we each give $500?" the new board member suggested. "We have to make a real investment to show we're serious."

Which made Caldamone the first official donor to Operation Happenis.

There was one more project to finish even though we had no spare time for it. I had witnessed the ascent of hypospadiology from a rabble of operations that no surgeon could master, toward a holy grail where all surgeons could use the same few operations to repair every hypospadias. A new textbook devoted to the surgery of hypospadias would aid that quest, since articles in urology journals were limited to a single topic, book chapters were too short to cover the breath of the subject, and the only available textbook described a chaos of operations that rarely made the penis normal. I started writing a new book during my final year at the university, taking advantage of the free time I gained by not being the division chief.

I had done this once before. Seeing how urologists were sometimes so overwhelmed by all the medical information available through the internet that they retreated to the comfort of familiar habits, I edited a textbook summarizing the best data available to resolve clinical dilemmas. It would be a resource that groups could leave on their conference tables for a quick review when there was uncertainty of how to manage a patient.

To do that I outlined each chapter, listed questions that various conditions posed, and then enlisted the help of our group to research the answers. Next, I wrote drafts, or revised those from my partners, before gathering everyone for a weekend retreat to my beach house for a final polishing.

Springer published *Pediatric Urology: Evidence for Optimal Patient Management* in 2013. One year later the company mailed the only report I ever received, informing me that the book was selling in the top 50 percent of similar textbooks, whatever that meant. Following the norm in academic publishing, Springer pocketed whatever profit there was, and the authors each received a free copy of the book we wrote.

For this new textbook I first gathered information, thumbing through all those photocopied articles in my Seattle file cabinet and updating those with fresh PubMed searches on the computer. Then, I got up early every morning before going to the hospital, and stayed up late every evening after work, typing a few new paragraphs. Some weekends I drove to the coast, exchanging the hours of travel for the solitude to plow ahead without distractions. Now a walk along the edge of the tide cleared my mind to work a little longer.

"The textbook needs a uniform message," I explained to Bush at the outset, "rather than the usual lists of options that imply there are lots of ways to get the same best results. Because, obviously, there aren't."

That meant she and I would write the entire book, rather than follow the usual practice of inviting different authors for each chapter.

And given our recent experience with traditional publishing, Bush and I also decided to publish the book ourselves and dedicate all its profits to grow the coffers of Operation Happenis.

I wrote the first draft. Bush redlined the text before passing it back to me for revisions. I made the edits and sent the manuscript back to her to finalize.

"It needs a lot more pictures!" she insisted during the editing. So, we wrote a list of key findings and technical maneuvers to photograph during surgery, which were cropped to size and then inserted into the text.

We produced a textbook that dispensed with the MAGPI and Mathieu's flip-flap and replaced them with TIP, since it alone could make any distal hypospadias into a normal penis. A book that challenged the conventional wisdom that it was better to make the urethra in proximal hypospadias from a skin flap instead of a skin graft. The first textbook which devoted an entire chapter to describing how to manage the abnormal penis skin that is an integral part of all hypospadias.

Whitney took the final versions of all the twenty-three chapters and formatted those Word documents into the layout of a standard textbook. Next, she found a self-publishing company to transform the electronic text into words on pages bound within a hardcover.

And then we all wondered what our many hours of labor would become. If we made a profit, I could imagine our example showing the way for our always cash-strapped professional societies to fund their own activities by self-publishing future textbooks and journals. In fact, I wondered why no one else had suggested that. But the puzzled looks that answered my proposal to our officers said, once again, that I was thinking differently.

◀ CHAPTER 17 ▶

I Feel So Betrayed

Her son was born with distal hypospadias. It was noticed in the new-born nursery during his first physical exam, but the doctor at the hospital reassured Mom, "He has a minor problem with his penis that's easy to fix." She had never heard of hypospadias and was not really certain what a newborn penis was supposed to look like, but she was relieved her son was otherwise healthy.

The pediatrician repeated the exam during her son's first office visit and confirmed the diagnosis.

"Don't worry," he told her, "He has a minor case, and I know a good surgeon who'll take care of it."

She followed his recommendation and made an appointment with the pediatric urologist. He took a brief look at the penis and then explained, "Your son has distal hypospadias and needs a minor operation to fix that. Surgery is successful 95 percent of the time."

Three years and several operations later, his "minor" hypospadias was finally repaired.

"I feel so betrayed," Deb Smith told me as her eyes filled with tears of anger and frustration. "Everyone told me this was a minor problem, but there is nothing minor about your baby having so many operations on his penis." She dabbed her eyes with a Kleenex. "I'm especially upset that we live so close, but our pediatrician never mentioned you." Now guilt forced out more tears. "I should have done my research instead of just listening to him."

It was a familiar story. I knew that one out of every twenty distal TIP repairs I did developed a complication needing another operation.

But I also knew that one of every five patients who came to me needing a salvage repair started life with distal hypospadias.

There is no minor hypospadias, and no minor hypospadias repair, I thought as she spoke, reminding myself of a lesson I taught trainees at the university and surgeons worldwide. Because there is nothing minor about a surgery in which dissection just one or two millimeters in the wrong plane can be the difference in success and failure.

"We certainly have complications too," I told Deb, hoping to ease her guilt. "And you shouldn't blame yourself for following the advice of your pediatrician and a board-certified pediatric urologist."

"Maybe. But when things didn't go well and I heard about you, I asked my pediatrician and he said he knew about you and your practice." Deb cried no more tears when she added, "Since then I've learned that he and the urologist are in the same hospital network,[43] and that's why he referred me to him. Not because he was good at hypospadias or had the same experience that you do."

I might have ended the conversation there with an upbeat, "Well, at least it's all turned out OK," or a reassuring, "It's good that your son won't remember all this when he grows up," but glossing over the hurt would not heal her anger and guilt.

"Maybe you can take this bad experience and make something good out of it." I suggested, tentatively. "So many moms go down the same path as you did. Maybe you can somehow let at least a few of them know what can happen."

Bush and I were both in the audience at the European Society of Pediatric Urology in 2015 when the intense Fred van der Toorn went to the lectern to present results of the Dutch Hypospadias Study. Bush advised the researchers as they organized this assessment of distal hypospadias repairs done by surgeons at the major medical centers around the Netherlands. Now they reported that pediatric urologists were not as good at this operation as most assumed. After analyzing outcomes from more than 800 operations, the researchers discovered that only

---

43. The *hospital network* referred to here is a group of physicians employed by a hospital, who are expected to refer patients to each other even if there are specialists with greater experience and better results available outside the network.

10 percent of the surgeons achieved success 95 percent of the time. Instead, nearly 20 percent of patients had complications, as did almost half the boys operated by two urologists.

I was disturbed but not surprised. Half of the patients who traveled to PARC had unsuccessful repairs by other pediatric urologists, and I heard over and over that the original surgeons assured parents that distal operations were almost always successful. I requested the reports by the first surgeons and read technical errors in most of them, steps that could have been done in a better way which might have prevented the complication.

There were fistulas in boys whose new urethras were sewn with one layer of stitches instead of the recommended two, or who did not have dartos laid over them to separate the stitches making the urethra from the stitches closing the skin above it. There were cuts and gashes through glans closed with deep stitches through the skin, rather than stitches completely under the surface. There were others whose glans dehisced after being sewn with a single stitch instead of the three I use. I read that surgeons decided not to incise the entire urethral plate, fearing internal scarring, and then rolled a neourethra that was too narrow and created the obstruction they were trying to avoid.

This news was foreseen by a colleague who once told me, as we stood in the door looking at our fellow pediatric urologists seated at a national congress, "If there are thirty different surgeons, there are thirty different TIP repairs."

I replied, "But there aren't thirty different ways that all give the same results."

These operative reports proved that was true.

The same month as the ESPU, an article was published that looked at the most influential papers written on hypospadias since 1945. I headed the list of authors. Together with Bush, I have written more articles on hypospadias than anyone in history, not counting book chapters or the textbook we had just finished. These articles and book chapters and that textbook all described how to do each step of a distal TIP. I have also operated in more workshops than almost any other pediatric urologist and organized the only live surgery hypospadias course beamed across the US and around the world by webinar, to show how to do those steps.

So, if I achieved success in 95 percent of my patients, and both told and showed others exactly how I do the operation, why did so many surgeons do things differently when that caused more complications?

It was Bush's first invitation to a surgical workshop that finally convinced me the traditional academic model of teaching and learning is broken. First, she texted me some touristy pictures of her finger touching the peak of a pyramid. Then she sent a few emails about all the redo operations they scheduled for her.

"I lectured on fixing it right the first time, but nearly every surgery they had me do was some disaster case," Bush explained when she returned, showing me photo after photo of scarred and twisted penises. "These were all *distals*," she emphasized, as I continued scrolling through them. "Finally, on the last day, I did a first-time repair, and the questions and comments from the audience were like I was never there." She was quiet a moment, before wondering, "Maybe they weren't listening because I'm a woman?"

"No, I'm pretty sure they knew that when they invited you!" I laughed. Then my eyes narrowed as I looked into the past.

"You know that I've been to Cairo several times, as have other surgeons, like Pippi, and probably Bracka too. The Egyptians also watched all our webinars, so they've seen how to do things right." I looked up from the pictures and agreed with her. "These are really awful."

Of course, we had no way to know if the boys she saw during her visit had the typical results of surgery done by the hands of her hosts, or if they were specially selected for her to repair because they had such terrible problems. The paradox of being a specialist is the uncertainty of whether the patients you see are like most patients, or outliers. Those patients shown to the visiting professor very well could be the worst of the worst culled for the expert to sort out, although Ziada told us he came to Dallas for our training because his colleagues in Cairo did not do TIP right.

"Regardless," Bush argued, "it's still wrong what's happened to those boys. Their penises will never be the same."

And that is the tragedy of surgery done wrong by any surgeon anywhere in the world to the organ that defines masculinity, that gives so much pleasure, that is so integral to life for both men and women. Bush could straighten their curvature and move their meatus to the tip of the glans, but no one could exorcise the scars from the skin or make the glans smooth again.

"You have to say it would've been better for those boys in their culture if they had only been circumcised," she concluded.

And what about the others with a penis just as damaged who she did not repair, because there were too many and not enough time to schedule them all? Their surgery had been recommended so they could stand to pee and not look different from other boys. But afterward they still had to sit to pee and hide their penises from friends in the locker room and lovers in the bedroom because it looked so different.

"What's sad is that the Egyptians are not uniquely terrible surgeons," I replied as our conversation came to an end. "This happens everywhere. You'll see."

I always seem to tune in to the middle of interesting stories on National Public Radio. Like the day I drove up the tollway from Dallas to meet Kim Hines for the hospital tour and caught part of a report about a surgeon who discovered a better way to fix club foot. Rather than multiple operations that might leave it scarred and stiff, Dr. Ponseti told his orthopedic colleagues they could apply a series of casts to gradually move the foot into place. That was in the 1950s. They ignored his advice for years.

"Then a mother in Michigan had a daughter born with club foot and was told that surgery was inevitable," the NPR story continued. "She decided to do some research herself and used her new dial-up connection to get on the internet." The narrator explained how she read about Dr. Ponseti and decided to go to Iowa, where he still practiced—well past a typical retirement age—to learn more about casting. It worked, and she was so thrilled that she told other moms about it on the World Wide Web.

The reporter wrapped up the segment telling listeners that today, the American Academy of Orthopedics recommends casting as the *treatment of choice* for club foot, because of those moms. I imagined the unspoken rest of the story. That Ponseti must have published the usual medical articles describing his technique and results. How he most likely was invited onto panel discussions at national meetings to explain why surgery was not needed, after several prominent surgeons first debated which operation was best. Certainly, he must have written chapters for textbooks and demonstrated casting during visiting professorships. In other words, I suspected Ponseti tried all the traditional academic ways to convince surgeons to do the right thing. But it took moms to make them listen. Four decades later.

Moms like Deb.

But Deb's frustration was not only that the first urologist considered her son's condition so minor that he did not bother with the details of the operation. She also felt betrayed by all the pediatric urologists who listened as moms told them over and over that they never heard of hypospadias before their sons were born yet did not act through their Society for Pediatric Urology or the American Urological Association or the European Society of Pediatric Urology to spearhead public awareness campaigns.

"Other parents should not feel the fear and isolation I did from not knowing about a common birth defect," she complained.

I certainly heard all this from other parents too. One family started the conversation several years after I repaired their son's proximal hypospadias.

"We'd never heard of hypospadias before," Mom said, as Dad nodded agreement. "Neither had our parents. And we didn't feel comfortable talking about our son's privates with friends, so there was no one to talk to."

Dad continued their story. "It was especially hard during the surgeries, because we had to come up with reasons why he was going to the hospital and would be out of childcare for a few weeks."

"The internet told us that hypospadias is pretty common, so we knew there had to be other parents out there facing the same things that we were. We just didn't know any of them to talk to." That was mom speaking again, looking away toward her son playing on the floor as she described their isolation one more time.

In this new practice, I also came to realize that hypospadias affects not only the boy and his parents, but even his brothers and sisters. One mother emailed ahead of her son's reoperation:

It looks like his father will be bringing him alone. I'm going to have to stay at home with his brothers, who are mad that their vacation had to be canceled. They refuse to go with him to another operation.

Another described how a younger sister became distraught when her brother went to the hospital, knowing from past experience that he would come back home bandaged and hurting.

"I guess even a second grader can be embarrassed about his brother having penis surgery," a third mom told me. "We've always been very open about the hypospadias affecting his penis, using the correct words for those things, but when a neighbor asked what kind of operation Ryan was going to have, Theo answered, 'Something on his back.'"

Academics failed to teach me this. Rather, as an academic surgeon at Children's, I saw far too many patients during clinic hours to hear these stories. When I picked up a chart labeled New Patient: Hypospadias, I sighed with relief, since I was usually behind schedule and considered this a straightforward diagnosis needing only a brief explanation before picking a date for surgery.

I had no idea that when a mom asked, "What causes hypospadias?" she actually wanted to know, "Did I do something to make this happen?" I never had time to listen to a mother of a boy whose surgery was unsuccessful tell me, "The guilt I feel is suffocating." Or to hear parents admit that worry about their son was stressing their marriage. Or to be startled by a five-year-old screaming, "I hate my penis!"

After nearly thirty years of doing and teaching hypospadias surgery, the patients in our new practice were showing me how much more I, and our profession, still had to learn.

◀ CHAPTER 18 ▶

Abnormal Anatomy Increases the Risk for Abnormal Function

Needing a community to discuss their worries, some moms joined Facebook groups. But sometimes the posts they read made their anxiety worse.

"Everyone say a prayer for us. Johnny's going back for the third time to close his fistula and we're really hoping it's going to work this time." "Our urologist said everything looks fine, but I think he still has chordee." "I see those scars and have to wonder how his penis is going to grow and if he'll have any feelings in it."

At the least, comments like these raised doubts that surgery would be as successful as their urologist promised. For some moms, they were enough to question if a repair should even be done.

After consulting the local pediatric urologists and Facebook, one mom traveled nearly twenty-four hours from Australia to hear my advice.

"Because if the operation is cosmetic, we'd prefer not to make a decision for him," she said, as I opened her son's diaper to begin the examination. "His dad and I think it'll be better to wait until he's older when he can decide for himself."

I showed Mom the urinary opening perched on the edge of the glans, and not enclosed by it as the meatus should be.

"Most boys with this anatomy will have trouble aiming when they get older," I explained, sketching a diagram of the normal anatomy that makes the stream go straight.

I had already responded to an emailed picture of her son's penis and recommended surgery, but she was still uncertain and wondered if seeing it in person might change my mind.

"I took him to two surgeons back home who both said he might be just fine without surgery. They told me the operation would be mostly cosmetic." A look of uncertainty spread over Mom's face, and then she added, "I've heard about fistulas happening, and I just can't face the possibility of him getting a complication for a cosmetic operation on a part that only a few people are ever going to see."

I acknowledged it was unsettling when specialists gave different answers to the same question. But teens and adults with the same anatomy as her son told me it was a struggle for them to stand to pee. And also that the appearance made them worry what a lover would think the first time they saw it.

"Every man wants to have a normal penis," I summarized. "Try to imagine when he's sixteen years old. Who's he going to talk to about his hypospadias—certainly not his friends, and he probably won't have a girlfriend. That leaves Mom and Dad, and he sure won't want to talk to y'all about his penis!"

"But what is the chance that *my* son is going to have problems peeing or be ashamed of his penis?" she asked, confused by the conflicting opinions she had heard.

"Well, it's possible that he won't," I admitted, telling Mom that neither I nor the other surgeons she consulted had the data to definitively answer her question. "But abnormal anatomy increases the risk for abnormal function. And every teenage boy and girl today knows what a penis is supposed to look like," I concluded, holding up my cell phone.

The type of repair a patient receives should not be an accident of which surgeon he happens to consult. Neither should a recommendation for or against surgery. Ideally, urologists everywhere should use the same criteria to make this decision, and a published article[44] described an objective standard that everyone could use. Glans fusion, the distance

---

44. "Normal anatomy of the external urethral meatus in boys: implications for hypospadias repair," was published by the *British Journal of Urology International* in 2007.

measured from the bottom lip of the meatus to the raised edge around the glans, that not only defined normal anatomy, but also the abnormal anatomy justifying repair. Because the glans acts like a nozzle on a hose to focus the urine stream.

But I knew that when I mentioned this to colleagues, someone would ask for longitudinal data showing how many boys with no glans fusion grow into men whose urine sprays or have a negative body image if it is not repaired. Of course, those surgeons already know that no one knows that answer. Because learning it would require convincing parents to not only leave the hypospadias alone, but to also bring their sons in periodically for evaluations throughout childhood and beyond puberty to document how many have problems aiming their urine stream and how many worry about their penis looking different, and accomplish all twenty-plus-years of this study without *creating* anxiety that there is something wrong that requires a doctor to examine their privates and ask how they pee and what they think about their penis, over and over, year after year.

"So, the critics don't have any data either," I complained to Bush as I tried to improve some slides for an upcoming conference. "The best I can do is prove that most of the men we see with abnormal anatomy spray or have other problems as a result."

I copied and pasted a picture of a man before surgery with a deep cleft splitting open the head of his penis, and another picture after repair made it normal.

"What those really show is how the little differences in what they look like as infants become really big differences when they grow up into men," she pointed out.

"Yeah, that's true. But at least glans fusion is something objective, with published normative values, that we can measure in the office and use to predict who's most likely to need surgery," I replied.

Bush listened and nodded, but the look on her face betrayed a search for a better answer, something unexpected that others would struggle to argue against. She stared past me and then pulled out her phone and started searching.

I returned to the draft of my lecture while she typed and scrolled.

Then she held up her phone toward me. "Here're two pictures to add to your talk. I'll email them to you."

I opened a photo of a baby's face with a cleft lip, and another of a baby's hand with an extra finger.

"No mom's not going to get those fixed!" Bush declared. "Even if cleft lip and polydactyly don't cause any functional problems. You need to ask your audience why we would treat a penis with a birth defect different than a lip or a hand with a birth defect?"

And Bush was not done.

While I downloaded the new pictures, she googled *cosmetic versus reconstructive surgery*, which led to the websites of several plastic surgery societies worldwide that all gave the same explanation.

"Listen to this," she said, reading from her phone. "The American Society of Plastic Surgeons defines cosmetic surgery as 'enhancing and reshaping *normal* body structures.' Reconstructive surgery 'treats body structures affected aesthetically or functionally by *congenital defects.*'" She smiled and said, "That's it! No one knows the difference between cosmetic and reconstructive surgery better than the plastic surgeons!"

Bush was quiet for a moment before adding, "Urologists have to stop saying 'cosmetic' when the operation is 'reconstructive,' otherwise they just confuse families with the idea that the surgery is all about vanity."

Further complicating these discussions were rumors circulating that repairs done in boys would have to be redone anyway when the penis grew larger at puberty. Unlike the obscure origins of most gossip, I could trace the roots of this hearsay back to the energetic Italian urologist renowned for the Barbagli stricture repair. Not surprisingly, men diagnosed with strictures flocked to him, and a few of those men had hypospadias repaired when they were children.

"Warren, I see these men with chordee or a fistula or persistent hypospadias that any urologist can recognize," Guido Barbagli told me during breakfast at a hotel in Amman, Jordan, waving his hands as he spoke. "But, Warren, there are other men who think everything is fine for many years, and then they start straining to urinate. We find a stricture in them."

Naturally, Barbagli wondered why this might happen. But he did not research their past to read how their operations were done, to confirm that most had flap repairs prone to this complication. Nor did he check for the penile curvature that at least some of those men likely still had, pulling on the reconstructed urethra until it eventually scarred. Rather, he looked at the constricted end result and reached a unique conclusion.

"Warren," he said, with the glance of a conspirator, "they have sex!"

I smiled at the excitement Barbagli could not express fast enough with either his words or his hands.

"Because their urethras do not have the cushions like normal ones," he hurried on, rushing to complete his theory. "You know, Warren, that the spongiosum[45] is like an air bag!"

Now I was trapped in his enthusiasm, anxious to hear where this led.

"An air bag that fills during a car crash!" he finished, leaving that image hanging in the air, the explanation incomplete, as he stood and sped off to give his lecture convinced the point he made was obvious.

"He thinks that sex traumatizes the neourethra and makes it stricture," I told Bush, after solving the riddle.

Barbagli published these musings, and like the whisper that changes as it is passed from person to person down a line, soon pediatric surgeons everywhere started talking not about strictures, but about new fistulas and new penile curvature that suddenly everyone knew happens at puberty. And not from sex, but because the "rapid" growth of the penis in teenagers stresses their scars to pull tissues apart and bend the penis down.

Except that was *not* what we found in the teens and men who came to Bush and me. I recalled only one teenager who developed a fistula years after a hypospadias repair, which was easily closed. But not a single adult said his penis was straight until it bent during puberty. Or that his opening was at the tip of the glans until it came back open during puberty to the way it was before his surgery as a child. Because patients do not go to bed as boys and wake up fully grown men. Rather, that "rapid" growth happens slowly over several years, and operated tissues grow along with all the others.

---

45. *Spongiosum* is a cushioning layer on the urethra to protect the urinary channel.

"Bones grow during puberty after a kid breaks them," I often reminded worried parents.

I reviewed my notes on the adults we saw with hypospadias complications after earlier repairs in childhood.

"Look at this," I said to Bush. "Just as we thought, most of them came with problems left over from childhood."

After their surgeons, or their parents, either did not see the problem, or kicked the can down the road until it could not be ignored any longer.

"But we have a second group of older men who developed new symptoms well after puberty from strictures, just like Barbagli said. And they all had flap repairs, which can do that, and not the graft repairs that we do."

"Even though graft patients have sex too," Bush surmised.

Despite assurances that hypospadias repair is reconstructive surgery, and that when it is done right the results can last indefinitely, there was still that worry about scars stunting the growth of the penis and decreasing feelings the man has during sex. I answered an email from one mom:

> The only incisions we make are in lines most men have—from the circumcision and down the middle of the underside of the penis. Those will all grow with him, just like other scars from surgery in children. If penis scars didn't grow with the penis, then all those men who had newborn circumcisions would be in trouble as teenagers!"

I told another mom nervous that sensation will change after surgery that we ask teens and men if they think their sensation is less, or if they have a numb spot after we operate.

"That almost never happens," I reassured her, "and when it does, it usually gets better over a few months."

Even men who had as many as twenty operations said their feelings seemed normal.

Every now and then a mom asked all these questions and listened to all my answers and then said, "I'm relieved he has distal hypospadias and that you can fix it with one operation. I was worried about scars affecting his growth and sensation, so I'm glad to hear those don't really happen. Dr. Snodgrass, we've done a lot of research on this and, if we decide to have it fixed, you and Dr. Bush are the only surgeons we want to do it."

That mother who flew from Australia for an office consultation told me this, but I knew by the hesitation in her voice that the discussion was not over.

"I just don't feel comfortable making this decision for him," she said, again. "What if he is one of the few who does have a complication? What if he grows up and is upset that he had surgery on his penis? He might be one of those men who has a spot with less feeling. I don't think I could live with myself if something like that happened."

There was no more medical information to give her, and the choice is up to the parents. I ended our conversation with a final observation.

"You might consider that a decision you make *not* to do surgery is also a decision you're making for him before he can decide himself," I said with a shrug.

A decision that also has long-term, maybe lifelong, consequences.

◀ CHAPTER 19 ▶

It Really Did Affect My Feeling of Manliness

"It's finally gotten to where I can barely pee," explained a burly fifty-year-old man whose grey mustache drooped around the corners of his mouth.

He had traveled from Clovis, in New Mexico across the border from Lubbock.

"I put up with it for years, but when it started slowin' down, there was no choice but to do somethin'. So I went to a urologist who stretched the openin'. That helped for a little while, but then it got slow again."

"Yeah, those dilations[46] never last very long," I commiserated. "And they hurt, so we don't do them."

"They do hurt, that's for sure! I asked about surgery, but the urologist said there are lots of complications and he didn't want to do it," the patient continued. "He sent me to a specialist way over in Albuquerque who said he could fix it, but he was only willin' to bring the openin' up to near the head. He said it'd be just fine like that, but that would leave it not far from where it was when I was born."

I knew that meant he had seen an adult reconstructive urologist, specialists who manage various urethra conditions, including, occasionally, a man with hypospadias. They generally seem content to leave those men with an opening at the base of the glans, converting whatever they had into a distal hypospadias. Or else they simply cut a small

---

46. *Dilations* are an ancient practice that use a metal instrument or a catheter inserted down the urethra to temporarily stretch open a partial obstruction from either meatal stenosis or a stricture.

meatus larger without doing an actual repair. I nodded as the story went on.

"But I figured if I was goin' to do more surgery, I'd rather get it fixed right. I did some research on the internet and found you."

He described the challenges he had faced for as long as he could remember just to pee standing. How sometimes it came out straight, but other times sprayed in different directions that he could neither predict nor prepare for. When he was younger, he pressed close to the urinal to keep the errant stream off his pants, or the shoes of someone standing to his side. But as scars gradually constricted the meatus, the splattering got worse, and now he had to hold his free hand in front to catch the urine and direct it toward the drain.

"Doc, I just want to pee right."

Examining him, I could see that his eight operations as a boy left the meatus right where it was at birth, only scarred tight from all the attention surgeons gave it.

"I already emailed you that this is going to take two more operations," I reminded him after the exam. "Tomorrow we'll be cutting out all that scar, so you'll pee better right away. We'll replace that with tissue from the lining inside your lip, and when that's all healed in six months, we'll roll it into your urine channel all the way to the tip of the head, where it should be."

After clinic I told Bush about this man we were going to repair the next afternoon.

"I can't imagine what it's been like for him, peeing into his hand six or seven times a day, every day, for years and years."

How he said his parents gave up when none of the operations he had as a child worked. That he saw an adult urologist when he was a young man who told him nothing could be done, and another more recently who advised him to live with dilations. How desperation finally drove him over 500 miles for us to operate because something had to be done, and he wanted it finally done right.

I predicted adults like this man, still struggling with their birth defect, would find our practice when few other websites mentioned both "hypospadias" and "men". Because men with never corrected, or poorly corrected, hypospadias wander through a no-man's land between pediatric urologists who do most of the hypospadias repairs but do not treat adults, and adult urologists who treat men but are not experts in hypospadias surgery. That is why Bush and I named ourselves PARC.

The journey for most of these men began with an appointment to see an adult urologist, who probably had given little thought to hypospadias since a residency rotation through pediatric urology years ago. Who likely recalled how confusing it could be for even those who routinely did hypospadias surgery to choose the right operation, and worried about the potential complications if he tried to repair one now. Most of those adult patients told me they were discouraged from having surgery during that earlier consultation, and instead were advised, "You should just learn to live with it." This despite the fact they made that appointment to see a urologist because they were already tired of living with it.

I once wondered if hypospadias was a sufficiently troublesome condition to lure me away from treating the terrible pain of kidney stones or the life-threatening risk of cancer. Seeing infants with hypospadias, I never pictured the life they would grow into if they are not repaired or have lingering complications after their repair. Rather, I could almost understand the sneer of a urologic oncologist who once told me, in front of an audience of laughing adult surgeons, "You pediatric urologists sure make a big deal out of moving the meatus a few millimeters!"

But who could imagine peeing into his hand to aim the stream into the toilet? Who could endure having a metal instrument shoved up his urethra over and over year after year to force a constriction open enough to empty his bladder for a few days?

It was not easy trying to help patients like these at the university, where I had no office at the adult hospital. Instead, I met them during my busy clinics at Children's, after they sat uncomfortably out of place in a waiting area filled with children, and then had little time to hear their worries accumulated over a lifetime. It was also an inconvenience to do their surgery, since I had to navigate the confusing pathway from Children's through Parkland and then across the street into Zale Lipshy, the university's adult hospital, to do their repairs in an OR where I worked only when I had an adult with hypospadias to repair. At least the staff tried to make me feel at home, but there were times when some needed item was not available during the operation, and they had to send a runner over to Children's to get it.

I did not see very many men with hypospadias during my fourteen years at the university. Not because there were few men who needed surgery, but because those who did simply could not find me since the university would not authorize a customized website to let those patients know I could help.

Here was another example of the contrast in my new life that I could now schedule men in my clinic at different times than the boys, and then do their surgery right across the parking garage in a hospital that welcomed both kids and adults. And that I now had the time to patiently listen to what hypospadias had done to these men, learning more lessons that academics did not teach me.

While most adult patients had complications following childhood repairs, others never had surgery. Some said the pediatrician thought their case so mild that it was not worth their parent's time to consult a pediatric urologist about it. Most reported their parents took them to a specialist, who then sent them away with the prediction that surgery would only be cosmetic.

One man in his twenties made a video proving his hypospadias was something worse. I watched as his stream spread into a fan angling straight down toward his shoes and the bathroom floor.

Others wrote emails expressing their frustration:

> Sometimes my stream will split in two, causing it to completely miss the toilet as both streams are going opposite. Or the "stream" can sometimes be very spackled. Pinching and trying to adjust my head helps at times . . . but I don't use the urinals unless I know the bathroom is empty.

> The slit is too long. Especially lately it results in erratic spraying when I void causing a mess.

> To be honest, I am tired of urinating wrong.

Most of these men reported their stream was straight at least some of the time, but it often deflected or splattered, and that unpredictability caused them to shy away from public urinals and instead sit on the toilet if others were in the bathroom. Even then, one man described how embarrassing it was to call his wife from time to time to bring him fresh pants at work when he got distracted or let down his guard. I could not help but wonder what if she brought the wrong color and his co-workers noticed?

And it was not only urination that was affected. Some of these men with distal hypospadias said their penis bent when it was erect, and pictures they took showed it curved down or to the side at various angles that ranged from thirty to as much as sixty-five degrees. I routinely asked if it hurt them to have intercourse, and routinely heard it did not.

"You're asking the wrong person!" Bush lectured me. "You have to ask the woman if it hurts, or if there are positions they avoid because it's not comfortable."

An email from a wife confirmed she was right.

> Sex has become a physical nightmare for me, and he also looks deformed.

A few men did have pain, despite straight erections. The first time I heard this I could not find anything wrong during the man's physical exam, other than his hypospadias. Then another with the same problem told me he also had that pain when he soaked in a hot tub. He pointed right to his meatus, and I finally realized it was the exposed lining of the urethra that was hurting these men. The pain went away after surgery.

But the greatest misery these men suffered did not come from soiling their clothes or finding their sexual positions were limited. An email explained:

> I was so embarrassed with my condition. I was timid to be intimate with any girlfriend because I was afraid I might hear the dreaded words, "What's wrong with your penis?" That would have been devastating for this young man. Even as a grown adult the embarrass-

ment never goes away, and I would consciously avoid any situation that might expose my deformity.

For another man, this fear proved real. He told Bush what happened when his girlfriend broke up with him.

"She was mad, and her final insult as she stormed out of the house was, 'I don't want a man with a broken dick!' I haven't had a girlfriend since, and I don't think I can until I get this fixed."

These experiences sent me back to my files to read again what others had published about men with uncorrected hypospadias. One article said many of them were not even aware that anything was different, and another reported they had grown accustomed to their penis and the way it worked. Both questioned if boys with distal hypospadias really needed to have surgery in the first place.

But the men I was seeing were all quite aware of their defect, and none of them accepted their splattering stream or bent erections or different and embarrassing appearance, even though most were middle-aged and had lived with hypospadias for more than forty years. Despite being called an expert in hypospadias, I had no idea the impact this birth defect could have throughout a man's life.

And now that more of them were coming to our practice, I could not help but see that the experience of surgery and recovery afterward was very much different in men than in boys. All the men wrestled with their decision, especially after their initial consultants told them to expect a lot of problems afterward. They also had to plan their surgery around work and decide how they would explain that time off to their coworkers and bosses. Most of them registered high blood pressure when they arrived for their office examination, which shot even higher when they checked in for surgery the next day.

Although the TIP repair I did in men was the same as in boys, it was very different. Every step took longer. Artificial erection required several large syringes of saline injected through a big needle to get the penis hard, in contrast to the few ccs quickly injected through a small needle in boys. Blood vessels in adults were larger and bled more. At least double the number of stitches were needed to sew the urethral plate into the new urethra. And their penis skin was less resilient.

As Bush explained, "Everyone knows that skin wrinkles as we get older, which means it's not as elastic as when we were young."

We sent boys home shortly after their operation, but Bush and I kept men in the hospital longer. In fact, we learned to keep them still in bed for several hours afterward and then sent them to their hotel in a wheelchair with strict instructions to stay in bed all night. That was especially important after more extensive reoperations, because if a nurse helped them up or they got out of bed for some reason, bleeding could start and fill the scrotum so that it swelled and ached and worried the man despite assurances it would all resolve back to normal on its own. In a few men the scrotum grew so large that we could not wait on nature to heal it and instead took them back to the OR to remove the blood and clots, which we almost never needed to do for a boy.

Then there were the erections men have in their sleep at night. Painful engorgements that woke them frightened their stitches were pulling apart. I reassured them the sutures would hold, but the best relief I could provide was a Valium to swallow at bedtime to make them a little dopey and a little less concerned. Because no medicine stops erections. Even though boys have erections after surgery too, theirs do not hurt nearly so much.

And men suffered more when the operation was not a success. A short, balding thirty-year-old pleaded with me to add him to a workshop program in Alexandria, Egypt.

"I'm not in charge of the meeting," I replied. "You'll have to speak to the organizer, but I don't think we have enough time."

"Please, sir, you must do my surgery! I have no other hope. I have too many operations You did one yourself, sir Then I had a leak and no one can fix it I pee on myself and it has ruined my life A woman won't marry me like this When the last operation did not work, I heated a nail with a flame and tried to burn it closed myself sir I don't think I can go on living with a broken penis," he blurted out in a spasm of despair, desperate to make his case in the seconds he had before someone shooed him away.

"*I* operated on you? In Egypt?" I asked.

"Yes, sir. In Benha. Fifteen years ago."

Then I remembered. The teen whose parents paid the organizer extra on the side to ensure their son would be operated by Snodgrass during a live-surgery workshop. The case that I protested needed a Bracka repair just when I was learning to do grafts and was not ready to teach that operation to an audience. Especially not in a pubertal teenager whose grown penis would make the surgery much more difficult. But my host would not relent.

The operation returned to my memory from a distant past, the details still vivid. Cutting back the man-made urethra through strictures and hair until finally reaching healthy tissues in the scrotum. Needing a very long strip of graft that I took from the teen's left cheek, before I learned I could take a longer graft from inside the lower lip. First sewing the graft to the meatus and then stretching it toward the glans, opposite the direction I do now. Returning to the mouth to take another graft because the defect was too long and too wide for the one to fill it. Then realizing I did not get enough the second time, either, because I was inexperienced. Having to go back into the mouth a third time for one more piece. A hundred surgeons watching me sweat.

"We know this man, professor," one of the local surgeons interrupted my thoughts. "Hadidi did his second-stage operation many years ago, but he developed a fistula that came back after another operation to close it. When Hadidi moved, two other surgeons tried to close it too. When he heard you were coming back to Egypt, he insisted on meeting you."

I was not optimistic about simply closing the fistula for a fourth or fifth time, but there was no time left for anything more complex before Bush and I had to leave for the long drive to the airport in Cairo.

"He is desperate. The driver can go faster to get you to the airport."

Which left us little choice but to squeeze him into the very end of the workshop.

Bush and I were learning that a recurring fistula is a sign of a deeper ailment, usually curvature of the penis that was not made straight or scars under the skin from the prior operation that strain at the wound with each erection. But this man's penis was straight, and we found no tethering scars under the skin. So, we searched for some other tension. Bush picked up the tissues with her forceps and stretched them, released her hold, then grasped again in another place and pulled in another direction until she found the problem.

"Here, cut across that," Bush told me as she held a tight band near the fistula.

I scissored where she directed.

"That's it!" she exclaimed and then checked again that the tightness was gone. "Look, it was a scar where two pieces of graft came together."

I stitched the fistula closed, and then we rushed to the car waiting outside.

"I'm not sure that's going to work," Bush worried as we hurtled down the highway. "He might need a patch graft where that scar was."

"We did the best we could, and it'll work, or it won't," I answered in my binary reasoning, slightly annoyed at her second-guessing our operation when it was over and there was nothing more we could do.

A few months later I clicked opened an email as filled with blessings and gratitude as the man's begging had overflowed with despair. For the first time in his life, he was a man—finally able to stand to pee and confident now to find a wife.

That Egyptian was fortunate that his fistula stayed closed. One forty-three-year-old, still suffering from his birth defect despite ten attempts to fix it, came to me for help.

"At least my operation worked to get his meatus to the tip of his glans," I told Bush. "But he developed a fistula, and my operative note when I closed it says the tissues looked ischemic,[47] so it's no surprise the fistula recurred. We'll have to do something to improve his vascularity so we can close the fistula again and expect it to heal."

That question sent us to the internet, searching for treatments to restore blood supply to tissues damaged by surgery.

"You would think there'd be something using stem cells," Bush said, "but everything I'm reading sounds more like snake oil."

---

47. My operative report said the internal tissues looked white, meaning they were *ischemic* from poor blood flow.

Then she looked up injuries to fingers, knowing that the blood supply was similar to the penis, starting at the bottom and working its way out to the very tip, where it is most tenuous. She wondered if orthopedists or plastic surgeons had found ways to improve vascularity to that critical region, but learned they dealt with it by simply cutting off the finger.

"Well, that's not an option for us!" she huffed.

I found nothing, either. After more than a week of googling and searching PubMed for "wound healing" and "stem cells" and "revascularization" between cases and in the evening after work, Bush remembered a faculty surgeon where she trained who quit her practice to start working in a wound care center. Treating patients with hyperbaric oxygen.

"That might be the answer," Bush told me. "From what I'm reading, HBOT increases tissue oxygen and stimulates neovascularity.[48] It also releases stem cells. Sounds like that's exactly what your patient needs!"

I managed to convince the reluctant insurance company to pay for several dives[49] before we operated again, even though I had no proof that HBOT helps to heal the wounds of hypospadias. Bush and I were both impressed that the tissues appeared healthier at the next operation and pleased that the fistula stayed closed. For the first time in his entire life, Raul could pee from the tip of his penis.

The stories all these men told rounded out my explanation to parents with vivid images of how the abnormal anatomy of hypospadias causes abnormal function. Their worries, their shame, their isolation became cautionary tales to the opinions that dismissed distal hypospadias repair as only cosmetic.

I continued weaving these observations into lectures for our colleagues, too, sharing experiences that pediatric urologists might otherwise never know in their practices limited to boys. I am sure that some listened, but others argued that the men contacting PARC Urology were not typical, but a few unusual fish culled from a large sea. It

---

48. *Neovascularity* is the new supply of blood flow.
49. Hyperbaric oxygen treatments are referred to as *dives*.

really should not matter how many or how few men with lingering hypospadias suffer these miseries. Rather, it was important for urologists to know the potential consequences of this birth defect if it was not corrected, or not corrected right.

In the meantime, patients kept telling me again and again what a middle-aged and married father emailed after Bush and I repaired his distal hypospadias:

> I have only recognized after the surgery what a powerful psychological effect this had in me. I cannot express to you the feeling of normalcy using a public urinal with a straight, normal stream. It really did affect my feeling of manliness.

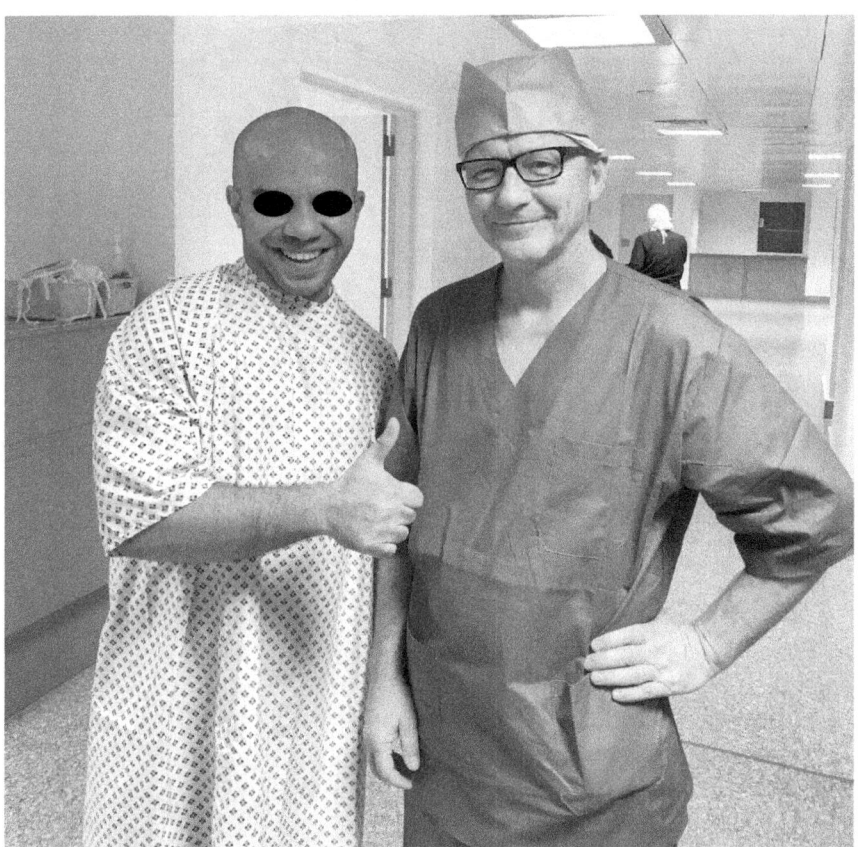

The Egyptian whose fistula Bush and I closed.

◀ CHAPTER 20 ▶

We Want You to Help Us Get Better

It was sheer coincidence that the boxes carrying the newly printed and bound textbooks arrived late in the afternoon the day before our flight to Prague. That evening we packed books on the bottoms of our suitcases and into the sides of our computer bags and then paid excess baggage fees to fly another couple of suitcases filled to the maximum weight allowed to haul the entire first edition to the meeting.

Fortunately, Bush prearranged a limo pickup from the airport, since there was no way we could herd those bags through the metro and then down cobblestone streets, or stuff them all into the trunk of a petite European cab. Besides, it was a rainy and cold October day, and we were happy to be delivered straight to the doorstep of the hotel and assisted inside by the doorman.

After moving in, we found a nook sheltered from the wintry gusts that accompanied each guest into the lobby and relaxed at a small table holding cappuccinos to warm our hands. It was our first opportunity to sit together and marvel at the new book, to admire its hard covers, feel its glossy pages, and regard its many color photographs. It was my dream to write an entire textbook about hypospadias, and now we held that book, one year after the new practice began and just in time to debut it at the 2015 ESPU annual congress.

It was worth flying them all from Dallas to Prague and then lugging them from our hotel across the city to the convention center to show them off at the largest gathering of our small world, and to save our foreign colleagues the considerable costs of shipping them a heavy book from Texas. Bush and I wrestled one suitcase full to the convention center the first day, and during a coffee break spread a few books on a table outside the auditorium where friends stopping to say hello could see them.

Word spread quickly, and by the second break a crowd pressed around our table wanting to thumb through the book, buy a copy, and then have us sign it. Our first-day supply was flying off the shelves, so to speak, delayed only by the cumbersome workarounds Bush had to devise to convince the Operation Happenis website to approve credit cards with foreign zip codes.

Fortunately, she anticipated a demand for our autographs and packed Sharpies in the suitcase, a lesson learned during her Cowboys Cheerleading days to never go to an appearance without one. She even planned ahead what she would write, scrawling in bold black and barely legible print, "Happy Hypospadias-ing!" I simply signed my name under hers.

The next day we brought more books. But when we set them out again on a table near the exit from the auditorium, an ESPU secretary asked us to move farther away to avoid any appearance of some impropriety. So we did, and brisk sales resumed. Then another secretary asked if we were licensed for sales, but admitted she did not know if a nonprofit had to be licensed the way commercial vendors were. Later that day an officer of the society worried the ESPU might be reported for some violation but was not sure what that violation might be. To be safe he asked us to relocate again into the midst of the product vendors, the reps who sold catheters and cystoscopes and Deflux, and so we did. It did not matter where we settled, colleagues wanting a book quickly found us.

Maybe there really was no problem, except that Bush and I were doing something new. Normally, a textbook would be sold for profit by a registered publisher at an assigned booth in a designated space rented at the convention, to be shipped to the buyer later. We did not have a publisher, or a booth, and no one knew if there were regulations covering medical textbook sales by a nonprofit because no one knew if a nonprofit had ever published and sold and then handed the buyer a textbook before. The AUA gave certified nonprofits like ours a booth for free at its congress, but the ESPU had never been asked for one and the books arrived too late for us to think of making that request.

Hypospadiology was an instant bestseller, the last copy of the first edition sold as we stood in line before dawn at the airport waiting to check in for the flight home. Buyers got a state-of-the art description of hypospadias repair sold at a discount, and the sellers funded the startup for our nonprofit. Everyone won, although one officer branded me a maverick for refusing to follow the rules.

Enthusiasm for the textbook proved surgeons wanted an authoritative reference to help them manage the uncertainties of hypospadias. One describing the key steps in operations and filled with photographs to help see what the surgery should look like step-by-step.

While the textbook filled an important niche, we had not forgotten that words and pictures cannot teach the same lessons that surgeons learn watching other surgeons operate. Our new hospital had cameras mounted in the surgical lights like we had at Children's, but not the audiovisual techs working in the OR to shoot and edit videos that we had before. It also did not have an auditorium where surgeons could assemble to watch live surgery, or the ability to project a live surgery course worldwide over the internet.

Meanwhile, our costs to travel for workshops and demonstrate surgery went up significantly after leaving Children's, even though the hosts who invited us still paid for the airline tickets and hotel rooms and all our meals. Now there was the added expense of all those supplies we carried to show what surgery looked like when we did it in Dallas: the sutures, catheters, bandages, and all the surgical instruments that we first thought we would buy through Operation Happenis, before we listened to our patients and repurposed its mission to making the public more aware of the common birth defect that most people have never heard of. Consequently, Bush and I paid those costs for workshop surgeries out of our own pockets. And we were no longer salaried by a university but only from the revenue our work earned, which dipped every time we were not in Dallas earning it. Not surprisingly, we found ourselves scrutinizing invitations a little more closely.

But I like to say that smart people find a way to win.

"We can videotape our operations and upload them to YouTube," Bush suggested one day, already excited by the possibilities. "The young surgeons we're trying to help all check out videos on YouTube before they do an operation."

Not that winning is easy. We could center the camera on the operative field but could not focus our attention on the operation and also fill the roles of those AV techs we no longer had—balancing the mikes so that my louder voice did not muffle hers, adjusting the lights to avoid a glare on the field, watching that one of us did not block the view with our head.

Worse, the unedited videos of operations that could last more than two hours often took Bush as long as eight hours to upload the HD files. But neither of us had the time, the tools, or the temperament to edit them shorter, so we paused the recordings at various times during the surgery and then risked losing the entire film if the circulating nurse hit stop by mistake, creating an entirely new file when we resumed taping.

Furthermore, just as our website describing hypospadias had been shoved several pages off the front page of a search by the SEO of major institutions, our first postings on YouTube were buried under the popularity of other surgical videos and accessible only from the keywords Bush tagged on them. It was several weeks after she uploaded the first videos before a few "likes" and an occasional comment appeared from people who discovered them.

She kept checking and eventually found more signs that people were watching from the messages they left. "Nice work." "Thanks." "Very helpful." Some decided to subscribe, and within a few months we had enough to open the PARC Urology channel and house our videos together. Soon there were hundreds and hundreds of subscribers browsing for the next upload.

Despite the costs we still traveled to selected workshops, including a third trip to Ecuador in early 2016. Bush and I were both impressed the first time we visited two years earlier when our host opened the meeting with a slide showing his own results repairing hypospadias. I could not recall another conference in more than a decade of travels that began with the organizer admitting that he needed help.

"This is why we invited Dr. Warren and Nicol," a smiling Jorge Garcia Andrade explained to the audience of pediatric urologists seated before him, and to others linked by webinar throughout South America. "We want them to help us get better."

We followed his introduction with a lecture on "How to Get It Right the First Time." Bush and I shared a single presentation; I reviewed the key steps in TIP repair, and then she described how to do two-stage grafts.

It was exactly the information the local surgeons wanted. While Bush and I lectured and operated, Andrade and his colleagues compared how they were doing these same operations, seeing a range of major changes and minor adjustments they could make to improve their results.

And surgeons might not have been the only people watching the course. Andrade explained that our visit was part of a drive by the Health Ministry to improve care for poor children in the public hospitals, and, he had heard, the President of Ecuador was keeping an eye on the proceedings from a monitor inside his residence.

"Maybe the president will be inspired by all this talk of surgeons fixing their mistakes to fix the Mitad del Mundo!" I laughed.

During our first visit, we took a cab outside of Quito to see this monument straddling the line dividing the earth into north and south. Except that it does not quite stand on the equator, which we realized when we could not steady eggs on the heads of nails, water still turned counterclockwise going down drains as it does in the southern hemisphere, and we could close our eyes and walk and not lose our balance. It turned out that the true center was two football fields away.

Bush and I returned the next year and Andrade announced his results were already better. At least for distal repairs. He confessed they were still struggling to repair proximal hypospadias, and, on this second visit, we focused our lectures on these more difficult operations emphasizing again the best way we knew to do two-stage grafts.

And this time we went to the equator, to the real line down the middle of the earth where Bush quickly discovered eggs can perch on the heads of nails, we watched water drop straight down a drain, and I fell into the northern hemisphere when I tried to walk that line with my eyes shut. We could see the false monument in the distance, where buses poured out tourists eager to visit the place declared in good faith during the 1730s to be the equator, and still proclaimed the center of the earth today despite irrefutable evidence to the contrary. "It's just another example of how hard it is to challenge tradition," I mused.

"We want to thank Nicol and Dr. Warren for coming to Quito for a third visit," Andrade said, opening our final workshop. "They have taught us many lessons, and we have watched them operate so we can do the operations like they do." He looked off the stage down to us sitting on the front row of the auditorium. "This time, my friends, we have some more questions to ask you, and some challenging redo cases for you to teach us one more time!"

And this time we brought our new textbook to leave behind a reference manual. We presented one copy as a gift to Andrade and sold a handful of others to interested surgeons. But the price for a hardback book was beyond the means of some, who we steered to a more affordable version on CD.

After the meeting ended, the flight back to Dallas seemed a little shorter, we felt a little less exhausted, and we returned home a little more optimistic thinking these visits to Ecuador might become a template we could use for workshops in other places.

"It's like those Bangladeshi surgeons," I reminded us. "We can't go everywhere three times. But we have to make time for people like Andrade who want to do better."

We taught the same lessons in the hypospadias course we gave each year during the annual meeting of the AUA, Bush eventually replacing Pippi-Salle when he scheduled a return flight home a day too soon. One surgeon who attended was Irina Stanasel, a fellow who heard me say that the Byars flaps her faculty were teaching for proximal repairs had given every one of my patients complications. She returned to Texas Children's and asked permission to wade through the charts of boys who had that operation.

Stanasel discovered their outcomes were nearly as bad as mine.

Over 70 percent of those boys needed three operations, or more, to complete a two-operation repair. She emailed me a draft of the manuscript they wrote, and I was impressed that her mentors found the courage to publish honest results quite different from the impossibly good results that others previously claimed.

Their article appeared in the *Journal of Urology* in August 2015. It was followed two months later by a similar report with similar results from Boston Children's, shepherded to publication by Marc Cendron who heard me warn several times about Byars flaps at the PUWF.

Then a year and a half passed, and a third article was published in March 2017 by the surgeons at CHOP, the program John Duckett made famous, who wrote that they, too, encountered many complications after two-stage repairs. I noticed they also mentioned doing one-stage transverse islands in some of their patients and had many more complications than Duckett ever reported.

I suspected that years earlier, when my first TI failed disastrously, and I heard that others were also struggling with that repair. So when Duckett died, I suggested his successors tell urologists how many proximal hypospadias he repaired with his transverse island, and how many of those developed which complications afterward. Routine details that surgeons need to know but which Duckett never reported, at least not to today's scientific standards. Months later they told me they stopped their review of his work when it proved "the gods have feet of clay."

Only after twenty years passed and two other reputable centers published less than stellar results, did the heirs of Duckett admit those one-stage transverse island flaps that he wrote had 85 percent success actually had 85 percent complications when they did them. Perhaps because of that, they also reported doing a two-stage repair in half their patients with proximal hypospadias, which must have sent Duckett spinning in his grave after he argued so long and so passionately for all hypospadias to be fixed in one!

I read on and saw there was another major change mentioned in a single sentence buried in the Discussion. While Duckett championed plications to straighten almost any degree of penile curvature, his successors now wrote that they no longer used them for anything more than the slightest bend. I found it curious they made this sea change without greater fanfare. No doubt they were struggling with patients who Duckett plicated returning bent, just as I found recurrent curvature after straightening my own patients with plications during proximal TIPs.

I showed the paper to Bush. She looked through it shaking her head.

"You asked them about those plications and TI repairs years ago. Now they rename Duckett's TI operation the IT and mention only in passing they've quit doing the plications he recommended."

I shrugged my shoulders, as though to ask what anyone could do about it.

"Yeah, weren't they clever," she sneered, "protecting Duckett's reputation since they keep theirs so closely tied to it." She looked away from the article and directly at me. "How many boys around the world have been hurt by surgeons who keep doing what Duckett said, yet CHOP still hasn't come clean. They should be ashamed," Bush rendered her verdict, disgusted by the games men play.

Meanwhile, she and I were analyzing results from our version of the two-stage graft repair I learned from Bracka. Although the plastic surgeon taught me the basics—how to harvest the graft, quilt it to the penis, secure it with a special bandage, and then roll it into a tube during a second operation six months later—there were other important steps I had to devise myself.

Like making the penis straight. Bracka did "chordee excision" that usually leaves the penis bent, which led me to make three corporotomy incisions across the bend to get it straight.

Bracka also took the shortcut of sewing the first layer of the urinary channel with a running stitch. Since his records were disorganized, he could only guesstimate that few of his patients developed fistulas afterward. In contrast, I knew from our database that placing the first layer of stitches one by one worked much better.

Then, after making the new urethra, Bracka waterproofed it with dartos, while I published that tunica vaginalis prevented more leaks.

Since all these technical changes improved results, they were important to highlight so that other surgeons could make them too.

"That's the reason the operation needs a new name," Bush declared after reading the latest draft of the manuscript we were writing. "We can't simply call it a 'two-stage repair' because that could be either grafts or flaps, and we can't call it a 'Bracka,' because it's not the same operation he did."

I agreed, and then asked, "So, what do we call it?"

This time it was her project to name an operation, and like I had done many years before, she toyed with several ideas to make an acronym from the essence of the procedure.

"What about this?" Bush finally suggested, after filling a wastebasket with rejected scribblings. "STAG, for *Staged Tubularized Auto-Graft.*"

"That's a mouthful!" was all I could think to say. But the name grew on me, especially since I could not think of another. Ironically, after all her musings, the *Journal of Urology* left STAG off the title when it published our article in 2017.

I was certain STAG would be welcomed by surgeons frustrated by the complications inherent in flap repairs. After all, our patients had less than half the problems reported in those articles from Houston, Boston, and Philadelphia. Not only that, but STAG transformed proximal hypospadias into the normal penis that flaps rarely made—longer and straight with the meatus enclosed within the glans as it should be.

It happened that the Society for Pediatric Urology scheduled its 2016 Fall Congress in Dallas during the time when we were finishing our manuscript.

"What a great opportunity," I said, "to showcase the operation for surgeons who'll be traveling to Dallas anyway."

But the largest space in the hospital could only seat around ten visitors. So I first emailed the urology chiefs in Houston, Boston, and CHOP inviting them, or a colleague, to attend free of charge with breakfast and lunch included. Those ten seats all filled, but not with any of the chiefs I personally invited.

Still, I remained stubbornly optimistic that the contrast in results between STAG versus any type of flap would persuade others to rethink their practices. Optimistic until word started trickling to us through patients and colleagues that those three reports on Byars flaps were having the opposite effect. Rather than prompt introspection, they *re-*

assured surgeons! If the urologists in the best programs in the US had complications in over half their patients, how could other surgeons hope to do better? And if no one could do better, then expectations were set too high.

One mom related the advice of the pediatric urologist she consulted before traveling to Dallas, who said, "We won't go in swinging for the fences!"

In response, I sharpened the lectures I gave. The highlights remained, "We are not as good as we think. We can do better. All hypospadias can be repaired by TIP and STAG. Here are the key steps for each of those operations. Please check your own results." But now I showed pictures of penises crippled by distal repairs, and I filled another slide with the misery of bent, scarred, strictured, and hairy penises after failed proximal repairs.

Then I stopped and abruptly changed the topic, remarking that everyone listening had flown in a plane.

"Did you google your pilot?" I asked, knowing, of course, that none of them had.

"No, we all buy tickets based on cost and convenience, never worrying if the pilot assigned to that flight will take us to the right destination and land us safely."

I showed a photo of a row of pilots standing in line that I found on the internet.

"These men have different personalities and natural abilities, just like surgeons, but their training makes them all perform within a box of acceptable outcomes." I summarized those as safe takeoff, safe flight to the destination, and safe landing. "If someone deviates from these," I continued, "a full-scale investigation is done, lessons are learned, and the pilot who strayed outside the box might not fly again." I paused to let that message sink in. "And that's why flying is safe."

The next slide declared in black and white "BUT HYPOSPADIAS REPAIR IS NOT." I contrasted surgeons to pilots for the audience of urologists. "We don't have standardized training. There is no box of expected performance. There are no investigations for results outside the norms." Then I concluded, wistfully, "Maybe, someday, surgeons will be as professional as airline pilots."

But I had one final point to make:

HYPOSPADIAS REPAIR HARMS MORE CHILDREN

THAN ANY OTHER PEDIATRIC UROLOGY SURGERY

I debuted this message in Portugal, repeated it in Cyprus, carried it to China, smuggled it into Iran, proclaimed it in Peru, explained it in Egypt, heralded it in England, and lost the moment to tell it in Greece when weather delayed my flight. I am still waiting for an invitation to deliver it to an American center.

Bush and I are ready to help, but first someone simply has to ask.

◀ CHAPTER 21 ▶

Should Our Team Have a Captain?

As soon as our small workshop ended, workers removed the HD camera from the overhead light and our operating room was shut down for remodeling into a cath lab.[50] This seemed an odd beginning for the women's and children's hospital that HCA[51] promised when they bought Forest Park. As did our introduction to the new chief physician in charge of emergency services, who explained to Bush and me the plans to greatly expand the sleepy little Forest Park emergency room into a big-city trauma center.

There had been rumors of shaky finances before we moved to Forest Park, which grew into undeniable signs of belt-tightening when vendors complained their bills were not paid and nurses whispered their paychecks came late. Somehow, though, the managers managed to keep supplies stocked and the hospital operating until it finally sold to HCA a year and a half later.

Soon after that, Bush and I were invited to dinner with the CEO and his Chief of Development at the III Forks Steakhouse in Plano, driving past the Capital Grille and Bob's Steak and Chop House and Perry's Steakhouse and Grille which were all much closer to the new Medical City Frisco. We were immediately escorted into a private dining room.

"Dr. Bush. Dr. Snodgrass. Thanks for joining us. Please, take a seat." Mr. Grasse beamed the smile of a politician as he waved his hand invit-

---

50. *Cath lab* refers to the place where heart catheterizations are done to diagnose and treat heart conditions, mostly in the elderly.
51. *HCA* is the Hospital Corporation of America, based in Nashville, Tennessee.

ing us to our places at the table. "Would you like a cocktail, or maybe a glass of wine?"

I soon noticed the wait staff knew Grasse's routine and easily anticipated his orders. If I had taken a moment to connect the dots, I might have read the signs of our future in this meeting held near Medical City Plano, which now managed Medical City Frisco even though it was sixteen miles and a full hour's drive away in workday traffic.

As our steaks were served, talk moved from an introductory exchange of pleasantries, and a polite curiosity about the operation named Snodgrass.

"According to market research done by our corporate headquarters in Nashville, Frisco, Texas, is the premier location *in the entire country* for a woman's and children's hospital!" the new CEO explained, sounding enthusiastic.

"That's right!" his Chief Development Officer agreed. "And we see the two of you as key players in that transition!"

We certainly did our part for business, transferring our entire practice to Medical City Frisco since it accepted patients covered by either commercial insurance or Medicaid. That, at least, was one improvement over the Forest Park days when we had to travel to other facilities to operate on boys insured by the government. It was certainly more convenient for us to work at just that one hospital, with its operating rooms on the same floor as our office in the building a quick walk across a parking garage. I could run over between cases to meet new patients arriving for surgery the next day. And we could both drop in to check a bandage or examine a wound to reassure parents before they flew back home afterward. Soon Bush and I were the most reliable surgeons at Medical City Frisco, operating there every day and already scheduled to continue operating there every day for weeks into the future.

Nevertheless, only a few months later we were pushed out of our operating room, intentionally located right by the PACU to transfer our infant patients more safely, when the hospital decided it wanted a cath lab and that adults undergoing heart catheterizations should be closest to the recovery area. Then we saw the head nurse guiding adult orthopedic surgeons and spine specialists through the OR asking what additional equipment and supplies they wanted to relocate their practices.

"I'm still not seeing any sign of that women's and children's hospital," Bush complained, meaning both literally and figuratively, after another tour group passed by. "And they still haven't replaced the HD camera we lost when they moved us into this new OR. The latest videos I posted on YouTube weren't sharp enough for surgeons to see the details."

Meanwhile, only two years after we opened PARC Urology over 80 percent of our patients flew in from outside Dallas and beyond Texas to see us. Bush hung a map of the US on the wall where the nurse took vital signs, and soon there were pins stuck in more than half the states showing where those families travelled from. A short time later she bought a companion map of the world.

In the early months, parents would contact our office and I would email them back asking for some basic medical information and a few pictures they could send to me directly at a secure address. After studying those, I wrote them a detailed explanation of what was wrong and what we recommended to make it right. I knew that most of them were getting opinions from other centers, too, and had to be wondering what was special about PARC that warranted a trip to Texas.

While those long emails were tedious for a man who once quit typing class, I had time to write them when there were not many inquiries. But as the ads we could finally afford and the SEO of our website attracted more interest, it became increasingly difficult to respond to everyone promptly and thoroughly.

"Why don't we schedule the out-of-town patients for telemedicines?" Whitney proposed with a shrug. "That way you can just talk, and they can watch while you explain what you plan to do."

Chaney Renfro, our receptionist, handled those arrangements: scheduling the appointments, setting up a computer in one of the exam rooms, logging on the parents, handing me a chart with copies of our emails, listening outside the door after I went in and sat down and greeted the family to be sure the connection was working.

I settled comfortably on a small sofa glancing through the chart to refresh my memory, and then looked up at the parents as I began our discussion. I immediately realized this was a better solution than laboriously typing out long messages, and I soon fell into my usual routine to explain what I saw and how Dr. Bush and I would repair the hypospadias if they decided to come to Dallas. It was as intimate as a consultation in person, without the distraction of their son demanding attention in the exam room.

I quickly learned the parents' two most common worries. "What happens if we get back home after surgery, and he has some problem that needs a doctor?" "How will we follow up after his surgery to make sure everything is all right?"

"We repair hypospadias using two methods that almost never need urgent attention afterward," I explained. "An urgency happens when there is a blockage from meatal stenosis or a stricture that we see in less than one percent of our patients," I continued, citing our data, before assuring them that if their son was a rare exception, I would call a nearby pediatric urologist to help. "So far I haven't had to do that since we started this practice."

It was also easy to monitor their son for complications after surgery. "If you lived in Dallas, you would bring him back in for a clinic visit. I would ask how he's doing while you undressed him. You would answer that you think he's OK, but you want to know what I think. I would take a look and then tell you to close his diaper, that everything looks fine. We can do that same evaluation by you sending me a few pictures, and maybe a video of him peeing if you think he has a fistula."

Afterward, I dictated a clinic note, circled the appropriate diagnosis and procedure codes, and handed the chart to Whitney to schedule both the operation and a preoperative office consultation the afternoon before. She looked at the calendar for the day the family preferred, and then at the day before to estimate when I could walk over to the office between cases, do the physical exam, and confirm the final plans with them while the hospital turned over the operating room for the next surgery.

I did nearly all the telemedicine consultations in the beginning, because it was my name the families found in their research. After navigating the difficult passage into a typical children's hospital clinic to see an overbooked and hurried academic urologist, my prompt email replies followed by a relaxed telemedicine conversation, and my clear and practical explanations backed by a decade and a half of data collection, assured many I spoke with to make travel plans to Dallas.

In fact, this whole experience was the opposite to what many parents encountered during their initial, local consultations. A live person answered the phone in our office, rather than a phone tree that always began with that irritating admonition to hang up and call 911 if this was an emergency. A timely reply came from the doctor, and not a nurse responding a day or two later to ask for more information. The telemedicine consultation was arranged soon, versus a hospital clinic appointment made as early as possible more than a month from now. Most importantly, there was ample time to ask their many questions when they met me on the computer, in contrast to the rushed moments with the first urologist they'd waited so long to meet.

I was happy to devote the added time for these telemedicine consultations. Bush worried that our new process left her sidelined where she would not routinely meet these families from out of town even though she was part of the surgical team. We decided to discuss the details of operation we just did together with the family afterward to highlight her role.

But doing those operations together was something else new that we had to learn. What parts of the operation would we each do? How would we decide what to do if the next step was not clear, or when we disagreed? Should our surgical team have a captain? Neither of us had seen two faculty work together day in and day out during our training. The closest similarity was the occasional operation done by two surgeons from different specialties, but they usually did their parts separately, arriving when it was their turn, working with their own assistants, and then leaving when they finished. I knew that Devine the urologist and Horton the plastic surgeon combined forces to repair hypospadias years ago but I had no idea how often they operated together or how they made decisions.

Bush and I made ourselves equal partners in PARC and carried that idea into the operating room. We both realized our model was not going to work if I managed the operation while she assisted, following my commands. Bush often said she knew I was a talented and precise surgeon, one of the very best she worked with during her years of training. But none of those best, including me, sensed the arrangement of the skin on the penis and how it was going to shift when it was cut in this direction or in that, or could tell when it was going to fit back together easily and when it was destined to cause trouble at the end of an operation that had not even begun, like she did.

"It annoyed my mentors in Chicago when their trainee suggested they cut the skin at a different angle, especially if they finally did it and saw that it was the right move," she told me one day, with maybe a hint of sadness. "Just like it did Pippi that time when I assisted him during the course and whispered he could get the skin closed without a skin graft if he took out that one stitch that was tethering it."

I remembered that moment, and how Bush finally took scissors and cut that stitch herself when Pippi-Salle refused, and then everyone could see the skin would now close without a graft. I also recalled my own training to manage the skin. How my mentor simply left the room when the urethra was made and the glans closed, leaving it to the devises of the resident and fellow to finish the operation while he went to the doctor's lounge for coffee and a slice of homemade pie. Probably, I surmised, because nothing about the penis really looked right in those days of Mathieus, and even a perfect skin closure would not make it look better.

So I mostly taught myself how to redistribute the extra skin on the top to the deficient areas underneath, and how to lower the scrotum and distinguish it from the penis in boys born with the scrotum hiked up high on the penile shaft. It was ironic that my very first publication on hypospadias described a different way to close the skin that I proposed one day to my teacher in the OR.

But it was not immediately obvious to me that Bush saw this better, especially not in those first months when all she could see was that something was not right but had not yet tested the intuition that insisted she do maneuvers to close the skin that she had never seen anyone do before. Bush had to convince me to let her try ways that I had never seen tried before either. And then she realized that she needed to mark the skin at the very beginning of the case, too, to set things up for the very end. Soon she decided to also make the initial incision, because sometimes what she marked was not exactly right and she needed to adjust the cut as she was doing it.

Then, when I finally picked up scissors and forceps to begin work under the skin, Bush might sense tension within the tissues that I did not feel, and would tell me to cut out a piece of dartos down by the scrotum that was pulling on the glans, or would fish out a tiny bit of scar and hold it just so for me to incise to make the graft more flexible.

Soon Bush worried that the way I simply left those corporotomy incisions open after straightening the penis might leak out enough blood to irritate the skin, and advised we cover over them with some dartos. Which meant I had to change my dissection to save enough dartos to do that. Next she worried how the grafts I laid over those three cuts healed, and said we needed to start measuring their dimensions when we placed them and then again at the next stage before we tubularized them, to make certain they healed right.

Now I began to wonder if I was being relegated to the assistant's role. There was no harm in covering the corporotomies, and I was once again surprised I had never thought to measure something as important as grafts, but as one tiny change led to another and then to still one more, I had to worry that I was the one who the parents and patients would hold accountable if her suggestions proved wrong.

And that was especially true in the reoperations, where the stakes were higher and the margin for error even less, when there were bands of tension coursing through all the structures, and the skin was impossibly short and terribly scarred and contracted. One might say we had little to lose in these cases trying to fix the mistakes of others, but those patients contacted me desperate for a win.

We stood under the bright lights trained on the scarred end of a graft. Six months earlier we took a long strip from inside this boy's lower lip to reach from his meatus in the scrotum to the tip of his glans. Nearly all of that looked and felt healthy, except the very end of it laid within the glans which would make his distal urethra. We looked back at the picture we always take after placing a graft, and then again at how the graft looked now, and could see that part of it was missing and that there was a lump of scar in the middle of the part that remained.

Bush marked the glans wings where we normally cut them and extended those blue lines down along the perimeter of the entire graft, where we would ordinarily separate the graft from the penile skin.

"I don't think we can finish his urethra today, looking at that scar," I pointed out, wondering why she was marking the incisions as though we could.

Bush took her forceps and stretched open the glans on either side of the end of the graft, testing its flexibility. "I don't know," she replied as she stretched the tissues again. "Most the graft is fine. I think we can do an inlay patch with some fresh graft into this scarred area and then go ahead and roll the neourethra."

"I'm not sure that's a good idea," I resisted. "I don't think we should take that risk and maybe end up with a distal urethra stricture."

"Well, you know our inlay grafts heal healthy 85 percent of the time," Bush argued back. "If this was my boy, I would take those odds to avoid another operation."

"But it's not your son, and the parents know we might have to repair this end of the graft and then finish his urethra in another six months. They won't be happy if we roll it today and it strictures and then we have to replace that part anyway."

Here was a dilemma like others we encountered from time to time: a situation where we both saw the problem and knew our results if we managed it one way or another but did not agree which road to take. An example of a situation when we both wished there had been role models to show how to make the decision.

"I've said before that when in doubt we should do the most conservative thing, so I don't think we should trust these tissues to make a urethra that will last a lifetime," I said, as my final answer.

"I just think an inlay operation would work," she defended her opinion again, "but it's your patient, so you decide."

And that was the best plan we could devise. It was not often that we reached this point of indecision, but when we did not agree on a course of action and neither could persuade the other, the surgeon who primarily managed the patient made the call. But we had to know if our batting averages were similar, and so I added a textbox in the database to record these disagreements for a future review once we saw the outcome.

We made our team work, because there was no other option but for it to work. Still, I wondered if we might gain insights from the experiences of the only other team I knew of, and proposed we fly to Richmond and talk with Boyd Winslow, a colleague who once worked in the same practice as Devine and Horton, albeit years later. Maybe Winslow at least knew stories told by those who saw those surgeons in action and could tell us if their team had a captain.

We met at a loud restaurant and strained to hear over the din as Winslow explained how the partnership began. But we could not really hear him answer how Devine and Horton divided the work, and when I finally asked how they resolved their differences in the OR he fell silent, eyed us suspiciously, and then asked if I was planning to write a book.

◄ CHAPTER 22 ►

You Are Rock Stars!

Six months after my first telemedicine, I looked at the schedule and saw the whole afternoon filled with them. I grabbed the first chart and walked into the exam room to start. I could see Mom already grinning through the computer screen with her husband standing nearby as I sat down.

"You are rock stars on the hypospadias moms' groups!" she greeted me.

I leaned back into the corner of my small sofa and smiled, wondering how many times a week parents told me something like that. "Is that how you found us?" I asked.

"Yes. We just weren't comfortable with the answers our local pediatric urologist gave us, so we went online. Everyone says you're the best!"

We had already exchanged information and a few pictures of their son's penis over our encrypted email server.

"So, as I mentioned in my email to you, your son has a urine opening that is both near the head, like a distal hypospadias, and near the scrotum, like a proximal hypospadias," I explained, using my fingers like pilots do their hands to illustrate. I told her there are two possible explanations: that his penis is straight but the scrotum is riding higher than it should be, or his penis is very bent down toward the scrotum. "Which operation we do will depend on the curvature; a TIP if his penis is straight, or a STAG if it is bent."

The wife responded. "OK, I understand that." She glanced from me to her husband to see that he did too. "Our first urologist just took a quick look and said Ryan has distal hypospadias. He told us it was simple to repair."

"And he might be right," I reminded her. "But it's actually more common with that appearance to have the proximal type and need two operations to fix it. At least the surgeon has to be prepared for that."

I waited a moment for them to process that information before continuing. "His exact anatomy is not so common. But we see several patients every month with that same appearance."

She looked at her husband again, and then back to me. "I'm just so glad we contacted you. It makes me sick to think the other surgeon might have gotten in there and done the wrong thing."

While I dictated a note, Chaney talked to the next parents, making certain both the audio and video were working.

"I can see you," she told the screen, in her soft Southern drawl, "Can y'all see me too?"

When the link was established, I returned to the sofa and opened a chart with our previous emails. "Good afternoon," I greeted them, "I'm just refreshing my memory for a second." I scanned through our correspondence and glanced again at the pictures they sent. Then I looked up at them. "OK, I remember now. Your son had one repair that healed with a fistula, and then two tries to close that. But it came back open both times and he still has a leak, right?"

I saw them nod their heads, confirming the story.

"Well, as you know, a fistula is the most common complication after hypospadias surgery."

They nodded again.

"But an operation to close the leak is nearly always successful, as long as the fistula is not the sign of some other underlying problem."

"Like what?" Mom wondered.

"Surgeons are taught there could be a partial blockage out beyond the leak—a stricture or meatal stenosis. But that's not what our data show."

They leaned forward, closer to the monitor, as though that would help them see and hear better.

I continued. "What we find most often is that the penis is curved," I said, holding my right index finger bent so they could see it. "That's not so obvious in these pictures, but it's most likely what he has."

"We thought he was still curved!" Mom exclaimed to the screen, narrowing her eyes. "But the first urologist insisted it couldn't be, since he fixed it."

"I read the operative note. He did a plication, putting a stitch here to pull the penis straight," I explained, pointing my left index finger to the bent middle joint on the right. "That works in the operating room, but if there's just thirty degrees of bending, and that's not much," I added, demonstrating it with my index finger, "then his natural erections after surgery can overcome that stitch." I went on to say how tension from recurrent curvature pulls the fistula back open.

"That makes sense," Mom sighed, realizing now why the other surgeries failed.

I dropped my hands from camera view and looked at Mom and Dad. "Unfortunately, that's not widely known. The second surgeon who tried to close the fistula didn't check to see if the penis was straight. At least the operative note didn't mention him doing an artificial erection."

"That's so frustrating!" Mom interrupted. "I told both surgeons that we thought he still had chordee."

"That's right," Dad agreed, speaking for the first time.

"So neither of them even checked to see when they operated on the fistulas? That just makes me furious." She wiped away angry tears.

"As I said before, recurrent curvature is the most common problem we see when a fistula recurs. But it's not unique to your surgeons. It's a bigger problem from how we've all been taught to straighten the penis," I explained.

Then I resumed. "Assuming he does have curvature, it'll take two more operations to fix things." I saw them leaning in closer again. "Almost certainly we'll have to cut across his urine channel, and then we'll make the short side of his penis longer."

I held up the index and middle finger of my right hand pressed together, with the left index finger fit into the groove they made. "That's what the penis is, two erection cylinders and the urinary channel surrounded by skin."

Then I showed with my fingers the three reasons the penis can be bent: short skin underneath, a short urine channel, and erection cylinders that are short on their underside.

"We don't say 'chordee' because that lumps those all together," I went on, telling them what our colleagues have heard me say for many years, yet still ignore. "We'll release the skin and any scar tissues from his previous operations, then peel away the urine channel," I said as I curled my left index finger down and away. "If he's still bent, then we'll know that the sheath around the erection cylinders is short."

I paused. "If it is, then we have to make some incisions into the sheath to let it stretch longer. Our data prove that works in nearly all patients."

I made three cutting moves across the bend in my finger penis, and then held it up straight.

"So his penis will be longer, and we'll need to build him a longer urinary channel. That tissue will have to come from inside his lip, since he doesn't have a foreskin anymore."

"Is that going to hurt?" Mom interrupted, again, surprised by this news. "Will he be able to eat?"

"He'll eat fine," I reassured her. Then I resumed my explanation. "We sew it down flat on the underside where the opening is," I said, using my fingers now to show where the graft would go, "so that new blood vessels can grow in and make it part of his penis. Then, in six months when that's all done, we can roll the graft into his new urine tube, all the way to the tip of his penis where it should be."

"Wow," Mom said after a moment's reflection, looking into the screen past me. "Two more operations."

"Yeah," I confirmed, knowing how painful this is for parents to hear. Then I leaned toward them.

"His chance of having another complication is higher now, since he's had several operations and so the blood supply to the end of his penis is probably decreased." I told them, "We want these to be his last operations," and saw them shake their heads in strong agreement.

"So we need to improve the blood supply. The only treatment that does that is hyperbaric oxygen." I then described how their son would enter a cylinder and watch videos for the hour and a half that each session lasts. "Moms find that easier if they tell them it's a spaceship.

"The pressure and 100 percent oxygen help force more oxygen

into the tissues, release stem cells, and stimulate new blood vessels to grow," I continued. "We're told that takes twenty dives. He'll go every day, Monday through Friday, meaning this will last a month."

Mom and Dad stared silently into the monitor. I waited patiently while they mentally calculated the time this would require on top of their already overfilled schedules. Time that would have to be found that does not exist in their lives right now. Time in addition to taking his brother and sister to school, time beyond the demands of their jobs, time they need for grocery shopping, and making meals or picking up fast food to-go. More time piled onto all the other time they have already devoted to their son with hypospadias and have not made up to his siblings, who are starting to resent all the attention he gets. Time before the time, and money, they will have to find to travel to Dallas and stay in a hotel for a few days to have another two, or more, operations.

"Well, we'll just have to make this happen," Mom sighed.

The next consultation was also for complications after an unsuccessful surgery. Another urologist did a TIP repair on a boy with proximal hypospadias, who then developed meatal stenosis so severe that he was only able to pee in drops. The patient ended up in the emergency room, where a different pediatric urologist on call had to urgently cut open the blockage. Now his urinary opening was back down on the shaft of the penis.

"We talked to the doctors, and both of them said this will be difficult to fix and that we should not get our hopes up," Mom opened the discussion. I noticed it was nearly always mom who bore the weight of this condition for the family.

"What did you understand that to mean?" I asked.

"That it's too risky to try to make his opening all the way back out on the tip. Both of them said there are more complications that way and that it would be better to just make it at the bottom of the head."

"So what do you want to talk to me about?"

"We did our research and read that you're the best. We want to know what you think," she answered, while her husband nodded before excusing himself to check why their son started crying.

"Well, we always fix the urine channel all the way to the tip. Otherwise, you're just making proximal hypospadias into distal hypospadias." I remembered the warning another mom heard about swinging for the fences trying to repair severe hypospadias. "If you leave the opening at the base of the head, then at least some of those babies will grow into teens and adults who will have trouble standing to pee because they spray."

"Do you see cases like my son's very often?"

I smiled, gently, to reassure rather than impress. "Over half our practice is boys like Nathan. Boys who were born with proximal hypospadias and now have complications after surgery by other pediatric urologists. We do reoperations several times every week."

"That's what we read," she told me. "When I mentioned your name to the second surgeon, he told me that if we really wanted Nathan to be fixed right, we should come to you."

But only after you asked, I thought to myself.

"Well of course you want him to be fixed right," I replied. "Wouldn't any mom?"

The last family called from tomorrow, half a world away. I had already corresponded with the parents by email after they sent medical records and pictures. But they wanted to see me and talk directly to me.

"Doctor, thank you so much for all your help. We are so frustrated with the hospital system here!"

Prenatal ultrasound found their baby was not growing properly, and, on closer inspection, that the genitals were not normal. Amniocentesis was done, and the report the parents copied to me said "male karyotype, no clinically significant abnormalities detected," meaning the baby was a boy.

Nevertheless, after he was born, the neonatologist took one look down there and declared the child had "ambiguous genitalia," meaning it could be either a boy or a girl. Endocrinology was consulted and a battery of tests were done. The chromosomes were checked again, and again confirmed him to be male. Although the prenatal ultrasound did not see a uterus, the radiologist reading a second one after birth was less certain, and so an MRI was ordered. That report was unambiguous: two testes in the scrotum and no uterus. Then a pediatric urologist was added to the team.

Despite identifying hypospadias with two testicles, the urologist agreed with the endocrinologist that more testing was needed to decide if their boy should be raised as a girl. And even when those tests proved his penis grew after he was given testosterone, the consultants still were not convinced. They insisted the family dress him as a girl, imagining the shame they would otherwise feel when they changed diapers around other parents, or picturing what it would be like taking him to swimming classes where he would change in front of other boys. After trying that for three months, they could not imagine putting their boy into dresses any longer.

"Dr. Snodgrass, we cannot express how confused we were when we were told before Vihaan was born that the tests said he was a boy, and then after he was born, they said he might really be a girl! It was horrible. What were we supposed to tell our family, or our friends?"

I have heard this story many times. Perineal hypospadias with the opening near the anus, is the most severe, and the least common type. Sometimes, the genitals do look feminine at a glance, but there is a penis and usually the testicles can be felt. And so it's a boy, and most often a boy with no other genital problems that modern testing can find.

"You're right, I cannot imagine it," I sympathized. "Unfortunately, doctors sometimes use that term 'ambiguous genitalia' too loosely. There was nothing uncertain about your boy with perineal hypospadias and testicles they could feel."

"Yes, doctor. But even when the tests kept saying he was a boy, they still weren't sure. The endocrinologists said he has a penis but might not think like a boy."

"Well this problem comes up because perineal hypospadias is so rare," I explained. "It happens in probably 250 boys in the US every year out of two million newborn boys." Because of that, I told them, pediatric urologists do not encounter it very often, and neonatologists and endocrinologists see it even less. "But boys with even the most severe hypospadias still consider themselves boys."

"We told them that you said that—"

I interrupted before she could finish. "I have *never* seen a boy with hypospadias and testicles grow up and say he was a girl. And the most recent publications say that when a boy like Vihaan is raised as a girl, he is likely to want to change back when he gets older. So it's not just my opinion."

"Yes, we understand that. But the urologist was really pressuring us. He said Vihaan would have a very small penis and would never be able to stand to pee or look like a man."

"His penis is normal size now, just bent," I replied. "And it will be longer when we straighten it."

I closed the laptop with a sigh from exhaustion, made worse knowing that so many parents remain so confused about hypospadias even after consulting with specialists. No doubt that helped explain the explosive growth of our practice, and the need to keep adding slots for these telemedicine consultations. And since I could start those in the late afternoon and finish after the office closed and most the staff went home, Bush and I could spend more time in the operating room. Which month-by-month filled with more hypospadias repairs.

Another year passed and then Whitney stopped me in the hallway.

"I updated your calendar while you were doing the telemedicines," she told me. "Did you realize the next available time for surgery is three months from now? Y'all are totally booked up 'til then."

I flipped through the schedule and saw that she was right.

That evening, Bush and I met for dinner to review our practice.

"It's time," she said to my slight grimace. "No, it's time," she insisted. "We have to write a letter to the pediatricians letting them know we're closing our practice to everything except hypospadias."

This was her vision nearly four years ago when we opened the doors to PARC Urology. I wanted to believe but could not share her faith in something that I thought had never existed anywhere before.

"Devine and Horton had maybe the closest practice to what you're talking about," I would say when she raised the topic. "But hypospadias was never all they did, and whatever they created together, it didn't last.

"Think how long it'll take for word-of-mouth to send new patients to us," I told her at the beginning. "And we won't get many from our colleagues, either," I predicted, recalling that as far as I knew, my own mentor sent only a single patient to Devine and Horton. "They don't think we know anything that they don't know.

"We can't even count on the local pediatricians," I went on. "They didn't refer to us when we were at Children's because of that town-gown thing, and now that we're not, many of them still don't refer to us because they're already used to referring to someone else." I paused a moment, and then added with a smirk, "Or they can't even if they want to, because they've sold themselves to hospital systems that tell them which specialists to refer to."

From time to time in our beginning a new patient would arrive from outside Dallas who was not referred by another doctor and had not seen our internet ad. I always wondered how they found me.

"I asked a moms' hypospadias group for some recommendations," was the common response. "They gave me a list with several names, and you happened to be the closest to us."

Deb was one of the first moms who recommended Bush and me to other moms. Gradually, more joined her; moms who, like her, were devastated by the failed operations their sons endured. Moms who were shocked to learn how few hypospadias surgeries most pediatric urologists do. Moms who felt their surgeons did not spend enough time to really explain the condition, the repair, or the possible complications. Moms, like Deb, who learned that most of those surgeons do not know their own results for the operations they did on their sons. Moms, like her, who hoped they might help other moms avoid all the heartache and guilt and frustration and anger they suffered for their sons.

Then there were moms who consulted social media groups before agreeing to surgery, especially those whose sons had proximal hypospadias. Maybe they sensed a hesitation, or a reluctance, in the first surgeon who examined him. Sometimes that surgeon told them outright the repair would take several operations and that they should not hope for the penis to look normal in the end. A few moms thought to ask how often the surgeon repaired hypospadias like their sons', and began searching for another opinion when they heard, "Oh, maybe two or three times a year."

And there were moms who were not satisfied with a ten-minute consultation for their son with distal hypospadias. Moms who described how the urologist hurried into the room, asked a couple of questions, and then did a moment's worth of an exam. How the doctor then consumed all the remaining minutes talking about surgery before wrapping it up by saying, "If you don't have any questions, we can go ahead and schedule him," before rushing back out the door.

Moms who just wanted it done right the first time, or wanted it finally done right after so many tries by others that did not work.

Soon I heard that some parents found me by googling "best hypospadias surgeon." And by our fourth year, Bush and I were hearing that the networks of moms rarely mentioned other surgeons anymore. It was a new version of the club foot saga. Surgeons might not listen to another surgeon, but moms listen to other moms.

We typed our letter and sent it to the pediatricians, and the new openings in our practice made by giving up general pediatric urology immediately filled with more boys, and men, with hypospadias.

◄ CHAPTER 23 ►

It's All a Matter of Pride, Isn't It?

Who becomes a surgeon, slicing a knife through the skin of another person, injuring someone's body with the aim of making it better?

Men confident they will succeed, despite the risk. Men who, like all men, inevitably have an off day, or make a mistake, but forge ahead past those signs of fallibility, like athletes who miss a clutch shot and immediately focus on shooting the ball again. Strong-willed men who take command in the operating room.

I witnessed the swagger of Duckett, the calm assurance of Gonzales, and the easy humor of Pippi-Salle in the face of challenge.

"That's the whole problem," Bush complained, after texting me yet another article comparing men and women surgeons. "Women are better surgeons and men can't accept that!"

It is not that women have better fine technical skills than men, although many do, or that women take fewer risks than men, although that is usually true too. "No," she explained, "it's that women don't have the *ginormous egos* that you male surgeons have!"

I showed the mistake of a surprised look.

"Don't act surprised!" she demanded. "You are the most competitive person I. Have. Ever. Met!"

My look shifted to disbelief. I have always taken pride in not being that stereotypical surgeon, strutting and preening to impress others with his virtuosity. Rather, I have always stressed that I have no special gift. Always encouraged other surgeons that they could have the same results that I do. And I told her so again.

"Yes, that's true," she conceded. "But that's just another type of pride. And pride was the biggest obstacle we had to get past to make this practice work."

It was time to scrub, so I tied on my mask, adjusted my loupes, and rubbed on a handful of sanitizer as I walked toward the scrub tech to gown and glove. Then I arranged drapes around the genitals painted a golden brown by an iodine prep, screwed in the light handles overhead and focused the beams onto the field, asked the anesthesiologist to lower the table an inch, and then extended my left hand for the first stitch.

I love this ritual that begins every operation. The comfort of the known before confronting the unknown.

Bush took her place standing opposite me, on the other side of the table. She held a hemostat in one hand and scissors in the other, ready to clamp and trim the tails of the stay stitch I pierced through the glans that we use to maneuver the penis. I slid a metal sound into the meatus to judge the thickness of the surrounding skin, and then she marked lines on the penis tracing where to cut. I held the penis taut while she made the incision. Then she held the cut edges up with fine-toothed forceps so I could snip the tissues underneath, freeing the skin and peeling it back to deglove.

We do every operation like this, marking and incising, holding and cutting, passing the stay stitch back and forth. We have played this music together hundreds of times, and surgeons watching the monitor in a workshop can only tell whose hand is operating and whose is assisting at any moment because I favor the left and she uses the right.

Her rebuke still echoed while we worked. After years of telling nurses and residents and fellows how to help while I decided what to hold, where to cut, and how to stitch, now I shared control and had to learn to follow her commands. Most often, she is right, but I have to remind myself of that so I do not lapse back into my former role.

I suspect she reads my mind, and that day there was proof. She turned to a visiting urologist, who hoped to copy our model in Mexico, and explained, "It was hard at first for him to see me as equal. But I have to give him credit, because he did, and that's why we're successful. I'm not so sure that other male surgeons I've known could have done that."

Then she drew two more lines down the glans, and I cut to separate wings away from the urethral plate. We both picked up the edges of the plate with forceps and stretched it gently taut. Then I incised down the middle with scissors, the maneuver that made me famous, and because there was a visitor watching, she narrated.

"You have to incise *deep*, deeper than you think, all the way down to the corpora."

I made the urinary channel, sewing the edges of the urethral plate together into a tube, while she watched to ensure the first stitch was not too close to the far end, which would make the opening tight and maybe cause a blockage. The urethra finished, she raised a flap of dartos to lay over it and separate its stitches from the ones that would close the skin above. Then I sewed the two wings of the glans together over the new urethra while she tested the surrounding tissues for any tension that might want to pull them back apart.

Satisfied, she took the skin of the penis and pulled and twisted it; measuring with her eyes, and once with a ruler, the lengths she needed to make it all symmetrical encircling the shaft. I am always amazed watching her smooth out a lump or cut into a hump or aim the scissors down to move the skin up. After four years of watching, I can sometimes anticipate her next move. But I know I have just memorized her steps; I'm not seeing what she sees.

I was silent while she made her decisions. After she cut the skin and began to sew it together, I looked to the visitor.

"Schoolkids in the US take aptitude tests that have these diagrams of boxes opened flat with dotted lines that you are supposed to fold up in your mind and pick the shape they turned into."

The surgeon nodded his head that he knew those tests.

"I could never see the answer, so I always checked 'B' and went to the next question! But for Dr. Bush, the right shape was so obvious that she didn't even have to think."

Once she aligned the skin margins, I helped sew them together. I threw a stitch or two and then finished my thought.

"She has a gift. No matter how hard I try, I will never see how tissues move the way she does." After a pause, and smiling behind my mask, I added, "Now I know what it was like for world class golfers to play beside Tiger Woods."

"Who's actually going to do the operation?" a mom asked during our preoperative consultation. She had not realized a fellow would be assisting, much less doing some of the key steps, the first time her son was operated for distal hypospadias.

"Hypospadias repairs always need an assistant," I told her. "Dr. Bush and I do all our operations together. We don't have trainees or surgical nurses assisting."

"But who is the main surgeon?" Mom persisted.

I smiled at her, knowing she had done her homework after her son's "routine" repair resulted in complications only made worse by another surgery that eventually led her to Dallas for a final attempt to fix his penis.

"We don't work that way," I answered. "There are parts of the operation that I do and parts that she does. We've been working together literally every day now for over four years, so we know who does what."

Her face betrayed a hint of uncertainty. At her first consultation the surgeon only spoke about his experience and success and did not mention there would be others participating in the operation. The second time she specifically asked if a trainee would assist and he answered, "Yes, of course, it's a teaching hospital, but they'll only do what I let them," shooing away her concern with a wave of his hand as though it were an annoying fly.

I doubted trainees caused this boy's surgeries to fail. But I knew from my years at Children's that sometimes a surgeon will change the operation to show a trainee something different. Or the surgeon will focus more on instructing the trainee than watching for pitfalls as the operation progresses. Occasionally, a chatty resident distracts the surgeon, or asks a question during a critical moment when the surgeon needs to concentrate fully.

In the end, and for whatever reasons, most complications result from errors made by the surgeon. "That's another advantage Dr. Bush and I have operating together, since we both have years of experience and can watch to make sure the other doesn't make a mistake," I explained.

Maybe that stitch is just a little too far from the last one, leaving a tiny gap that might leak into a fistula. Maybe one more little snip will relax tension in the glans wing and prevent postoperative dehiscence.

"Trainees might not even recognize an error, much less be comfortable pointing one out to their teacher!"

But more important than monitoring each other is our recognition that the two of us working as a team are better than either of us working with an assistant. I have seen more than she has. She sees spatial relationships that I will never see.

Most pediatric urologists do nine distal repairs for every one proximal hypospadias repair. Eighty percent of the repairs Bush and I do are for proximal hypospadias. Most pediatric urologists do one reoperation for every five or so first-time repairs. Reoperations are half the surgeries that we do. Most pediatric urologists do only one or two hypospadias repairs each month. Bush and I do three every day and operate four days a week.

The best results in complex operations, like hypospadias repair, come from surgeons who do them the most. Yet no one else has specialized his or her practice as we have. No other center has declared one surgeon, or a surgical team, to manage proximal hypospadias and reoperations like I did earlier at Children's.

I mentioned this to a US colleague who happened to visit Israel when Bush and I were there operating.

"There's not enough proximal or redo cases here for all the pediatric urologists to share them and still get good results. So the Rabbi guides those patients to us," I said, explaining our trip. "Of course, it's the same problem in the US. There aren't enough patients for everyone, but centers refuse to specialize complex hypospadias."

"Well, that's certainly true," the surgeon admitted, knowing that his program, ranked as one of the top five by *US News*, spread those operations among all the faculty. "But I have to say that it would be hard to give those cases up even knowing that results were better," the young urologist, who specialized in robotic surgery, confessed. "I like doing hypospadias."

We spoke to the parents after completely redoing surgery in their son, who'd already had four operations by a renowned pediatric urologist trying to repair his proximal hypospadias. "Just as we predicted, the reason his repairs kept coming back open was because his penis was still bent. Seventy-five degrees in fact," I began the explanation and held up my index finger mimicking what the penis looked like when all the scarred skin was released. "So we made those three cuts on the underside that we discussed yesterday, and now his penis is finally straight."

Mom wiped away tears she could not restrain, relieved that progress had been made at last.

Dad's frustration was angry. "So that other urologist totally screwed this up," he said, barely raising the last word into a question.

"What he did is very common," I replied evenly. "Most surgeons straighten even that much bending with plications, and probably the most common proximal repair is Byars flaps, like he did."

"We see this all the time," Bush confirmed. "Literally every week, from all over the US."

"So why don't those other surgeons do what you did?" Dad persisted. "My son's operations didn't accomplish anything."

"Well, that's the key question," I admitted.

"But it's not just us saying that repairs like your son had don't work very good," Bush interrupted. "Three major US centers recently published they had lots of complications doing Byars flaps."

"Yeah," I agreed, and shifted to her tack. "I used to do that repair too. But every one of my patients had a complication, so I quit doing it."

"But those centers are *still* doing Byars flaps!" Bush interjected. "He's not telling you that we organized a workshop here to show how we do proximal repairs and invited the chiefs of those programs to come . . ."

"But none of them did," I finished her sentence with a shrug.

"Why not?" Dad asked, incredulous, his anger growing. Mom had no more tears either.

"We weren't really surprised," Bush said, matter-of-factly. "Dr. Snodgrass is invited all over the world as a visiting professor, but almost never in the US . . ."

Now it was Dad who interrupted to answer his own question. "So it's all a matter of pride, isn't it?"

I had already reached that conclusion and tweaked my lectures yet again. I downloaded a picture from the internet that cropped off the face of a surgeon standing with his arms folded across his chest. Then I asked why surgeons keep using operations like Byars' flaps that have many complications. Or why they cut corners on the key steps of a TIP that lead to more complications. With another click of the mouse a caption appeared under the picture reading,

PRIDE

"I'm as good as anyone."

But there is more than the ego of individual surgeons. The next slide showed cartoon drawings of different castles representing pediatric urology centers scattered across an outline of the US.

I told the audience, "These feudal states all teach and do what they want. The same boy with a bent penis might have chordee excision at one, dorsal plications at another, a single corporotomy with a corporal graft at a third, or three corporotomies at a fourth. The urethra might be repaired with a Duckett tube or Byars flaps or grafts from the foreskin or the mouth."

I clicked the mouse and a caption under the map defined this chaos as:

INSTITUTIONAL PRIDE

I clicked again to make a textbox appear with the message:

The hypospadias repair a boy gets should not be an accident of geography!

Then I concluded, reminding the room filled with surgeons, "Moms expect the best care possible for their sons, and it's our professional responsibility to provide that."

Or sometimes I let a final slide speak for itself:

Every child is a child of God. We must treat them all the best that we can.

However I ended this lecture, I left and returned home wondering how many of the seeds I cast fell onto fertile soil. And disappointed that my own colleagues in the US rarely hear it.

◀ CHAPTER 24 ▶

They Don't Feel Comfortable
Saying "Penis" on the News

"Doctors! I've managed to get you an interview on Channel 8 news!" Whitney announced one afternoon several months after we organized Operation Happenis. "I know someone at the station, and they're interested in the angle of 'Dallas Cowboys Cheerleader becomes a famous surgeon.'"

Bush straightened her office, and then her hair, for the interview, plotting how she could bring hypospadias into the story. It would be our first chance to call public attention to the most common birth defect that almost no one has ever heard of.

The reporter and his cameraman arrived and crowded into her office, focusing on squad photos, an autographed football, and other souvenirs displayed in her bookcase while they asked about her journey from cheerleader to surgeon. Inevitably, they had to ask what kind of surgeon she is.

"I'm a pediatric urologist who specializes in hypospadias surgery," came the ready answer.

Which made them ask, "And what is hypospadias?"

"It's a common birth defect of the penis, where the pee-hole opens lower that it should be."

Mission accomplished! She announced her interview on Facebook and waited for it to air on the evening news. Bush hoped that her mention of hypospadias would be picked up by other outlets and begin a discussion about the condition. Instead, the story highlighted how the demands of cheerleading for the Dallas Cowboys taught her how to manage the demands of medical school and residency and a surgical practice that included repairing birth defects.

"*Birth defects*," Bush repeated the next day, frustrated at the edit.

"They don't feel comfortable saying 'penis' on the news," Whitney explained, after talking to the reporter. "He tried, but his editor wouldn't let him."

"That's so frustrating!" Bush responded.

"And ironic," I added, "considering how many commercials during the news talk about erectile dysfunction and feminine hygiene products."

There was no time to pursue this disappointment, as we struggled with the billing company and our insurance payments trying to stay afloat. And no sooner did our finances stabilize than those at Forest Park began unraveling.

When HCA finally took over, we had to recredential our work in the new hospital, reauthorize insurance for our patients preauthorized at Forest Park, and renegotiate our office lease originally sublet through the now defunct hospital.

But as the doors to Forest Park closed, a new door opened for Operation Happenis when the public relations department of Medical City Plano decided to produce a feature on hypospadias. This time the story would focus on actual patients and use animation to illustrate their birth defect of the penis. There was an initial flurry of action to discuss what stories to tell, which boys to film, and where to market the final product.

And then nothing happened. Weeks dragged into months with no word from the producer, while our phone calls for updates went unanswered. An occasional word through the grapevine suggested the project was over budget.

More time passed, and then, just as mysteriously, Bush received an email with a link to the video for her to review and approve.

"It's perfect!" she told me. "And they decided to feature Deb's son."

Not only that, but the PR department worked its contacts and convinced Channel 8 to run this second feature, and this time to say the word *penis*.

The story ran on the evening news, following a tease by the anchor about a common birth defect no one had heard of because it happens below the belt. But this time the reporter explained that hypospadias affects the *penis*, with an illustration showing the urethra opening lower than normal. A graphic emphasized how common hypospadias is, for a birth defect, based on numbers Bush thought to calculate at the last possible moment.

"Hypospadias occurs in twenty-seven boys born each day, versus twelve children with a cleft lip and sixteen with Down's syndrome," said the narrator.

This time, I could say how ridiculous it is that a common problem is not discussed because people are embarrassed to say penis. And Bush could emphasize there is surgery to make the abnormal penis normal and know the word penis would not be edited out again.

We were excited to learn our message was picked up by other outlets, envisioning ripples in the pond caused by this first stone. One of those spread all the way to the UK, where Bush found a British newspaper that devoted several inches to the story.

And then it died. Bush begged the producers to advertise the video to other markets but heard that the corporate bosses in Nashville were nervous promoting a feature about penises.

We had better luck with the CDC,[52] using Operation Happenis to request their birth defects website simply say how common hypospadias is. It was a small victory, but one which might reassure moms of boys with the condition who searched the site that they were not alone.

But letters to the Dallas branch of National Public Radio, and others to the March of Dimes, went unanswered.

After creating the charity, Bush and I learned it is not easy to make this little-known birth defect better known. Yet we continued to hear from parent after parent how distressing it was to be told their newborn son had a penis birth defect which neither they, their parents, nor their closest friends had ever heard of before.

---

52. *CDC* is the Centers for Disease Control, which operates a website informing the public about birth defects.

We also realized these newly aware parents needed a website providing accurate medical information. Although social media guided more and more parents to PARC Urology, the questions they emailed me proved that those forums have the potential for spreading misinformation too.

"Is this cosmetic surgery?" "Will the operation decrease his sensitivity?" "If we have his hypospadias repaired now, will the surgery come apart when he grows at puberty?" I answered these over and over, but the fact that moms asked them again and again meant word of mouth kept fears alive.

So we added this mission to the charity, to grow its website with descriptions and pictures of hypospadias and other penis birth defects for parents to read and trust. We do not know how many moms land on Operation Happenis and are reassured, but worry is a powerful emotion, and this was another way we could try to help parents cope.

Parents also asked how they should tell their sons about the hypospadias they had repaired. Both Bush and I responded there is no one way to explain to a boy how his penis was different when he was born, and how surgeons made it into what it is today. No perfect time or age or opportunity to begin this discussion. What we do know is that parents cannot shy away from telling their sons. Otherwise, they will think that Mom and Dad were too ashamed or too embarrassed to talk about it when they, inevitably, somehow, find out.

"You just need to be ready to explain in words that he can understand whenever the opportunity comes up, but before he gets to puberty and doesn't want to talk about his penis with his mother!" I would advise, knowing this was not much guidance. Bush would point them to data about adoption: how it was once hidden from children presuming they could not possibly understand the concept, but now experts agree it is much better to bring up the term and what it means when they are young.

Meanwhile, Deb's interview on the Dallas news made her realize there should be no shame or embarrassment talking about any body part, including the penis.

"It wasn't easy to explain to Maddox that he was going to have surgery when he got old enough to know something was going on," she told Bush months after his last reoperation. "So I've decided to write a children's book for parents to read to their sons to help them understand better."

"That's a great idea!" Bush answered. "And I know the perfect title for it: *How Down There Bear Got Repaired*," linking Deb's story to her own idea for a teddy bear with a catheter that boys could take out before their own was removed.

"Of course, the book will need a lot of illustrations, and I know someone we can ask who's really good," Deb continued.

And so Operation Happenis became a publishing house once again, releasing a second book two years after its textbook *Hypospadiology*. Now moms and dads could read to their sons what they were about to experience, or what happened in a past they do not remember. Not surprisingly, *How Down There Bear Got Repaired* also became an immediate best seller, at least within their practice, the story and its characters delighting parents and boys—everyone, it seemed, except Bush, who worried that the face of the bulldog surgeon representing her was exceptionally wrinkled!

Four years after creating the nonprofit, Bush and I finally hired the first full-time employee to grow Operation Happenis, donating her salary from our own paychecks. Moms told us they wanted to help other moms facing the unknowns of hypospadias in their newborn sons. Moms of boys who suffered complications volunteered to hear the pain and guilt they knew from experience that other moms whose sons developed meatal stenosis or dehiscence or recurrent curvature needed to express.

Someone had to organize these volunteers into networks to assist parents around the country, and, eventually, the world. Then someone had to match volunteers to parents who asked to talk to other parents about their son's perineal hypospadias, or his fistulas that kept coming open, or how to find the best surgeon.

The charity needed someone to again convince the media to discuss the common birth defect people need to know more about. It needed someone to solicit donations to buy the 750 *Down There Bears* that were the minimum required to custom order them. Operation

Happenis needed someone to design T-shirts and coffee mugs for others to wear to the mall and take to the office to spread the word about hypospadias.

We hired Brittany to build this foundation. But to match volunteers to parents facing similar problems, Operation Happenis needed information from PARC Urology that was protected by HIPPA. The letter drafted by an attorney to surmount that legal obstacle only served to persuade the most eager volunteers to reconsider their offer.

Meanwhile, Brittany struggled to find a vision for the scale of fundraising that would buy awareness, and instead focused on what she could see: small gifts from small businesses not remotely related to a birth defect.

After her brief tenure, those connections between parents who have experienced hypospadias and others facing its challenges were still waiting to be organized. Donations to the charity continued at the same slow trickle as before she was hired, and the monies needed to keep Operation Happenis alive still flowed out of the pockets of its founders. Meanwhile, every day another twenty-seven boys are born in the United States with a birth defect that most people still have not heard of.

But Brittany did claim one small victory in the ongoing fight to defeat this ignorance. After spending hours sparring with Instagram, she finally convinced them to allow Operation Happenis to open an account, even though the managers were uncomfortable that the charity's name said penis.

◀ CHAPTER 25 ▶

It's Time for Us to Go!

After Bush made the incision, I took forceps and scissors to dissect the skin away from the urethra. I began cutting the delicate tissues, but almost immediately noticed the scissors were dull. I tossed them onto the table without taking my eyes from the wound and asked for a new pair, extending my hand toward the scrub tech.

These aren't cutting either," I said after another moment, looking up at her. The tech told the circulator to open another one, peel-packed in the cabinet and handed it to me.

I tried it, but it was just as dull as the other two.

It was not safe to continue. The tech told the nurse to pull out all the scissors off the shelf, and when none of those were any better, to open another set of our hypospadias instruments to try the ones in it.

"This is crazy," Bush said as we stood helplessly still, unable to proceed. "When were our scissors last sharpened?" she asked the room.

The tech shrugged her shoulders. "They're supposed to come once a month, since y'all use them so much." She passed the last peel-packed scissors to me, and when those did not cut she had a sudden inspiration. "Get the plastics set," she ordered the nurse, who left the room to find an instrument set down the hall in the room where the plastic surgeons worked. "They use the same tenotomy scissors that you do," the tech explained to us while we waited.

And that finally solved the problem. After trying seven of our own scissors, only a pair used by the plastic surgeons was sharp.

Between cases the tech researched the matter, and before the next operation began, she whispered to us, "I checked the instrument logs. Your scissors haven't been sharpened in three months!"

We were fortunate to have that tech assigned to us that day. Those orthopedic surgeons who toured the OR and then scheduled some cases to try the new hospital were assigned the best techs and circulators to entice them to return. Even though Bush and I operated every day, soon we were working with nurses who did not know where to find the sutures and catheters we used, and techs who could not see to load our tiny sutures on Castro-Viejo needle drivers, left-handed for me and right-handed for her. Which meant our cases stretched longer, and we risked distraction from the task at hand to remind the nurse which cautery tip we wanted when we were handed the wrong one or instructed the tech several times to *please* cut off the second needle of the double-armed sutures while leaving them full length.

We worried about this staffing to the head OR nurse, the same director we knew from Forest Park and had strongly urged the new hospital to retain. But the situation only grew worse as the daily schedule filled with more orthopedists, as well as spine and bariatric surgeons, and the continuity Bush and I needed fell to one or two nurses and techs these other surgeons refused to work with. So we raised our concerns up the chain of command to the on-site administrator, and were soon staffed by travelers,[53] who knew even less where to find supplies or how to pass our instruments.

"This makes no sense," I tried to persuade back up the hierarchy, pointing out that travelers cost the hospital more money that would be better spent hiring new staff for our operating room.

I finally told Bush we needed to schedule another steak dinner when all our arguments fell on deaf ears. But now the CEO and his Chief Development Officer could not find the time to host two of their key surgeons again.

Then one afternoon one of our former techs relieved a traveler and immediately noticed two medications on her Mayo stand were mislabeled. It was an error that could result in a catastrophe, had the wrong

---

53. *Travelers* are temporary nurses and techs brought in to work shifts as needed.

one been injected into the penis. Bush walked downstairs to administration when the operation ended.

"There are safety issues for our patients when inexperienced staff are assigned to us," she told the head administrator.

"We'll have no choice but to investigate your disruptive behavior if you keep upsetting the staff," came the reply.

As we left the building that day I sighed, "Clearly, it's time for us to go."

We did not think we had to move far. A few months earlier Bush and I were among thirty or so other surgeons invited by Grasse to the nearby Bob's Steak and Chop to announce an investment opportunity. HCA planned to build a new Ambulatory Surgery Center directly across the street from Medical City Frisco, and they hoped to attract the surgeons' business, and some startup capital, by offering them a sliver of the profits not expected for several years.

Since all our hypospadias repairs could be done in an outpatient center, and the new ASC would be operated by a different branch of the company than the hospital, we attended the dinner and took forms back to the office afterward to report the CPT[54] codes we most commonly used and how often we envisioned working in the new facility. Weeks later, the regional vice president for ASCs scheduled a meeting with us.

"We've reviewed reimbursements for the codes you gave us," he explained, as he reached into his briefcase to find a chart comparing average payments to various specialties. He handed each of us a copy. "As you can see, payments for your services are below orthopedics, spine, general surgery, and even OB Gyn."

He gave us a moment to review the column of numbers arranged from high to low, before concluding, "We don't think you fit into our model."

I asked if the figures were gross or net, knowing that our supplies cost hundreds of dollars compared to the thousands, or tens of thousands, for orthopedic and spine operations.

---

54. *CPT* codes describe surgical procedures for billing insurance.

"These are gross payments," the VP admitted.

Before I could continue my cross-examination, Bush looked up from the figures and objected. "You haven't tallied ours correctly. You must have looked at payments for secondary codes as though they were the primary ones, and then averaged all of them together. Whatever you did, there's just no way that your reimbursement would be less than ours, since hospitals *always* make more than the surgeons!"

"That could be," the VP shrugged, without much interest. "We don't have any pediatric urologists in our entire ASC network, so we aren't familiar with your cases." He promised to recalculate the reimbursements.

But not with any urgency. We expected a revised report within days, but weeks dragged past before he returned with new documents.

"Well, you were right," he said matter-of-factly, without a hint of irony. "I guess you do fit in after all. We'll need your down payment by the end of the month."

"Hardly an enthusiastic welcome," I noted afterward.

Bush agreed. "First, they tell us we won't make them enough money, then they take weeks to figure out that we will and now they want our buy-in right away! Without giving us any floor plans or sketches of the building to show us the place will be kid-friendly."

"Or promise that we can have an OR to work there every day," I added. Then I thought for a moment. "I'll bet this explains our problems at the hospital. They probably weren't billing our procedures right."

We met the new CEO of Baylor Frisco for dinner at the Cowboy's Club, a private steak house located in the heart of the football team's training facilities.

"I'm intrigued by your practice," he began the discussion. "I understand that you have patients flying in from all over the world. That's amazing!" he smiled, with that same politician's friendliness that I suspected was a prerequisite to lead a hospital. He continued. "I'm looking to expand our services, and you two would fit right in. You know that we already have one of the largest birthing centers in the area."

So Bush and I filled out credentialing forms, and emailed our preference lists of instruments and supplies to the OR. Whitney faxed diagnosis and CPT codes to their billing department, and wrangled the pre-authorizations needed from insurers to do our first cases at the Frisco branch of a regional chain of hospitals. Robert Davis, the anesthesiologist who replaced Miller when we quit Children's, met with the head of anesthesia and reviewed their supplies, pleased they were already equipped for pediatric surgeries. Finally, we did a tour of the operating theater accompanied by the CEO and his assistant and followed by an entourage of nursing directors and supervisors.

"Watch out for those nurses!" an orthopedist warned us at lunch back at Medical City Frisco when he heard we were considering this move. "They'll write you up for anything."

But our first day ran smoothly, helped by a circulating nurse we knew from Forest Park. Smooth except for an obsession with paperwork that required every box on detailed forms be checked, including those of no relevance to our young patients.

"But infants don't smoke or wear SCDs[55] during surgery," I said, puzzled why our patient could not leave the pre-op area until those queries were answered.

"I know," the pre-op nurse agreed in a hushed voice, glancing to her left and right to be sure she was not overheard. "But it's policy—patients cannot go back for surgery until everything on those sheets is filled out. No exceptions."

Bush and I worried about this later, but decided to just check all those boxes until we could request pediatric forms be created and approved. We scheduled into the operating room whenever there was time available, waiting for administrators to reclaim unused bloc time[56] from other surgeons to squeeze our practice in. I heard that would take at least three months, and even then, it was not clear there would be enough to let us operate full time.

Which meant we still had to work at Medical City, still had to worry about the staff assigned to our room, and still had to open several packs of instruments to find one sharp pair of scissors.

---

55. *SCDs,* or surgical compression devises, are wrapped around the legs of adults during an operation to reduce the risk for blood clots to form.
56. *Bloc time* is reserved time for surgeons who use a facility regularly to schedule their operations.

On top of that, Whitney reminded us our office rent was about to increase, again, as it did every year. "It's going up to $10,000 a month."

"So $125,000 a year, just for rent," Bush signed, shaking her head. "For the convenience of having our office near a hospital where we're trying to quit working!"

"That's just for next year. It keeps increasing the next two years after that, and then the lease will be up, and we'll have to negotiate a new one that'll cost even more," Whitney added, insult on top of injury.

"And we all remember what a pleasure that was," I sneered, recalling we spent over $25,000 in legal fees negotiating our last contract just to convince the landlords to finally put up a Medical Office Building sign so patients could find us, and to remove a clause that allowed the owners three months to repair a leaking pipe flooding our office, or a cooling system that refused to cool, even if our space was uninhabitable until they did.

"I just don't see how we can afford rent that keeps increasing like this when our reimbursements for surgery hardly change," Bush complained.

"And when we get paid the same as a pediatric urologist fresh out of training, despite all our years of experience and all our published results that are among the best in the country," I finished her thought. "So much for 'value-based' reimbursement![57]"

"I'm sure that's why so many physicians are selling themselves to hospitals," Bush resumed, "but we've seen what that's like . . . how they treat you once they own you." She was quiet a moment, searching for a way to escape this straitjacket. "I think we don't have a choice in the long run. We're going to have to build our own office and then pay rent to ourselves."

Now I stared silently into our uncertain future. "I really don't want to go into debt toward the end of my career," I said, finally, ending the conversation.

But whatever the coming trials, the pressing need remained a place

---

57. *Value-based reimbursement* bases compensation on the quality of a surgeon's work rather than by traditional fee-for-service.

to work now. Then one day at Baylor the scrub tech fumbled a tiny needle off the Mayo stand onto the floor several feet away from the operation. She and the circulating nurse began a diligent search but could not find it.

It was déjà vu for Bush, who asked what the policy was for lost needles.

"We have to X-ray the patient," the circulator replied.

"Even when the tech saw it fall on the floor?" she wondered.

"Yes."

"Even for a tiny needle that probably won't show on an X-ray? Children's didn't do that," she protested, before continuing, with some drama. "It's a baby's genitals! We don't want our patient exposed to an unnecessary X-ray just because of a policy."

I stepped into the fray to separate the combatants, asking for a nursing supervisor to come review the circumstances.

"I'm sorry, but we have to take an X-ray," the supervisor confirmed, despite all the circumstantial evidence that it was not needed to protect the patient.

Fortunately, at that moment the circulator finally located the errant needle hiding on the wheel of the bovie[58] cart—well away from the operative field, and the patient, as expected.

"I told you they're crazy about their policies. I'll be surprised if they don't write y'all up for questioning them!" the orthopedist laughed when he heard our tale. "That's why I stopped working there."

"Looks like it's already time for us to move on again," I sighed, again, to Bush.

"You should come look at Legent," our orthopedic advisor suggested.

He sketched the background, how it was first named Destiny, built by a group of bariatric surgeons best known locally for the jail time they were serving after defrauding the feds. "Some investment banker from New York bought it and brought in a new management group to oper-

---

58. *Bovie* refers to the electrocautery used to stop bleeding, named for its inventor, William Bovie.

ate the ASC. I'm working there and I think there's plenty of time available for y'all too."

"At least they changed the name!" Bush smirked. "I mean, who names a hospital *Destiny*? That sounds more like a stripper!"

She had already visited Destiny during its bankruptcy a year earlier, the troubles at Forest Park and then at Medical City having warned the future might lead to some place we owned.

"It's way too big for us to buy," she reported to me at the time. "Which is unfortunate, since it's really nice."

Nevertheless, it could be our new home for now. Yet again we sent over the list of supplies and instruments we needed, submitted credentialing paperwork, and obtained new insurance authorizations to operate on our patients there. Bush also asked for a camera to resume filming segments of operations for our YouTube channel.

"It'll take us a little time to get these instruments," the manager told us as she looked over our request. "We haven't been doing pediatric operations, so we don't have the Castro forceps and needle holders."

"No problem," Bush replied, "We have our own for workshops when we go overseas. We can use those to get started."

Soon we were operating there all day every day. But we could not help but notice that we were the only surgeons operating on most of those days, the orthopedist who recommended the facility to us nowhere to be found, and the spine and pain specialists who typically populate ASCs only showing up for an occasional procedure.

Yet even though it was our work keeping the doors open, those new instruments we were promised still had not arrived six months later, and no HD cameras had been brought in for us to test. When I requested an update an administrator promised quick action, but within a week he no longer worked there. We began to seriously wonder if we would arrive for work one morning to find the building shuttered.

Then the Star called one Friday morning. "The Board of Directors met last evening and approved opening the facility to more specialties. Y'all are the first surgeons we're contacting to come work here!"

Bush hung up the phone excited. "I told them last year they should do more than just sports medicine if they really wanted to create a medical center of excellence attached to the Dallas Cowboys. My gut's telling me this is the right place for us," she beamed at me. "Certainly, they have the money to buy us instruments and a camera!" Bush could already imagine a marketing strategy by the Star highlighting the former-cheerleader-turned-internationally-known-surgeon, which might also increase public awareness of hypospadias.

A tour a few days later confirmed there was an operating room immediately available to accommodate our entire practice, and an adjacent one free for a second surgical team when Bush and I were ready to add partners. And both those rooms were already equipped with HD cameras.

The head nurse told us, "We can have your instruments and sutures within a few weeks, and one of our scrub techs worked with you at Medical City, so she'll be assigned to your room."

About the only downside was all the sports imagery plastering the walls in the waiting area, which at least was an improvement over the imposing picture of a spinal cord we insisted be removed from the waiting room at Legent.

One more time we filed the paperwork to be credentialled, and Whitney began reauthorizing insurance to approve us operating at the Star. Once more we had to organize a first day at the new facility, made easier by the experienced scrub tech. Yet again our cases ran smoothly, although the day ran late for me, and our staff, since I had to drive ten miles in rush hour traffic to the office afterward to meet the patients for surgery the next day, rather than see them between cases like I did working at Legent.

"That's going to be a problem," I told Bush when I finished at 7:00 p.m. "If we make the Star our home, we'll have to move our office over there too."

"Yeah, it's too far to run back and forth between cases to see patients," she agreed. "But the only offices available in that area right now are in the same building as the surgery center, and Jerry's[59] pretty proud of that space."

And even though we wanted to operate there more often after the successful launch, the Star was still negotiating contracts with most of

---

59. *Jerry* Jones, owner of the Dallas Cowboys.

the major insurance companies more than a year after opening,[60] limiting the patients we could schedule. Not only that, but in a surprising move, the board declared our single-price agreement for international patients, or Americans paying out of pocket when their insurance refused to authorize surgery in Dallas, would not pay the Star enough money.

"That's interesting," I answered when Whitney told me the news. "It was enough for Children's and Forest Park and Medical City and Presby Plano."

"Apparently Baylor nixed it," she replied, explaining that they managed billing for the surgery center.

"We were led to believe the ASC is run by a management company, with Baylor and the Cowboys minority partners," I protested.

"Whatever, we gave quotes to our international patients months ago. If they change the fees now, we'll have to pay the Star out of our own pocket."

After nearly five years PARC Urology was a successful practice searching for a place to practice. We could not take our adult patients into a children's hospital, and we found most adult hospitals were not very welcoming to the boys who filled most of our schedule. Ambulatory surgery centers offered the most hope, since our hypospadias repairs were all outpatient and ASCs could easily accommodate either boys or men. But ASC business models were all based on the work of other specialties, and our cases seemed an odd fit mixed among orthopedics and spine surgery.

"We're being forced to build our own ASC," Bush said, more out of frustration than aspiration, "Or buy one somewhere, even if that means mortgaging everything we own to get a loan."

"Even if we had the money, we couldn't do that," I reminded her, "since there's no way we could get insurance contracts."

---

60. The *insurance contracts* mentioned here are agreements between hospitals and insurance companies for payment, and typically take more than a year to negotiate.

◀ CHAPTER 26 ▶

Stories Are More Powerful than Statistics

"Did you see this article?" Bush asked as she entered the OR waving a Xeroxed copy. "It's an interesting study comparing stories to data for persuading people."

She set her computer bag down at the workstation and slid the report toward me as I glanced over at Davis, about to do a caudal[61] on our patient.

"What's the *Reader's Digest* version?" I asked, glancing at the first page while I tied on my mask.

"Bottom line, that stories are more powerful than statistics."

I thought about that for a moment, and then went to the OR table to position the boy for surgery.

"OK, you can prep now," I told the circulating nurse.

I put on my loupes and then rubbed sanitizer over my hands and up my bare arms.

"Does that mean dogma wins? That for all the talk about evidence, anecdotal medicine trumps evidence-based medicine?" I asked. "I can hear a lot of colleagues say I told you so!"

I walked back across the room to gown and glove as Bush sanitized her hands.

"It's not how you and I think, but it means we'll be more convincing if we weave more stories into our presentations," she explained.

But I was already doing that, telling the story of the middle-aged

---

61. A *caudal* is a type of nerve block commonly used in boys before hypospadias repair to reduce both the level of general anesthesia needed for surgery, and postoperative pain when the operation is finished.

man who peed into his hand so that he could stand at a urinal, or about her trip to Cairo where every patient was maimed from a distal hypospadias repair. And wasn't my slide contrasting the professionalism of airline pilots to the pride of a surgeon standing with his arms crossed another story making my point?

Surely those anecdotes helped me connect to at least some in the audience. Probably the younger surgeons still open to new ideas and nudged toward our algorithm by the thought of pee splattering everywhere, or boys crippled from surgeries done the way they, too, were taught, and were still doing. But the older surgeons, including many in charge of departments, were less likely moved by my stories of patients or persuaded by the data we showed. A visitor watching Bush and I operate told us how her chief was skeptical of grafts. So, when he reluctantly allowed a younger faculty to do a STAG repair for the first time and the graft partially contracted, he declared, on the spot, "We'll never do that operation again as long as I'm in charge!"

"And I guess that none of his flap repairs ever have a complication?" I replied.

I met one of those chiefs during a visit to South America in 2016. I began the meeting with a lecture called *Dogma to Data: Practicing Evidence-Based Pediatric Urology,* relying on statistics to convert my listeners. Afterward, one of the trainees walked alongside me down a hallway and confessed that he and the other residents, and the younger faculty, were anxious to test my lessons, but their boss would not allow any deviation from his decrees.

I remembered the article that Bush gave me, and that evening back at the hotel I added a new story—my own—into my next presentation for the following day. That lecture started with the data from the Netherlands and those reports from the three major US centers to emphasize that pediatric urologists everywhere are struggling with all types of hypospadias.

I reminded the audience that when the first operation results in complications, the next operation has double the risk for more complications. I showed that slide of the surgeon with his arms folded with pride. Then I asked, "How do we get better than this?"

And to make the answer personal, I changed "the mistakes surgeons make" to "the mistakes *I* make," and "the wrong things professors teach" to how "the wrong things *I* teach" hurt the patients of my students for years to come. I showed the 3Ps slide, and covered it with errors I found and corrected, after reviewing my own work.

Nevertheless, I did not read a new expression on the chief's face as I spoke, nor hear a change of heart in his comments afterward. I left that conference wondering if the seeds I planted could possibly survive in that hostile climate until the day a new chief might let them grow. *Probably not,* I told myself.

Yet, some months later, one of the younger faculty in that department found me at another meeting. "Your lectures made a huge difference!" he told me. "The chief has relaxed his grip and is even trying out some of the things you suggested himself."

Maybe I misread my host, did not sense his willingness to examine practice from a different perspective. But the resident who described life as his trainee had also not seen any hint in him of an open mind.

"It's no great mystery," Bush bluntly replied when I told her. "If the famous Snodgrass admits he has failures, then that chief doesn't lose face if he has some too."

And that might explain the response when Bush and I traveled to Alexandria, Egypt in 2017 for HypoAlex 4. I had been invited to HypoAlex 3 the year before but declined when the organizer admitted he had already invited another guest to argue for flaps.

"And that's exactly what he'll do," I replied, recalling the last time the two of us met. "You know what I'm saying is true. Blood sport between guest faculty might be entertaining, but it doesn't help surgeons who come to the workshop looking for answers to the problems they're having."

Of course, the show went on without me, and without me became a one-man performance filled with sound and fury defaming TIP. The surgeons who returned for HypoAlex 4 heard a very different message, delivered in a very different style. Bush and I taught pragmatically and backed our message with results published from both our own practice and from other surgeons worldwide. Results that proved our algorithm of TIP and STAG is superior to any based on flaps.

After laying that academic foundation, I again made the message personal. I told the Egyptians that Bush's trip to Cairo made us both realize that a boy in their country might be better off with nothing more than a circumcision, rather than a distal hypospadias repair that left his penis crippled.

"This is not OK!" I declared in a stern voice, looking around at the surgeons in the auditorium as I pointed to a slide showing several mangled penises. "You. Have. To. Change!"

I might have ended there in an earlier time, thinking such overwhelming evidence enough to convict professionals to do better. But now I knew it was not.

After a dramatic pause, I smiled, and, in a gentle voice, said, "And that's why y'all came to this meeting, to do better. Hypospadias surgery is hard, and we all struggle to get it right."

I then advanced the slide. The title read, "I'm not as good as I thought," centered over a picture of me operating in the middle of a bell-shaped curve. A list of my own mistakes from throughout my career filled the rest of the slide.

Then I encouraged them, "But I got better, and so can you. That's what HypoAlex 4 is all about."

After our lectures, the workshop continued with live surgery. We resolved in Ecuador to begin these courses with a distal repair, since those are most common. "Choose a patient that you think is *not* suitable for TIP," I now tell the organizer, "so we can show it works even for that anatomy."

Then we follow with a proximal hypospadias, demonstrating the three corporotomies to straighten curvature and the foreskin graft for a STAG repair.

"We really don't want to do any reoperations," I also inform the organizers. "The theme should be getting it right the first time, and that's why we only want to do first-time repairs." Otherwise, I know they will fill the schedule with their most difficult failures, as happened to Bush in Cairo, but they will not learn how to avoid making them.

We followed this program at HypoAlex 4, plus the fistula closure we added on at the end for that man desperate for help. From our perspective, it was a routine workshop using our new format, made memorable for us by the pigeon we were served on the Thanksgiving holiday we missed back home because there was no turkey in Egypt.

But it was not a routine workshop from the perspective of the surgeons who attended. Those looking to do hypospadias better heard Bush and me describe how to do the best operations known in the best way that we know, and then everyone saw those operations done live, step-by-step.

And everyone at HypoAlex 4 witnessed firsthand something unique: hypospadias repair done by a surgical team. Bush and I moved almost effortlessly through the operations, performing our roles smoothly and efficiently, each taking the lead for one step and then assisting on the next, going back and forth until the work was done. No one watching could doubt that two skilled surgeons working together have the greatest likelihood for success doing hypospadias repairs. There is so little margin for error.

A year later our host insisted we return for a repeat performance at HypoALex 5.

"You started a revolution here!" Sameh Shehata exclaimed. "Your message was like an explosion in our minds, and everyone is changing to what you said!"

"That's an interesting compliment," I told Bush. *With just a hint of hyperbole!* I told myself. Because no lecture, no live surgery convinces everyone, and I knew there had to be some left unmoved.

There will always be that human reaction by some surgeons to push back against a fresh idea, to resist a challenge to the ways that comfort them so that they can get up in the morning, plow steadily through the day, then go home to their television and a drink or two in the evening and lose no sleep at night wondering if they are doing the best that can be done for the children who are brought to them. What is best, and who decides, they might ask, only to resent my answer told with either data or a story.

A year later I flew to London, invited by my old friend Roland Morley, the first surgeon ever to visit and watch a TIP repair when I was still a general urologist in Lubbock. Mr. Morley[62] had since become President of the Urology Section of the Royal College of Medicine, and in that capacity organized a program that included a lecture by me.

I climbed the stage and walked to the podium in a lecture hall of the Royal College of Medicine, incongruously packed with surgeons. This time I began my presentation by telling the audience, "I did not google the pilot when I booked my ticket to come here." Then I introduced my new theme contrasting the performance standards required for pilots to the lower expectations for surgeons.

Toward the end I told my own story of pride. How I ignored Mike Mitchell's advice to sew the urethra in two layers, until I recognized my many fistulas and then was willing to change. Next, I asked how many boys would have been spared another operation if I had just listened earlier?

Afterward, one of those ESPU officers who once accused me of flaunting the rules at the meeting in Prague now commended my humility.

"Once again, you were right. Those stories do help," I told Bush, recapping events when I returned.

An email came from the AUA in the winter of 2018, and I read an invitation from the executive secretary to debate Mark Zaontz, a surgeon at CHOP, at the upcoming national congress in May. Both of us would defend the statement "Hypospadias: My Way Is Best." I did not know whether the secretary or the SPU came up with this theme and this title, but I recognized a symmetry in the idea. Me, the champion of TIP and grafts, debating CHOP, the center built on flaps. My view that even the most severe hypospadias should be made into a normal penis, versus their teaching that the standard for success should be lower. My data versus their reputation.

But it would not be a real debate with opening statements and follow-up rebuttals, or questions posed back and forth by a moderator. Time was too short and the topic too broad. I was given ten minutes to summarize lessons learned over thirty years.

I spoke at a plenary session just once before, in 2006. Then I was

62. *Mr* is the British designation for a surgeon.

given twenty minutes to highlight new developments in hypospadias surgery and riffed off the title of one of Duckett's last articles to present "The Current Hype in Hypospadiology: Part 2." It was an honor that might not come my way again, and I worked and reworked my presentation describing repairs without flaps, and then practiced saying it out loud again and again until my words flowed smoothly from slide to slide.

It was even more likely that this time thirteen years later would be my last opportunity to address American pediatric urology gathered in one place. A last chance to reach colleagues who might never invite me to speak in their centers. I had half the time, but so much more knowledge to share than when I spoke those many years before; so I had to decide the most important points to make and then work and re-work the presentation to get it right. Bush reviewed the drafts and suggested fine tuning. Then I practiced the speech out loud, first timing myself to be certain I did not talk past the limit, and then lingering over each slide until I made the right comments with the right emphasis consistently.

Because now I knew it was far less important *what* I might say about TIP and STAG, or performance standards for surgeons, or the 3Ps for self-improvement, than it was *how* I said it. On this stage and before this audience I would not be teaching so much as performing. I already knew I would take an extra Inderol that morning to calm my pounding heart, so that I could speak without a breathless anxiety, or in a loud voice compensating for my nerves that might sound condescending. And I knew that I should close with the story of my own pride and the boys who suffered from my mistakes until I learned to do better. Finally, I knew that I would pause toward the end and say as humbly as possible that I am not special.

I sensed all this before organizing my speech. Bush confirmed my intuition. "Do you remember you're an INTJ?" she asked, recalling the Myers and Briggs personality test we both took several years earlier.

Bush typed search terms on her phone, and then read to me from Google.

"That means you're very smart and curious to test common wisdom. You're open to change when there's proof you should, but you're also confident in your own decisions." She looked up at me. "Well, that's all true, and it explains how you discovered TIP."

Then she added, "Well, that and those three corporotomies . . . and how we both evolved the Bracka into STAG."

Bush thought for another moment. "And that's just in hypospadias, not to mention that you changed from how you were taught to do hernias and orchiopexies, reflux, and neurogenic bladders."

I shrugged my shoulders.

"But it also says here that others think INTJs are arrogant and set in their ways." She looked up from her phone toward me again. "Isn't that crazy! Considering they're actually quite changeable." She scanned the article silently for several moments, before reading out loud again, "It goes on to say that people accuse INTJs of thinking the rules don't apply to them. Like what they said to you for selling books at the ESPU!"

So here was a chance to say to those who found me rigid and arrogant that I am not better than they are. A fleeting moment to unravel years of their resentment. I prepared knowing the irony that if roles were reversed with my critics they would stand at the lectern and proudly declare the operation with their name is obviously the best.

But I also knew the history of hypospadias surgery is littered with operations that were once the best, until something better came along. And even if my operations endure into the future, what is fame after you die?

I prepared knowing I am an imperfect messenger, but the only messenger telling surgeons the raw truth that repairing hypospadias harms more boys than anything else we do; and I'm the only one describing a systematic process for everyone to do better.

In the end, the title of the lecture was perfect. I am convinced that my way is best, not because of the operations I use, but because I am never satisfied that I have achieved the best.

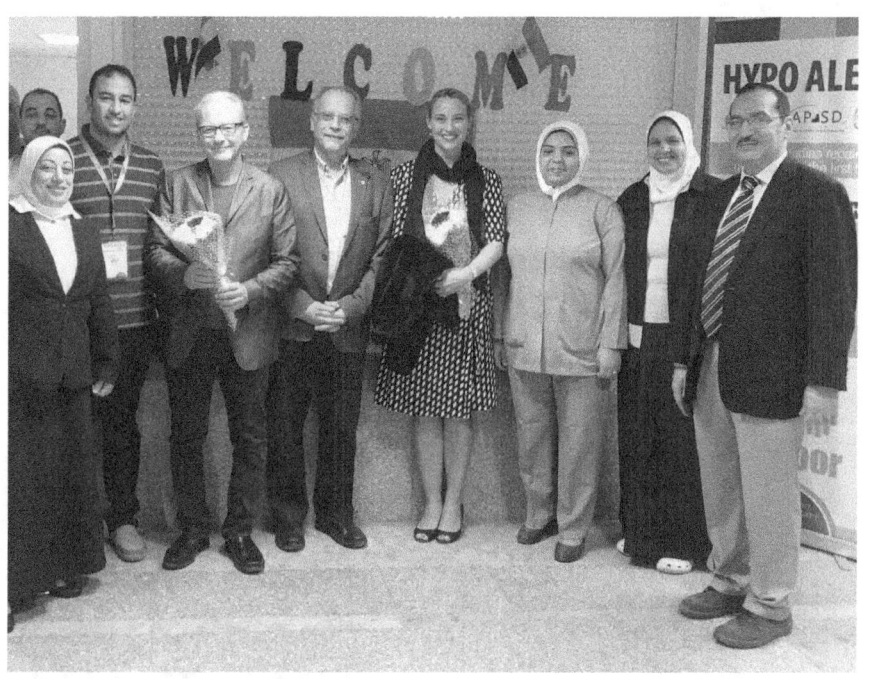

Shehata is standing between Bush and me at HypoAlex 4 in 2017.

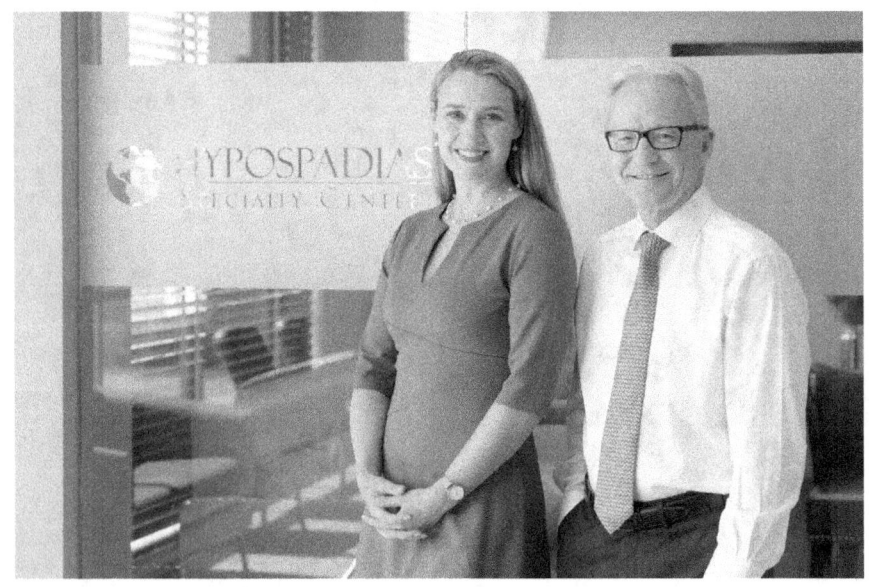

Bush and I at the entrance to the Hypospadias Specialty Center office, 2020.

STAC REPAIR

Hypospadias Specialty Center

◄ CHAPTER 27 ►

Maybe You Can Afford Your Own Shangri-La

Bush opened the meeting. "We need to build our own ASC. We want to have our offices and ORs all in one building, and we're thinking it'll need two operating rooms for when we hire another surgical team and grow our practice."

Dan D'Amico sat on a white cushioned bench across from us in Whitney's office, smiling.

"Is that feasible?" I asked.

"It could be," Dan replied, brushing his salt-and-pepper hair back through his fingers. "You might be able to make it work with two ORs doing hypospadias surgeries," he smiled. It would just depend on if that would generate enough revenue to cover expenses."

"Whitney tells us your company already has a contract with Blue Cross," I said, in a question.

"We do," Dan confirmed. "We're working on the other big three, but those should happen soon."

"How'd you manage to get in to talk with them about contracts?" Bush wondered out loud, knowing that we would never get an audience with an insurance company to discuss our payments.

"Good timing," Dan answered. "I went to Blue Cross not long after Forest Park closed. That out-of-network model[63] was shutting down everywhere and big hospital chains were buying up ASCs that relied on it.

---

63. *Out-of-network* refers to services done for a patient not covered by an insurance contract, which meant the patient paid more and the surgeons and facilities made more.

I told them we could run ASCs for less than the contracts those hospital systems were negotiating."

"Not having contracts is what's made us have to work in some hospital or someone else's ASC," Bush explained. "But we just haven't found the right place." She paused, but that thought was not finished. "Despite all their lip service about patient care, some cut corners on supplies and instruments, while others are more obsessed with following policies and procedures than doing what's right for patients." She glanced over at me before resuming. "We can't find a place that'll give us good help even when we operate there every day. It's been really terrible. No wonder so many physicians burn out!"

This was a much-abbreviated version of her full speech recounting our travails after Forest Park closed. Left unsaid were our always rising costs and never increasing reimbursements. And her lingering medical school loans consolidated into one federal program whose high interest rate was nonnegotiable. It made me sad to hear Bush warn her own children away from the path that led her through medical school and residency and fellowship into a practice doing what she loved with skill that was internationally acclaimed. *Yes*, I agreed silently, *it's no wonder that so many physicians burn out.*

Dan returned the discussion to the original topic. "Would you consider buying an existing ASC, if one was available?"

"Sure," Bush answered for us.

"OK, first I'll look for something we can buy. If there's nothing on the market, then we'll look for a building we can renovate an ASC into."

Dan went on to explain how much that cost per square foot, not counting all the equipment needed to outfit an operating room. "There's always the option to build something, but property values in Frisco are through the roof, so that adds even more to the bottom line."

He smiled at us again. But I noticed that it was different, somehow, from the smiles of those hospital CEOs who invited us to steak dinners.

"Whitney's been telling me about your practice. She says you two operate all day every day, and that your patients come here from everywhere. If you operate that much, maybe you could afford your own Shangri-La."

That first meeting was in May 2019. Two weeks later Bush and I went on a cruise in the Gulf of Mexico with our families. We barely escaped from port before Whitney texted, "Dan's found an ASC for sale, on 121!"

Bush showed me the message. While excited by the news, I was irritated that texts reach even to the middle of the ocean.

"Highway 121 . . . I bet it's that Faith Surgical Center," Bush mused, recalling the large green sign no one could miss driving to the airport. She texted Whitney back, who confirmed that was the place.

"Good location," she told me. "It's closer to the airport than our current office and right off the highway. I've driven past it a zillion times."

"Yeah," I agreed, "I know where it is. It might be perfect for us."

When we returned to Dallas, Dan explained he had his eye on this building for years, and even tried to buy it once before. He called the owner after our meeting, who told Dan he had just decided to sell and had not even put it on the market.

"It's a *great* building!" Dan said. "It's only ten years old, and it matches *exactly* what you're wanting." His huge smile underlined his words. "Best of all, it's *distressed,* and the seller just wants out." He shifted to the conspiratorial look of someone about to share a delicious secret. "So he's offering it *under market value!*"

Cold air flooding out an open door diffused through the summer heat outside, inviting us to sip our wine on the patio at Cru. Bush chose a flight of French Chablis, while I swirled a full pour of Carménère around my glass. We toasted the prospect of a new home, though careful not to celebrate what might not come to pass.

Earlier Dan toured us through the building, inviting us with large sweeping gestures into the offices PARC Urology might occupy, then down to the entrance into the surgery center, saving the walk-through of the operating rooms for a dramatic finale. It reminded me of a modern Pompeii: every exam room, each office, the perioperative areas, and the ORs all left exactly as they were the day the owner changed the locks on the door when rent went unpaid for six months.

"You could literally start operating here *tomorrow!*" Dan gushed. "There's really *nothing* that has to be done to start it back running again."

"Except that the surgery center waiting room *has* to be updated," Bush corrected him. "It's way too '80s! The colors are hideous."

Both Dan and I recognized an opportunity to remain silent, our guide warily commenting, "That's what TI is for," and then explaining that money for tenant improvements would be included in the loan.

"My gut's telling me this is our future," Bush said, as we snacked on an assortment of cheeses at the wine bar.

"Your gut's told you that several times now!" I laughed.

"And it's usually been right," she replied, defending her intuition, "especially about Forest Park. Now we need a new home, and I think this is it. It's got everything we need to become a destination *center* for hypospadias repair."

That was true. The main office suite upstairs could house both PARC and Operation Happenis, with room to spare. Another space across the hall remained unfinished, which we could lease to a hyperbaric oxygen company. Meanwhile, there were two operating rooms in the surgery center downstairs, one for us and the other for a second surgical team we hoped to recruit soon, as well as a procedure room that could easily become a third OR.

"It just can't be an accident that doors kept closing, leaving us no choice but to keep looking until we found this," Bush continued. "I know you're worried about going into debt, but this is the only way we can do what's best for our patients, and we'll get to pay rent to ourselves! That alone is worth doing it."

I said nothing more, sipping my wine and recalling the last time we sat outdoors at Cru, with the administrator for the STAR who wondered why we stopped coming there.

"The scrub tech you keep assigning to us. We ask for a suture five minutes before we need it, remind him again to have that suture ready, and then when we stick out our hand for it, he doesn't even have it open, much less loaded. Even though it's on our card because we always use it. And that goes on all day," Bush answered.

"Why can't you give us the tech we had the first day there . . . the one we worked with at Forest Park?" I asked.

But we already knew the answer, which was the same everywhere we went. The best help went to the surgeons the administrators thought brought in the most money.

By the end of June, Dan was ready to present us a pro forma, 193 pages secured in a ring binder projecting revenues and expenses for both the building and the surgery center inside it for the first three years of operations. Page after page listed every cost we could imagine, followed by columns of numbers arranged month by month subtracting those costs from the gross income Dan calculated by matching our billing codes to the payments Blue Cross agreed to in their North Dallas Health contract.

Here was the repair of hypospadias without its art and science; stripped of the skill and knowledge accumulated case by case over many years, our tireless determination to improve operations and decrease their complications, and our commitment to operate together as a team even though we would make more money working separately. Hypospadias surgery revalued in the dollars and cents that businesspeople use to analyze an investment and bankers scrutinize before loaning the money to make it all happen.

Figures that totaled a bottom line predicting the partnership of PARC Urology and Dan's company, North Dallas Health, could buy and operate Faith Surgical Center; assuming Bush and I agreed to travel less and work more, since we would not break even until the end of the third week each month after a first-year startup in the red. She and I double-checked all those costs and calculations the best we could, and then sat with Dan for hour after hour revisiting his projections line by line trying to be sure that no expense was forgotten, and no profit overestimated. There was so little margin for error.

Next Dan gave the pro forma to several banks, letting each know who else had a copy, and arranged meetings after their reviews to discuss terms of the loans they were willing to make. One required a 25 percent down payment for the monies they offered. Fortunately, others asked for less cash up front, provided Bush and I personally guaranteed the loan since our North Dallas Health partners carefully calculated their own investment percentages to come in just under the threshold that required those guarantees that someone had to give.

Knowing the stakes, we went back through the pro forma yet again. We could read what the Blue Cross contract would pay, but had to be certain that those rates provided enough dollars to buy supplies whose costs we knew, those sutures and catheters and bandages we now purchased ourselves for workshops, plus those costs we never had to consider before. For breathing tubes and anesthetic gases and bags of IV fluids, for antibiotics and antiemetics and anxiolytics,[64] for gowns and gloves and surgical drapes, for nurses assessing the patients before surgery and recovering them afterward, for OR circulators opening supplies and for surgical techs passing the instruments, not to mention the cost of washing, sterilizing, and wrapping those instruments into packs and terminally cleaning the OR at the end of each day, and the bills for electricity and air conditioning and maintaining a back-up generator in case the power failed. All this to do three hypospadias repairs a day, which also had to cover the salaries of the receptionist to check in patients, the schedulers to book operations, the secretaries to pre-certify our work with insurance, and the billing specialists to collect the payments afterward.

I started waking up in the middle of the night worrying that Shangri-La would cost us everything. In those dark hours, fears of financial ruin stirred me nearly as restless as had the witch hunt years ago at Children's. Usually, Bush remembered some figure that put me back at ease the next morning. Other times I asked Dan to run through the projections again, over-estimating the costs for supplies and people, under-estimating payments from insurance, seeking reassurance that the model would work when the money went hard, the loan documents were signed, the keys changed hands, and Bush's and my personal guarantees for all the monies borrowed became real and inescapable.

"You almost qualify for a finance degree!" Dan punctuated the end of a Sunday afternoon pouring over figures the three of us had already scrutinized several times before.

"Except that medical school and residency don't prepare doctors *at all* for the business side of medicine," I grumbled.

---

64. *Antiemetics* are medications given for nausea and vomiting. *Anxiolytics* are medications to reduce anxiety.

Finally, after four months of this, the documents to purchase the building, create the surgery center and lease the office space, and the agreements to manage the building and to run the surgery center were finished, pending approval by attorneys for both PARC Urology and North Dallas Health. A bank had been chosen and the terms of our loan negotiated, generating more documents for the attorneys to review so we could sign to close the deal.

The principals already agreed on the broad strokes of these relationships. After making the largest down payments and personally guaranteeing the loans, the surgeons would become the building landlords, hiring North Dallas Health to keep it running—collecting rent, supervising janitors, replacing lights in the foyer, and servicing the HVAC units on the roof. The Blue Cross contract stipulated that North Dallas Health had to be the majority owner of the surgery center, which the businessmen would manage while the surgeons did the work that generated the revenue to pay the bills.

Dan wrote in checks and balances to nurture a long-term agreement, but our attorneys worried the scales weighed too heavily in the businessmen's favor. They red-lined every line of every document trying to protect their client's interest to the point that North Dallas Health nearly lost its interest in the deal. With no other options for our practice and concerned the owner would sell to someone else if we did not quickly come to terms, I finally told our lead attorney at the height of the turmoil, "It's your job to give us your best advice, but it's up to us whether we take it or not."

Meanwhile, Bush and I tried to picture the new signs we would hang on the front of the building. The large block letters of FAITH Surgical Center colored the same shade of green as our practice logo suggested we keep the A and transform FAITH into PARC. PARC Surgical Center. We also wanted a new name for our practice, this time something that said HYPOSPADIAS to announce what we now did all day, every day. A name to stand over the main entrance where it could be seen by the tens of thousands of drivers passing by on the highway. Prompting at least some who saw it to google the word most had never heard of, while reassuring others who knew that word, because they or their son had hypospadias, that they are not alone.

But HYPOSPADIAS was not easily captured in either a name or on a sign. Bush wrestled with terms that defined our new home and our mission, trying to fit them together aesthetically. She spent hours studying words and fonts and the three dimensions of letters, and then drove down the freeway looking at the colors of signs that were easiest to read both day and night. Finally, she was ready to preview some options.

"Our practice is bigger than the US, or even North America," she reminded me. "So I've been thinking about:

WORLDWIDE
HYPOSPADIAS
CENTER

or maybe

INTERNATIONAL
HYPOSPADIAS
CENTER

But I can't make either of them look right. 'Hypospadias' is so long that it's hard to balance it on a sign."

I was not enthused by either name. "'Worldwide' sounds like a shipping company, and 'International' reminds me of a diamond store," I objected, "or one of those oriental rug places that are always having a going-out-of-business sale. Maybe it's less important to advertise that patients come here from everywhere than it is to say that we're a specialty center for hypospadias."

She typed that out on her laptop and played with the words. "Here, take a look at this. It actually works!"

HYPOSPADIAS
SPECIALTY CENTER

And, with that decided, there was still more work to do after we finished long days of surgery, and worried about documents and squabbling attorneys and the final terms of the loan. Somehow Bush also found time for another total office makeover, choosing new flooring, fresh paint, updated countertops, matching tile, modern light fixtures, new furniture, and modern art for the new walls. I contributed the suggestion that she shop online to see if any of my daughter Laura's paintings would work in the lobby or family waiting rooms.

Word of our center taking shape inevitably leaked into the community, and soon nurses and techs sought out Dan to schedule interviews.

"I've been working for Dr. Snodgrass and Dr. Bush at Legent," a circulating nurse explained, "and what they do is something special. I definitely want to be part of this!"

A scrub tech told Dan, "I've done some hypospadias cases with other surgeons, so I watched their videos to compare. All I can say is that they're amazing, and it'll be a fun challenge to work with two surgeons at once."

Two other nurses applied to work in pre-op and post-op, telling Dan that we repaired their sons and now they wanted to help other moms stressed by the day of surgery.

The loan documents were finally typed and ready to sign near the end of October. We met Dan in Whitney's office to sign stacks of papers everywhere a sticky label pointed. In minutes it was done, until someone at the bank noticed a change in the Dallas Health hierarchy that made everything null and void until new papers were drawn up with the correct titles for everyone to sign all over again a week later.

And then it was time for a celebration, a moment for Bush and me to stand together with Dan and Whitney under the lights in our new OR for a toast of champagne and some photos. To marvel that six months earlier we worried where our practice would go when it did not fit anywhere. To remember our first meeting with Dan, and a text soon after that he found a place, this place, for sale at a price we could afford. To smile and hold the keys and not think about the debt and the personal obligations that handed us those keys.

Renovations were completed in early December, which meant Dan could schedule the state inspection for our operating license just before the holidays so we could open in the new year. Except that the inspectors were all booked well into January, although one was free to make an unofficial walk-through looking for any infractions. Dan expected none but the inspector found several, even though FAITH passed the last inspection less than a year before.

"You need a sink here," she declared, pointing to a corner between two nearby sinks. "And the code says you must have another toilet in the ASC," even though Dan could not find a regulation anywhere that said that.

The contractors were back within days and managed to squeeze in a small sink just large enough to pass the next inspection. But a surgically precise demolition was required to pry up the new flooring and jackhammer through the foundation to lay pipes for the toilet into a re-purposed exam room.

When that dust settled the inspectors were invited back, one finally arriving in mid-January almost three months after the clock started ticking on the six rent-free months negotiated with the bank while we got started. Dan predicted the survey would now be little more than a brief formality, yet the half-day affair stretched through the whole day as the inspector breezed without a word past the new sink and bathroom to march through each room counting outlets, lifting ceiling tiles, turning switches off and on, and in the process, finding a few minor faults which could have turned into a major failing had Dan not gathered an army of repairmen to make the mandated corrections in real time. Nevertheless, the inspector did not check off the box on a form to make our certification official before he was off to another survey.

We waited days that became weeks without that mark of approval. At least our employees used the time to organize all the paperwork and supplies and then practice checking in, pre-oping, operating, recovering, and discharging baby dolls, troubleshooting each step until everything moved smoothly and efficiently before real patients arrived. But we still waited for permission to open. Calls to the state office were placed on hold pending that inspection report, and even friends of friends who knew someone could not penetrate the veil of bureaucracy that kept us from working in our new center.

Then, on the fifth day in February, permission was granted just as mysteriously as it had been delayed. Despite the short notice, Whitney somehow managed to get single-case agreements[65] to do the first cases in the PARC Surgical Center the very next day. Once again, Bush and I walked out of one life to begin a new one, this time at the Hypospadias Specialty Center.

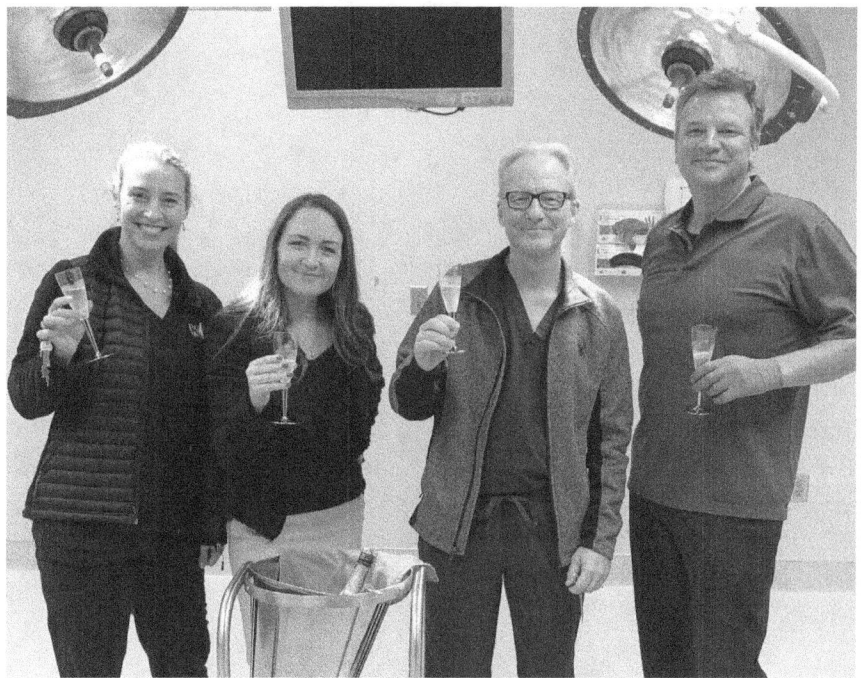

Bush, Whitney, me, and Dan toasting our new center in 2019.

---

65. A *single case agreement* is an authorization issued by an insurance company to an out-of-network surgeon or facility to provide services at an agreed-to rate for one patient.

◀ CHAPTER 28 ▶

Three Operations Was the Right Decision

We both looked up from the operative field and into each other's eyes, neither saying a word. Despite cutting away the contracted graft and all the scar we could see and feel underneath it, the penis was still bent nearly as bad as it was when we first operated six months earlier. Which meant the three incisions we made to straighten it had also scarred.

I recognized signs that the graft had shrunk during an examination in the office the afternoon before. Summoning the dispassionate look on my face that I once used to hide my disappointment after Mathieu repairs, I studied the boy's obviously bent penis and a scar running across the graft.

I hated these moments when I realized a graft had contracted, anticipating the discussion to follow with parents distressed to hear that Bush and I would have to repair, or maybe even replace, the graft. And that meant another harvest of tissue from inside their son's mouth, another six months of waiting and hoping it worked this time, and then another trip back to Dallas when they thought this time would be the last. News that was all the more difficult for families, like this one, which had only known failure and came to us desperate for success.

"You can see that his penis is bent again," I told Mom, looking up from my exam. "There's a scar here in the graft where it's almost certainly contracted." Then I pulled up the boy's shorts and hopped him down off the table so I could sketch a quick diagram of the situation on the exam table paper. "Tomorrow we'll have to cut across that scar and remove all the unhealthy graft," I continued, tapping on the drawing and pausing for her to process the words, and sigh. "But that should make his penis straight again, and then we can take a smaller graft this time to fill the space where it scarred," I explained with a note of optimism.

But that was not what we found. After releasing the scarred graft and the skin next to it, his penis remained bent because the sheath surrounding the erection cylinders had contracted too. A combination we had never seen before.

And that meant the corporotomies had to be done again and we would need another long piece of graft from inside his mouth—repeating the operation that did not work the first time and expecting it to somehow work now.

Bush broke the silence first. "I think we just make the corporotomies and then close his skin without grafting."

Which was exactly what I was thinking, spoken an instant sooner. I immediately nodded agreement, already looking back down to the operation.

But the parents were *furious* when we explained what we found and what we did and why we did it afterward.

"We did not fly all the way here from New York for this!" summarized their jumble of emotions hearing that this operation had failed just like all the others, and then learning there were at least two more operations in his future.

Several weeks later I opened an email from them, dreading what it had to say.

WE ARE SO HAPPY! FOR THE FIRST TIME IN HIS LIFE HE HAS A PENIS!!!

I clicked on their attachment to see that it was true. This penis was straight, and the skin around it looked healthy. In fact, the penis looked normal, except for the low meatus.

The skin easily opened six months later, and we placed more graft, which healed perfectly this time and then rolled into a healthy urethra at the last operation.

Bracka never taught me how to manage the disappointment of a failed graft. He must have had some grafts that did not take, because at least a few will shrink no matter who harvests them, where they are taken from, or how they are placed. But I never heard Bracka mention those or tell surgeons what to do next when it happened. I had to learn that on my own.

The Europeans, influenced by Bracka, used grafts more often than Americans and routinely claimed they healed with 100 percent success. Following one such presentation at the ESPU, I stood to ask how the surgeon achieved that, and then tried to follow up with a related question to make clear his long and convoluted answer. The moderator, however, interrupted and told me I had already taken more than my fair share of time at the microphone.

At least the HBOT we now used routinely in redo surgeries helped grafts heal, as Bush and I eventually published. But it did not *guarantee* a healthy graft.

Then another boy returned with a contracted graft, and I saw that the skin along its edges was also dramatically accordioned. That reminded me of Graham Humby's comment in his report about the first lip graft, how grafts need healthy skin around their perimeter to help nourish them while new blood vessels grow in. It seemed the demands of the graft were too much in this boy and damaged his penis skin.

The next day Bush cut away the ruffle of scar in the skin and I removed the scarred portion of graft.

"I think we should just close the skin without regrafting in this boy too," I said.

Six months later his penis was straight, and the skin was smooth and supple. Now the grafting we did healed.

The next time we straightened a penis and closed the skin without placing a graft to make the urethra, Bush asked what we should call this operation derived by dividing STAG into its two basic components done six months apart. I thought about the key steps and suggested "SAC, for Straighten And Close."

This time she was not enthused, and several minutes later countered with "The Triple C: Corporotomies, Cover, and Close." Now I winced, my opinion clear despite the surgical mask covering half of my face.

As we debated back and forth, Davis, our anesthesiologist, stood up, looked over the drapes, and proposed "Snodbush" to stop our quibbling. Whatever the name, this operation was quickly proving a god-send for our most difficult redo surgeries.

I returned to the PUWF in February 2018, looking forward to skiing the famous powder at Snowbird. But so much snow fell so fast and thick that the lifts shut down and I had nothing to do between meeting sessions but sit in my room and look out the window. So I opened my databases and pulled out the entries for patients who had grafts, segregating them into those placed onto a smooth surface and others placed directly onto corporotomy incisions to make the penis straight. Then I tallied how many in each group healed so that we could tubularize them. After checking the results twice I called Bush.

"Listen to what I found. We have nearly 95 percent success when we put a graft on smooth corpora," I told her, "but that drops to 75 percent when it's over one incision, and even lower if it's on two or all three incisions."

And that explained why enough of our grafts failed that I once declared to Bush in exasperation, "I'm going to specialize in first stages. You can do all the second stages!" Now we finally knew why that happened and had a solution for it: the Snodbush repair. I could not help but think back to all the grafts I had done for so many years and wish I had learned this lesson sooner.

It was not long before a boy who had never had surgery for his severe hypospadias fit our new criteria for a Snodbush. Now we faced a new question: what to do with his foreskin? We still wanted to use that to make his urethra, but we were not going to take that graft until the next operation. Bush decided not only to keep it, but also to reconstruct the foreskin around the glans to be certain there would be enough skin to use at the second stage. When he returned, his penis was straight and there was ample skin to make the urethra.

The next several boys healed the same way; the first operation making a normal penis except for its low urine opening, the foreskin graft healing supple and healthy after the second stage, and the final operation successfully moving the meatus to the tip of the glans. Never had all these steps worked so reliably in boys with severe hypospadias, and never before could we be so confident that we could make severe hypo-spadias into a normal penis.

I mentioned this new idea for the first time to a handful of trusted colleagues. Their responses were predictable, maybe even inevitable.

"I can't see any reason to do a repair in three stages."

"My grafts do just fine when I put them on corporotomies."

"What hubris to call it the Snodbush!"

Bush was more concerned what moms would say, before taking their sons to other surgeons promising to do only two operations.

"Maybe they'll think the risks of placing grafts on corporotomies are worth taking if they can avoid a third operation."

But I heard no complaints when I explained to parents of boys with proximal hypospadias that the first operation makes the penis straight more than 98 percent of the time, then nearly 95 percent of the urethra grafts heal healthy after the second operation, and the third operation brings the meatus to the tip without complications in a little less than 90 percent. Not when the other surgeons they consulted warned them not to expect too much from their repairs done in two stages. While not every boy needed three operations, it was the right decision when the urethra graft would otherwise be put over corporotomies.

Then one day I was explaining to a family how we decided be-tween STAG and Snodbush and realized it would be easier to under-stand if STAG became "STraighten And Graft," and Snodbush became "STraighten And Close," or STAC.

CHAPTER 29

That Meant More STACs and Fewer STAGs

"This is exactly how I did *not* want to start the workshop!" Bush hissed under her breath, looking up at the screen showing a boy with distal hypospadias and a bent penis. "We'll end up doing a STAG and lose the entire audience because they won't understand why we're doing a staged repair when there's a distal meatus."

We both walked into the auditorium that morning energized with caffeine, after flying halfway around the world to join two hundred other friends of Pippi-Salle in Doha, Qatar. The meeting was promoted as his last hurrah, and Bush and I were scheduled to lead off the live surgery with a distal TIP.

The screen changed to another boy scheduled for surgery at the same time in a second operating room. The camera angle made his penis look straight.

"That one's better," I whispered back. "Let's just examine both of them in the OR and then choose."

But both were curved enough that neither was a likely candidate for TIP. Resigned, we showed our patient to the audience over the closed-circuit TV and predicted what we already knew was going to happen.

"If he's bent thirty degrees or more after degloving, we'll cut across the plate and then do three corporotomies to make him straight," I explained, holding the penis so the audience could see the curvature.

"Meaning we'll probably be doing a STAG," Bush finished the prologue.

The protests she feared came immediately over the speaker from the crowd watching downstairs, though more a trickle than the torrent that washed over me years ago when I started that case in Sweden.

"Because we decide whether to do TIP or a staged repair based on curvature regardless of where the meatus is, even if its distal" she answered, while I stripped the skin down and we both saw the penis was still bent, as expected.

"We really needed to explain this in our lectures first," she complained to me when our audio was turned off for Pippi-Salle to talk in the other room.

We realized several years earlier that it was curvature that determined if a hypospadias should be considered distal or proximal, and not the location of the meatus nearer the glans or the scrotum as surgeons are taught.

A last-minute revision to the surgical algorithm in *Hypospadiology* tried to make that clear, and we lectured this insight at every workshop and AUA course afterward. But even in this era of instant communication, it can still take years for a message to reach its audience.

I did the artificial erection and Bush announced, "So that measures sixty degrees," holding up the goniometer to show the camera.

"Are you sure? It doesn't look like that much to me," an American in the audience challenged her.

"I would definitely plicate that," another surgeon assured the crowd.

A third added, "I've heard that the goniometer is not that accurate."

Those skeptics were happier when Pippi-Salle plicated the curvature he eyeballed and then declared looked less in his patient. Meanwhile, Bush and I continued working, moving through the complex operation. I did my parts and she did hers, alternating back and forth as we always do, the camera focused on the dance of our hands. While one assumed the lead the other described the moves to the audience.

And parried the criticisms. "As we'll explain in our lectures later this week, the most common problem we find in boys coming to Dallas after unsuccessful surgery somewhere else is recurrent curvature," I said as Bush marked where I would make the three corporotomies. "We recently published that happens in 85 percent after proximal repairs, which this really is," Bush added, as I took the knife. "*Eighty-five percent!* That's astounding," I emphasized, in case someone missed that point.

"And when that happens, you have to start all over," Bush explained, "but now without foreskin for the graft, and usually with very short skin on the shaft of the penis where the curvature has recurred."

I finished both the last corporotomy and her comment.

"It's hard to make a normal penis when that happens. We have to fix these right the first time."

Next, we moved on to suture the urethra just past the incisions and then to stitch adjoining dartos tissues around them to contain any bleeding, new steps she added to make the two-stage Bracka repair I had already improved even better.

That done, Bush pointed out the skin was a bit shorter on the left side, as it often is, and made a cut that I suspected no one in the audience foresaw, to make it longer. Then she aligned the skin to cover the shaft of the penis and finally cut off the foreskin for the graft, doing these steps in a different order than Bracka taught.

"There is no substitute for penis skin," Bush told the surgeons watching. "And if you do the operation like this, there's enough for both the shaft and the urethral graft."

"But you have to do it *just like that*," I repeated, knowing from experience that at least some of the surgeons in the audience were already "modifying" the operation in their minds.

Our second case was a more typical proximal hypospadias, and the only comment from the audience as we began the operation asked why we opened the skin down the underside rather than around the penis, as is traditionally done.

"Because he might need a STAC and we'll want to do a prepucioplasty to save the foreskin for the next stage," I answered, while dissecting the skin free from the underlying tissues.

This time there were fewer protests when Bush showed the goniometer reading forty-five degrees during the artificial erection and announced we would make the three corporotomies again.

"Even though he's less curved than the last boy!" she laughed, when the audio went to the other room.

But the bend was more distal in this patient, nearer the glans. I incised through the lines she marked, and then she pulled the urethra to show it would not reach past the corporotomies.

"And that means we'll do a STAC, since we've stopped placing grafts over those incisions."

"We've documented that grafts heal best over intact corpora," I continued the narrative. "So we'll save the foreskin for now, close the shaft skin, and then let these incisions heal. In six months, we'll use the foreskin to make the graft, then finish the urethra in a third operation in another six months."

"I don't understand why you don't make one larger corporotomy and then do a tubularized flap to make the urethra all in one operation," a voice from the audience protested.

"Because I quit doing flap repairs twenty years ago," I replied, while we kept working. "Duckett claimed he was *successful* 85 percent of the time, but it turns out that operation actually has *complications* 85 percent of the time!"

"Well, that's not my experience," came the prompt rebuttal.

It would have been quite reasonable for me to respond, "Then you should publish your results and tell us all what you do different that makes the operation work for you." But that was not going to happen, since neither this surgeon, nor any other, had responded to the articles from Houston, Boston, and CHOP to explain how to make flaps better. Almost certainly, this surgeon's results were not as good as he thought, because they almost never are when results are tallied.

I had no idea how many of the other surgeons watching still did flaps, especially among those who attended one of our earlier workshops at Children's or watched our YouTube channel. All I knew was that every single patient I ever repaired with a flap suffered complications afterward, and that all the recent studies confirmed grafts are superior to flaps to make the urethra.

In an earlier time I would have debated these facts against the challenger, trying to proselytize the audience and maybe even persuade my opponent. But I had learned these rebuttals only hardened the hearts of my inquisitors, and irritated those bystanders who judged them a personal attack rather than a professional parry.

I breathed deep and relaxed.

"All I can say is that I hear Duckett's own successors rarely do that operation anymore because they had so many complications," I responded, finally, in a tone chosen to suggest confusion over certainty.

That surgeon took the stage the following day and performed the single corporotomy and a tubed foreskin flap in another boy with proximal hypospadias. The moderator tempted me to take a microphone and argue against what I was seeing.

"These people are here to learn from you, so you must tell us what you would do differently, and why."

"I had my time yesterday," I demurred, keeping my seat in the far back of the auditorium. "And I'll have more time in the lectures tomorrow and Saturday."

During a coffee break for the audience, a surgeon asked when I did a STAG and when I did a STAC. A small crowd gathered to hear me explain that decision-making, drawing diagrams just as I did for parents. Soon more stopped to watch and listen. Then someone asked to take a picture with me, and suddenly everyone wanted a picture with me. I finally reached the table for coffee and saw that the break was over, and the coffee and snacks had all been taken away!

An electronic poll of the audience later that afternoon surprised me, when most answered they would have repaired this hypospadias the way Bush and I recommended yesterday. We managed a brief glance toward each other across the auditorium when the bar graph of the results appeared on the large screen, and I saw the hint of a smile on her face before she looked back toward the front.

Even though our grafts were unquestionably better when we stopped laying them onto the corporotomy incisions, we noticed that some patients who had a STAG nevertheless returned with scars and contractions. I thought a graft could damage the skin, but now I wondered if the skin we moved to cover the underside was not nourishing the graft. I reviewed their preoperative pictures, and saw these grafts contracted when there was not much skin on the underside of the penis in the first place.

Most boys with hypospadias are short of skin underneath, especially those with proximal hypospadias, and it is a standard part of a repair to move some skin from the topside to fill in the gap. But now we saw that those who had little penile skin on the underside were more likely to contract a graft, even when it was placed onto smooth corpora. Once again, I recalled the admonition from Humby and realized the skin we transferred to fill that deficit needed time to recover before it could help heal a graft.

And that realization meant we would do more STACs and fewer STAGs.

I smiled at the irony that I trained at a time when Duckett proclaimed all hypospadias could be repaired in one operation, and now, at the other end of my career, I was increasingly doing it in three. Not for all proximal repairs, but in those where the urethra would not cover the corporotomies or the skin on the underside was too short.

This seemed an easy concept to apply. Yet, as in all things in medicine, the extremes were easiest to define, and Bush and I struggled to agree when the line was crossed between skin that could support a graft and skin that could not.

◀ CHAPTER 30 ▶

Closed by the Contagion

"Did you see this?" I asked, looking up from my email. "There's a message from the Texas Medical Board, but it won't open on my computer."

This was odd, since I could not recall a single time in all my years practicing in Texas that the TMB sent out an email. Maybe that explained why it did not work. I googled and found that the governor had just ordered all elective surgery in all hospitals and ASCs stopped immediately.

"But we already have cases scheduled, including that family who's flying in from the Republic of Georgia this weekend for surgery Tuesday," came Bush's knee-jerk response.

"This says no exceptions," I read out loud.

It was Saturday, March 21, 2020. There was little premonition, and certainly no advance warning, that this was about to happen. We read the news when the coronavirus emerged from Wuhan, China and then arrived in the US on cruise ships and airplanes. We heard when it first showed up in New York before unleashing an apocalypse, and then listened to a podcast as an Italian physician described the battle raging against the virus in the emergency departments, hospital wards, and ICUs in the northern part of his country.

Ten days earlier I reluctantly canceled a trip to Cincinnati, a rare invitation to lecture US colleagues on hypospadias that I had been preparing for since December. But I was sixty-five, in that age group already designated at high risk from the new contagion. A day later the entire conference was cancelled, as was the remainder of the NBA season, and incoming flights from everywhere in Europe except the UK, an exception presumably made because the president owned a golf course there.

That same March 11, I gathered the ASC staff in the downstairs waiting room while Bush met the HSC staff upstairs to announce that everyone we were looking at had the virus. Or, at least everyone had to assume that everyone else did so we would all remember to keep our surgical masks on, stand six feet apart as often as possible, and wipe down every door handle and light switch, every chair and sofa, between each family coming into the office or the surgery center.

Sarah Williams, our equipment manager and back-up scrub, confirmed we had the supplies needed to continue operating for at least a month, and Missy Norris, the surgery scheduler, told us no one had called to cancel their operation. So we kept working with these added precautions, knowing that if either surgeon fell ill patients would be inconvenienced and twelve staff would be out of work. Bush and I knew our greatest vulnerability was in the OR, where the scrub tech stood beside me all day and we took grafts from inside mouths near where the virus landed in its victims. But we were not yet worried, since the first case of COVID-19 in North Texas had been confirmed only two days earlier.

Now the state closed and locked our doors just five weeks after our center finally received approval to open, sending everyone into shelter for at least the next six weeks. I was relieved that we still had a few rent-free months on our loan startup, and pleased when Dan announced he was going to convince the bank to extend the grace period another six months.

Bush and I decided to quarantine at the beach, where we could review data that we had no time to update during the several months devoted to buying and remodeling the PARC Surgical Center. Now there was a luxury of time that I had not had again since my year in Seattle. Which gave me a taste of the retirement I might never have, since my work was required to guarantee the bank note.

The newsfeed on my phone offered movie suggestions for people not reviewing spreadsheets to pass the time in lockdown, but my eye caught a story of greater interest than binging Netflix. How an earlier pandemic drove a young Isaac Newton from the university in London back to his home in the countryside, where he sat one day staring out the window and saw an apple fall from a tree in the garden. I figured Newton must have seen many apples fall from many trees over the years, but this time, with no tasks to finish or deadlines to meet, that simple observation became a cornerstone law of gravity.

Although not a project of similar magnitude, I decided I would also use this surplus of time to start work on the second edition of *Hypospadiology*. And I decided to post that story about Newton as an inspiration to others in a hypospadias email group that Bush and I recently started to use their time productively too. I was surprised when that prompted a terse reply from one colleague admonishing me for "seeking glory when our colleagues are dying in a pandemic."

I had not heard of a single pediatric urologist succumbing to the contagion, and I knew from prior experience that there is no glory in the hours I was about to spend finding words to describe the movements of surgery, and photos that would save a proverbial thousand of those words for each step.

Once again, I could look up from my computer to relax with views of the sea, but this time I was forbidden to walk on the sands along the shore and let the waters cool my feet because the beach was closed, with patrols enforcing the decree. Bush and I could wander down to a passageway through the dunes leading to the sea but go no farther. I declared this was also an opportunity to fill a lake that formed on this path with every rain and storm surge, and soon we were working on our academic projects every morning and shoveling sand every evening. I recalled the father of one of my German exchange students in Lubbock once commented that I seemed to always need a project, and now I had several for these extraordinary times.

Bush and I also researched all we could find in the news, from posts on physician Facebook groups, and the occasional phone call to anesthesiologists like Miller, to learn how others were coping with the pandemic and planning their reopening when elective surgery was allowed again. We heard that Children's was using the rapid test to screen every child for COVID-19 before urgent surgery and deciding from that what types of masks and gowns the staff should wear.

"Well, that's not going to work for us," I declared, thinking ahead to the risks we would face relying on rapid screening that was already known to be unreliable.

"I agree," Bush answered, "but that means we'll have to find a lab that'll guarantee a quick turnaround on the PCR[66] test."

Then we imagined every step in the process of moving a patient through surgery, like the staff did with dolls before our original opening, and found new questions that had to be answered before we returned to work. Who knew the accuracy of any test for the virus done by a tech bending down to the window of a car trying to swab the nose of a squirming baby? Was it possible that a boy might test negative even though his parents were spreading the virus whenever their masks slipped beneath their noses? What effect would surgery have on a patient so recently infected that his test had not yet turned positive, and what effect might the virus have on the surgery that we did? How likely was it that one of our nurses might show up for work feeling well with a normal temperature, yet be fully infectious before her symptoms appeared?

And what about the risks for families traveling to Dallas for surgery? Could they safely fly masked on a plane, and if so, how would they protect their child too young to wear a mask? What should we advise those who might be caught in a delay and need to remove their masks to eat and drink? Should we recommend families reserve an Airbnb, or could they stay on the ground floor of a hotel to avoid the elevator and ask the maids to stay out of their room? Where could families order groceries and have them delivered if they stayed in a place with a kitchen, and could they arrange deliveries from restaurants if they preferred to stay in a hotel?

Both Bush and I were well-accustomed to asking questions that had no clear answers, but now the ante was higher. We decided not to reopen until we found a lab to do the most reliable tests and report answers within thirty-six hours, at a time when many needed five days or more. We would swab not only the nose of the patient, but of his parents, too, and everyone else who entered the surgery center. That included our staff, who would have to test at least every other week,

---

66. *PCR* tests use a polymerase chain reaction to amplify viral genetic material and make it easier to detect.

and more often for the tech and circulator and anesthesiologist who worked close to us inside the OR.

We agreed we would brook no argument about masks from parents, and that all the staff who worked with patients would wear N95s[67] all day, every day. So, we had to be certain that Sarah ordered enough of those too.

Now the waiting room for the ASC that Bush spent hours refurbishing would sit empty all day. Patients and their families would be greeted at the check-in desk and then whisked into private waiting rooms remodeled from exam rooms in the original building design.

Finally, we typed all these decisions regarding safe travel to Dallas, preoperative testing for the virus, and masking and other precautions inside our facility into a COVID-19 information section to add to the website when we resumed work.

I thought the new chapters in *Hypospadiology II* would mostly be cut and pasted from the first edition, with updates here and there. I quickly realized that we had learned so much in the past six years repairing complex hypospadias every day that nearly everything had to be rewritten.

We still straightened penile curvature using either dorsal plications or the three corporotomies I devised twenty years ago, but now we measured the bending with a goniometer to accurately determine which to do. I still did TIP the same way, but less often now that the goniometer showed that some boys with distal, and most of those with proximal hypospadias had curvature measuring too much for that repair. These were better repaired by staged grafts, but I bogged down trying to write when it was best to do a STAG and when it was best to STAC. It was easy to say the urethra had to reach past the corporotomies to consider STAG, but it was much more difficult to explain when the skin could not help a graft heal and STAC was needed. After all, Bush and I were still fussing over that dilemma ourselves.

Compounding the problem was the fact that most future readers were still doing two-stage repairs using plications and foreskin flaps for severe hypospadias, and I knew those surgeons would resist any-

---

67. Tighter-fitting *N95 masks* provide better protection than do looser-fitting surgical masks.

thing that seemed so radical as a three-step repair with three corporotomies and a foreskin graft. Not to mention that to do a STAC meant other changes were necessary too. For example, no longer degloving the entire penis at the beginning of the operation or splitting the hood of foreskin to cover the penile shaft at the end.

I wrote the chapter on STAG and STAC as clearly as I could, but then admitted to Bush, "It's not perfect."

Two weeks after the governor ended the Texas lockdown, having found a lab near our center that promised a quick turnaround on PCR tests, and confirming we had a sufficient supply of N95s for us and the staff, Bush and I left quarantine and resumed surgery on June 1. We did not know how many patients would come, nor how effective our precautions against the virus would prove.

In the months that followed, one person in the Hypospadias Specialty Center upstairs was given the virus by her brother, fortuitously discovered by one of our routine screenings before anyone else was infected. A nurse downstairs in the ASC fell ill after her bridesmaid brought the contagion to her wedding but did not return to work until she recovered. We knew of no one, parent or patient, doctor or nurse or secretary, who caught the virus inside our center, and only a smattering of cases had to be cancelled at the last minute when a parent or child tested positive.

And no one working in either the HSC or PARC Surgical missed a single paycheck, thanks to the government's Paycheck Protection Program that kept our coffers sufficiently filled during the two months of quarantine.

But the lockdown, and then the masks and physical distancing and PCR tests needed to keep the virus at bay when we returned, cost us the momentum we anticipated when the new center opened. During those first weeks in February, we began each morning downstairs in the operating room and ran upstairs between cases to see the next day's patients or say goodbye to those returning home. The smiles we saw on everyone's faces walking through the building were even larger than those of the families who followed me out of Children's to PARC Urology.

One day a man walked into the surgery center and up to the receptionist to tell her, "My son had hypospadias, and I had to stop to say it's *fantastic* to see that sign over the front door!"

And we planned to add another sign to the face of the building, after convincing Dan and his North Dallas Health partners that it was not scandalous to label the new center with the word penis in letters large enough to read from the freeway.

"That's important," I told them. "Operation Happenis is an integral part of our work because we have to raise awareness about this birth defect."

"That's disgusting!" an official for the city declared when the sign company took in the paperwork for her routine approval. "We are *not* going to allow *that word* on a public building in The Colony."

"That's perfect," I said smiling when I heard we could appeal her decision to the entire city council in a public session. "Jennifer, please make sure some TV reporter covers it!"

Jennifer Bogdanowitz, our new OH director, brought to the job the passion of a mom whose own son had hypospadias repaired, and easily envisioned the coming scene. She would represent the charity, backed by a group of moms wearing powder blue T-shirts emblazoned with the Operation Happenis logo on the front and a declaration on the back that *It's Just Another Body Part*. They would hand the councilmen copies of our new awareness brochure, while she highlighted how common the birth defect is that affects the penis. She would describe the isolation she and all these other moms standing behind her felt when they were told their sons had it. She would inform them that their city was now home to the only center in the US devoted to hypospadias, and that families travel here from around the country, and the entire world, to have it repaired.

Then Jennifer would turn the microphone over to some of those other moms to tell their stories and express their indignation that prudish reluctance to say penis keeps this common condition hidden. Which would lead to the finale, when ten-year old Maddox would step forward with his mom, Deb, to announce that he was born with hypospadias, and that no one in this room, or anywhere else, should be ashamed or embarrassed or disgusted that his birth defect was on his penis.

Jennifer contacted a reporter who drove out well ahead of the hearing to film background shots for the segment they would feature, showing the Operation Happenis office with its paraphernalia and the outside of the Hypospadias Specialty Center with the blank space where the sign for the charity was supposed to go.

Everything was ready. I already considered this another victory in the making, like our best-seller *Hypospadiology* first turned down by a publisher, and the practice that became the Hypospadias Specialty Center turned away by a university, a few private hospitals, and several ASCs. After the city council's hearing, our Operation Happenis sign would either be installed on the front of our building, or we would use another denial to stir more indignation and spur more protests and call more attention to the common birth defect that involves the penis.

But then the pandemic closed Texas and canceled our moment. Jennifer had to return home to watch over her children now that it was no longer safe to place them in daycare. And, as the weeks turned into months that kept her in the house, she finally saw no choice but to re-sign from Operation Happenis. Nearly three years later she still has not been replaced.

◄ CHAPTER 31 ►

We Want to Make Sure
That You Do the Surgery

Even after several months I still was not accustomed to that N95 mask. The nose bridge was too thick and made it difficult to position my loupes. The straps dug into my ears and dislodged my surgical cap. The layers of fiber made my face sweat and my glasses fog and sometimes robbed my breath. And no sooner did I get one adjusted than the straps loosened, and it was time to break in another.

Other adjustments to the pandemic were easier. I was well-versed in telemedicine consultations long before the contagion made them fashionable. Our three separate family waiting rooms, one for each patient we typically operated in a day, kept everyone safely isolated. There was also a private lounge with a small kitchen in our office upstairs where Bush and I ate home-packed lunches between cases.

Organizing the upstairs staff working mostly from home was a bigger challenge. Those receptionists and schedulers could no longer simply lean back from their desks and ask someone nearby a question, and the text messages and emails they now sent back and forth quickly blew up my phone and flooded my inbox with chatter I did not have to know. But one of our secretaries had one of those "underlying medical conditions" that the news constantly reported increased the risk for dying from the virus. And since Bush and I had already explained each patient's surgery in detail by telemedicine, it was easy to decrease traffic in the office and limit the personnel on hand throughout the day.

We returned to work unsure how much work we would have. More than two months of patients had to be rescheduled from the lockdown, shoehorning them back in among others already scheduled throughout the summer months when school was out. That promised a full calendar, but how many of them would now be willing to travel to Dallas in the midst of a pandemic? How many of those would test positive and have their operations postponed at the last moment, when it was impossible to find a replacement to use their slot? And would Sarah still be able to find adequate supplies for surgery if production lines were disrupted and distribution systems were delayed by the virus?

I assumed demand for our services would decrease, with parents distracted by remote schooling, Zoom work conferences, home grocery delivery, and the time it took to sanitize every letter and box they carried inside the house before people realized the contagion spread through the air. So I was surprised by what they often told me during our telemedicine chats. Like the family in St. Louis I warned to expect two or maybe three operations to repair their son's penis still bent after a local pediatric urologist tried twice to straighten it with plications.

"That's what you said in your email," Dad responded. "We're ready to get this started."

I explained there would be six months between each operation and, if their insurance deductible was high, they could postpone the first one until January, or whenever their new year began, so that both, or all three surgeries, could be done in one calendar year under a single payment.

"Thanks for thinking of that. We do have a high deductible and it resets in May, so we'd be looking at waiting nine months to get started," Dad replied. Then he leaned over and mumbled something in a low voice to his wife before looking back at me. "We'll just go ahead, even if we have to pay the deductible twice. There's just too much uncertainty out there to wait."

"It's up to you, but as I said that it doesn't matter, medically, to wait until then," I reminded them.

"Yeah, but we want to make sure that *you* do the surgery," Dad answered immediately. And then I realized they were worrying I might fall victim to the virus before their son could be repaired if they delayed.

Although the clinical work resumed, it appeared our academic activities would go on a prolonged hiatus after the Cincinnati conference, and then the annual AUA and ESPU congresses, all canceled. Then Bush clicked open an email from Brazil. An invitation to Zoom down to Sao Paulo and lecture the residents and faculty there who were also locked down, and restless. She and I reworked our Get-It-Right-The-First-Time lecture, using the data we updated in lockdown and adding some new STAG and STAC photos. She tested the connection the afternoon before, and then we spoke as we did during the AUA course, back and forth from a single set of slides for an hour followed by questions.

It was an experience both familiar and foreign. The slides prompted the comments we wished to make, but there was no feedback from the audience as we spoke, no faces we could read to see if our message was connecting, no hands raised to ask a question or rebut a point. Only the sound of our voices speaking into a void. I was reminded of the late-night comedians now working from home, delivering their monologues to no audience and no response that they could see or hear.

The second time was easier, if only because we now knew the routine. Our host for the HypoAlex workshops invited us to Zoom back to Egypt, and this time Bush and I decided to complete our cycle of two Doing-It-Right-The-First-Time lectures with a final What-To-Do-When-It-Goes-Wrong conference, following the template we developed in Ecuador.

This time five hundred surgeons logged on to watch, the rest turned away because Zoom would not admit more. It was *four times* our usual pre-pandemic audience, with urologists not only from Egypt, but also from across the Middle East and around the world trying to get on. After all, no one had to pay or leave home to attend. There were so many questions at the end that I spoke some answers while Bush typed in others. And within days, our lecture was uploaded to the web for still more colleagues to watch.

Shortly after that we Zoomed to the UK and an audience of over three hundred plastic surgeons. The successors to Bracka conceived the idea and organized it, inviting me and Bush to challenge their lingering faith in the chordee excision and dorsal plication their mentor taught to prepare the penis for a graft. It was a unique audience calling for a unique lecture, and I approached the task as a lawyer might prepare his closing statement, laying out an orderly progression of facts leading to a sure conviction.

"You remember that article I read in lockdown that said it's easier to move people inches rather than miles?" Bush asked as she looked through my draft of the presentation. This STAG and STAC discussion has too many new steps for them."

Which returned to the problem I found writing about those operations for the new textbook. If pediatric urologists hesitated to make three corporotomies and then dissect the urethra deep into the scrotum to reach back over those incisions, plastic surgeons had never done any type of corporotomy or dissected a urethra so extensively. And despite their expertise with grafts, these disciples of Bracka were not practiced in saving foreskin from one operation to make a graft at the next since their teacher never reconstructed a foreskin.

"Make it something they'll think they can do," she advised.

Meaning a simple STAC. I pictured those steps for plastic surgeons, knowing they could deglove the skin and dissect the urethra to the base of the penis to make the meatus there. Once the penis was straight and the skin was closed at that first operation, they could later finish the repair with the two-stage urethroplasty they already did, using grafts from the mouth. The new step for them would be doing the corporotomies, and I realized I would have to focus on teaching that maneuver and convincing them that they could do it. Which was the same challenge we faced with our urology colleagues, moving them from the other ways they used to straighten the penis that all too often did not work or last.

Our host lingered before signing off after the lecture and the following discussion.

"Speaking for all the plastic surgeons, you certainly gave us a lot to think about. Can we count on you Zooming with us again?"

Zooms to Pakistan and Iraq followed, two places we would not have traveled before the pandemic. Altogether, we lectured in five countries in five weeks, reaching more than one thousand surgeons to talk about TIP and STAG and STAC, and the 3Ps. And to answer all the usual questions, such as the age we do those repairs, why we do not use testosterone, if you can do a distal TIP when the urethral plate is narrow, and how much those corporotomies will bleed. It was easily a year's worth of travel and teaching done in a month without the cost of being away.

And the finale was a Zoom inside the US to lecture the pediatric urology fellows, after I invited us by filling in an empty time slot on an email invitation sent out nationally. I revised our Getting-It-Right-The-First-Time presentation based on comments and questions from surgeons on the previous Zooms, and then tailored it for the trainees. Bush and I logged on early to verify the connection and asked the coordinator how many participants to expect.

"Usually somewhere between twenty and forty," she replied. "Hard to say now that everyone's back working again."

We spent the opening half of the lecture discussing curvature: why the penis is bent, how to make it straight, why chordee excision does not work and plications do not last, how to tell if the curvature returns—a radical departure from all the other presentations on hypospadias the trainees were accustomed to hearing that mostly discussed making the urethra. Next, Bush and I told the fellows that complications their patients will have are usually signs of mistakes they will make. Only then did we spend a few slides discussing technical details of our three operations, knowing the fellows could read those in our articles and textbook and watch them on our YouTube channel. I closed the hour telling the fellows again that they would make technical errors, and then I showed them a list of the ones I had made. Finally, I challenged them to use the 3Ps just as I do to find those mistakes and correct them.

This time there was objective feedback: an email filled with charts and bar graphs that reported fifty-two participants watched me and Bush live, followed by another 120 (and counting) who caught the reruns afterward. Our effectiveness in teaching was rated excellent by 100 percent of the audience.

"We're going to have to do more of these Zooms," I said, smiling as I looked at the report.

Months later, I realized we could link together a series of Zoom lectures, devoting each to a specific topic in managing hypospadias.

"We'll call it a Hypospadias Masterclass," I told Bush, selling her on the idea.

I could already see the outline of the course taking shape, the topics we would cover, key points we would make, and colleagues we might invite to guest lecture.

"We can make it better than all the visiting professorships we're not asked to do, and anyone can watch replays of our presentations on our YouTube channel."

A year later the least watched episode had over 2K views. Yet judging from comments I read on a pediatric urology email group regarding hypospadias, many of those tuning in to the Masterclasses must have been parents, or maybe trainees, but not colleagues, who still refused to listen.

◀ CHAPTER 32 ▶

We Have to Get Control of the Doctors!

"Your partners want the ASC to make more money," Dan announced, his head turned away from us and toward a screen as he fiddled with the projector. "I'm trying to pull up the financials," he explained, glancing briefly at Bush and me seated on the opposite side of the conference table.

"I thought we were doing okay," I grunted in surprise. "Especially in a pandemic!"

"That's what I said," Dan answered through a tight-lipped smile. After a moment's pause, he stared back at the projector and tried a few more adjustments. "I had this working just a few minutes ago before y'all arrived."

We watched while Dan typed orders ignored down the chain of command from his computer to the frozen screen. He rebooted, and then unplugged the projector, trying to force a reset.

Bush looked down at her watch. "We reviewed those not long ago, and our collections are *ahead* of the pro forma."

Dan shook his head in agreement and sighed, regretting his role as messenger. "But what they see is one OR sitting empty, and the other one not being used on Fridays. So they think we have to get control of the doctors to make the place run right!"

I recalled an afternoon a few days before the lockdown when Dan toured some pain specialists through the surgery center. The group walked past me without an introduction, their guide explaining later that PARC Surgical would not work for the visitors.

"They're looking for a place to take their patients with insurance,"

Dan said. "Since we only have a Blue Cross contract, they can't come here until the other contracts are done." Then he paused before adding, "But I'm not sure we want those guys anyway," and left that comment hanging unfinished.

We were told that negotiations for those other insurance contracts were well underway when PARC Surgical opened for business. But the pandemic slowed whatever progress had been made in this process which took up to a year in normal times to coax payments from insurance companies higher than their rock bottom rates.

Which meant Whitney had to continue her own negotiations with Aetna and Cigna and United Health Care to settle on single case agreements for each patient we scheduled who was insured by them. And then spend more hours on the phone convincing them to pay those fees once the surgery was done. Time that subtracted from her full-time job billing and collecting for us in the Hypospadias Specialty Center. As a result, we watched our practice revenues fall to lows reminiscent of our start-up at PARC Urology.

"I'm exhausted!" Whitney admitted to Bush and me in October five months after we reopened from lockdown, and following another weekend spent working through both the ASC and HSC accounts to keep them from falling further behind.

We told her to post a job for another biller to help, which only sucked more time that she did not have to wade through resumes only to find no one able to walk through the door and start working those accounts right away.

"North Dallas Health has to get those contracts done before Whitney completely burns out," I complained to Dan. "That's y'all's main job in this company."

But North Dallas Health was distracted, trying to grow its empire by buying more ASCs. Now we realized the significance of that last-minute change that demoted Dan from CEO to president of the company and made us have to sign the loan documents all over again. Because that move sidelined their best salesman, and the surgeons who previously worked at the bankrupt ASCs that their company bought after ours were not convinced by the new leadership to return, much less invest in the new ventures. Even with our limited understanding of the world of finance, Bush and I suspected that meant this time the businessmen had to personally guarantee the loans and write checks from their own accounts to cover losses and keep their investments afloat.

And that made them desperate for cash.

As the first year of PARC Surgical came to an end, North Dallas Health scrutinized the profit-and-loss statement, finding suspicions in the accounts receivable. Whitney patiently explained that payments for all those many single case agreements took longer to collect than would contracted fees that they still had not negotiated.

Not convinced, the businessmen cornered the accountants flinging accusations that someone had to be hiding money, which pushed the bookkeepers to the brink of quitting. When no more money was found, they demanded the raw data for all the outstanding claims—patient information, account numbers, billing codes charged and payments received, and all communications to and from the various insurances—so that they could track down the money themselves.

"We shouldn't give them those details," Whitney advised us. "Otherwise, they could harass our patients thinking they owe what their insurance is supposed to pay."

Bush and I needed little convincing, knowing how byzantine the process is to collect the money that insurance is obligated by its agreements to pay, and how Whitney had gradually learned during years of trial and error which rabbit holes to go down and which representatives at each company to contact to finally get paid what we were owed.

But the businessmen insisted North Dallas Health could help by working claims, and so Whitney turned over a small stack from the past due accounts to their billers, who worked for weeks and collected nothing.

"They have to stop harassing us," I finally demanded. "Dan, we're working as hard as we can every day, and that money will eventually get collected. Y'all will get your share when it is."

In fact, North Dallas Health was already taking a share every month, in management fees pegged to the ASC collections. In the beginning, Dan painted the big picture that the surgeons would focus on operating and his company would provide back-office support: hiring and firing, billing and collecting, human resources and regulatory compliance. At the end of the first year it was already clear they had neither the staff nor the expertise to meet these obligations, which meant our earnings paid twice for these services, once in management fees and again to employees who actually did the work.

As a result, the businessmen were well on their way to profits on their small investment, while the surgeons who operated all day every day received no dividend.

"Well, we said all along that it didn't matter if the surgery center made us any money, as long as it didn't cost us out of our own pockets," I rationalized, "since we've never been paid anything by any hospital or surgery center where we've worked before."

Bush would have added this to her list of reasons physicians burn out, but our personal guarantees on the loans kept us amply incentivized to continue working hard, nonetheless.

Meanwhile, we had not posted a new video to our YouTube channel since the day Medical City Frisco moved us from our OR to make room for their new cath lab. Bush and I knew these videos were an important pillar supporting our teaching to other surgeons, but we were also surprised to learn how many parents watched them, too, and then decided to come to us for their son's surgery. Consequently, we wrote an audiovisual package into our contract with the businessmen, anticipating a deal with Stryker who provided lights, cameras, and video systems to hospitals and ASCs throughout the region.

But Dan declared he found a better deal, smiling his broad grin as he told us, "It does *everything* that Styker's does, but at only *half* the cost!"

Except that the camera would not focus if there was any red color in the field, even though, in an operating room, there is always some red in the field. Various adjustments, added filters, and software updates could not sharpen the image during a back and forth with the company that dragged into several months. Then Bush simply asked one day how to white balance this camera that lacked the usual button that surgeons normally use for all cameras in the OR, and it finally worked.

Our excitement to resume videotaping was, however, short lived, when the system turned off after recording only a few minutes. More calls to the company, and then to local AV services found no one who could either convince the video recorder to work longer, or replace it with some other recorder that would.

"This is unbelievable," we told Dan. "It looks like the 50 percent you saved with this company no one has ever heard of is going to add that much more to the cost for a system that actually works." And take even longer to order and install, since the pandemic slowed both production and delivery of the Stryker system we finally ordered.

Then one morning Whitney texted urgently, "Have you looked at the bank account? North Dallas Health wrote themselves a check for $140,000!" Not a payment for services rendered, since they provided none, nor a distribution, since we were not paid our 49 percent . . . simply a withdrawal made by one of them walking into a branch office and taking it out in cash.

"They think they have the power to do that," Dan shrugged when Bush and I confronted him. "They own 51 percent of the company."

The checks and balances he wrote into the company agreement that said the ASC would be managed by a board consisting of me, Bush, and a North Dallas Health representative were, it turned out, trumped by a single phrase hidden in another portion of the agreement that stipulated decisions would be made by ownership. Or, at least, that was how their attorney, who wrote the document, interpreted it. Our first attorneys, who redlined every line, somehow did not catch this internal confusion that on one page said North Dallas Health always had the final word while several other pages made clear the Board of Managers, which we controlled, made the decisions.

The new attorneys we consulted also gave conflicting opinions. The first leaned back in his chair, his cowboy boots crossed on his desk and his hands clenched behind his head, and advised us, chuckling, "Many folks don't realize that it's harder to divorce your business partners than it is your spouse. Having said that, I'd love to take this before a judge." But before matters reached that climax, another attorney in the same firm led our next discussion and warned, "While you might have a strong case, y'all really don't want to put your future in the hands of a judge. You really should try to buy the businessmen out."

And for once our interests and those of North Dallas Health aligned. They wanted money; we wanted them out and were willing to pay them to leave, assuming we could agree on a price. Not surprising, their number was much higher than ours, but this decision would be guided not by our differing valuations, but by the fair market value independently determined by an appraisal company chosen by the bank.

Just as that process began, I received a call from Josh Wilson, an intense man who spoke straight to the point. "Mel tells me y'all need help. I have a lot of experience in the healthcare space, so I'm calling to offer my assistance."

A few months earlier I spoke with his wife, Melanie, for a telemedicine follow up after we operated on their son. He had no problems, which left us a few extra minutes to chat. Melanie reminded me she was a surgical biller and I laughed and said we were in the market for someone to help Whitney handle the load from adding the ASC to our practice billing.

"I'd be interested in doing that," Melanie volunteered. Her dive into our books found many opportunities for improvement, and she knew no one better than Josh for that task.

He proved to be another godsend at another critical moment, a businessman who could speak the language of business with North Dallas Health.

"I can definitely help you with the purchase of your ASC," he told me. "I've done many mergers and acquisitions, so I can make sure the asking price is right." Soon he took our places at the negotiating table to land a deal that we could never have gotten ourselves.

As the third-year anniversary of the HSC and ASC approached, it was clear we had not found the Shangri-La that Dan once painted into our imagination. But posts on Facebook that Bush read from other physicians across the country describing the travails of their practices also made clear the Shangri-La we had was a paradise few others find.

But then Josh managed to wrestle control of Parc Surgical Center from the businessmen, making it clear that the surgeons who earned all the revenue also controlled the finances.

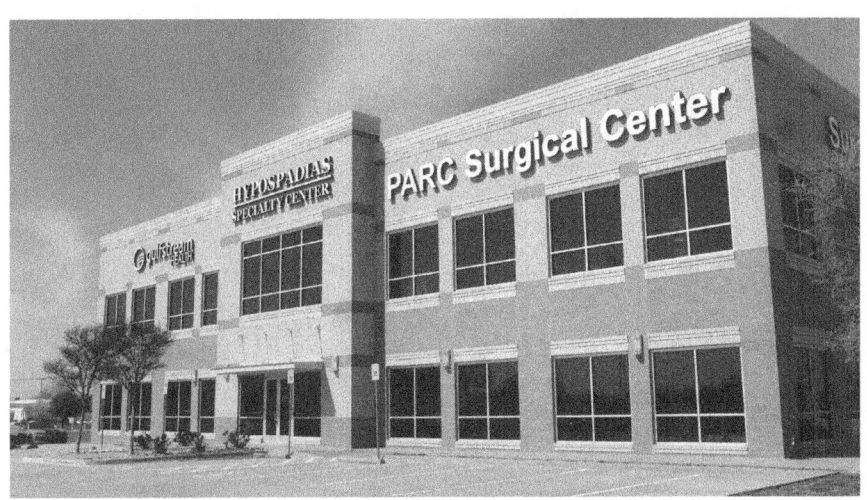

The first center for hypospadias repair.

◄ CHAPTER 33 ►

The Worries Parents Told Us

I tried to mention some of the worries that parents told us during Pippi-Salle's meeting in Doha—stories that taught the experts that this birth defect of the penis is more than the surgical exercises we debated at this and other conferences like it. Just a few words about the impact that hypospadias has on others that I did not hear at the university, and suspected these colleagues had not heard either. But I was immediately shouted down by that skeptic in the crowd who also questioned the need for staged repairs to correct severe hypospadias.

"Where's the data you're always saying we need?" the critic taunted. "These stories are not convincing!"

We had that data but were struggling to share it. Now, while we sparred with our business partners, Bush also found time to revise a manuscript that had already been rejected by both the *Journal of Urology* and the *Journal of Pediatric Urology*. She read back through the reviews, slowly shaking her head, and then finally sighed her exasperation at the computer screen.

"It's a *descriptive* study using a *validated* questionnaire with *260* respondents."

A study tabulating the concerns parents had been telling me for years, done so we could officially report them to other pediatric urologists. The fear when they learned their son had a birth defect that they had never heard of, and their isolation once they realized that neither of their parents had either and were unsure if they should discuss their newborn's penis with friends. The guilt they carried wondering what they might have done to cause this to happen, a burden made heavier if mom took progesterone to stabilize her pregnancy. Worry about their son's future, which did not end even when surgery to repair his hypospadias was a success. The frustration that surgeons did not spend enough time listening to their concerns, answering their questions, or explaining the surgery they proposed. The sadness most felt, and the anger some felt.

Our study was set into motion by the persistence of a mom asking me what caused hypospadias.

"No one really knows," I answered. "If you google that you might read about pesticides, or soy milk, and progesterone."

"Yes, I saw those, but I don't think I was exposed to any of them," she replied, puzzled. "No one else on either side of our family has hypospadias, either, as far as I know."

"That's typical," I said. "Usually, the family history is negative."

"So why do you think it happened?" she asked again, staring at me through her computer screen.

"Well, there's other associations, like older mothers or IUGR[68] . . ."

"I've read all of that too," Mom interrupted, "and I still can't figure out why this happened." Then she looked away. "I feel so guilty that my son was born with it."

And that confession opened my eyes. She was not researching the etiology of the birth defect. Mom was asking how *she* caused hypospadias to happen to her son.

The next time a mom posed that question, I smiled gently and told her that no one knows. But then I continued. "I wonder if what you really want to know is if you somehow caused it?" and was surprised to see tears immediately well in her eyes as she reached for a Kleenex, embarrassed by the emotion suddenly pouring out.

That happened again with another mom. It was always the mothers who asked what causes hypospadias, and I routinely gave the same answer. She could not restrain her tears either.

"I'm so sorry," she apologized as she wiped them away and quickly

---

68. *IUGR* is intrauterine growth restriction, meaning the baby's growth before birth is less than expected.

regained her composure. "I've been so worried that I was somehow responsible."

Clearly, this fear lurked just under the surface, gnawing on many moms, and some dads, whose sons had hypospadias. Soon I decided to raise the issue even when the parents did not ask.

"Maybe this doesn't apply to y'all," I would say, after explaining the surgery I proposed. "But many parents worry that they did something to cause it, or didn't do something to prevent it, so I wanted to mention that his hypospadias is not your fault." And nearly every time they would look at each other and then nod their heads agreeing. Most of the moms cried.

I recalled a review of hypospadias published in 1917 by the surgeon Carl Beck, who mentioned the condition occurred in 1of every 300 boys, citing the prevalence recorded by Napoleon's surgeon general from induction physicals in the early 1800s.

"That's the same number reported today," I started telling parents, "but in a world that did not have pesticides or progesterone."

These conversations finally sent me on my own Google search to better understand how birth defects impact parents. I read that the reactions I was seeing are typical, as both moms and dads often wonder if they are the reason for their child's problem. In fact, this response is so common that a scientific questionnaire had been written and tested to capture their feelings. Questions posed to parents of children with other birth defects, such as those involving the heart, Down's syndrome, cleft lip and palate, and spina bifida, but not hypospadias even though it is more common than each of these.

"That's a perfect project for your son," Bush declared when I first mentioned it.

My youngest studied political science as an undergrad, and then spent the next few years cycling on teams in both the US and Belgium before ultimately deciding to attend medical school. But first Phillip had to go back and take two years of biology and chemistry and then earn high enough marks on the MCAT.

Now the third generation Snodgrass was in medical school and already feeling drawn toward urology; an attraction which seemed preordained when he encountered a man with gangrene of his scrotum, another in severe pain from a kidney stone, and a pregnant woman with fever from a urine infection, all during his first night in the emergency department. That stirred sufficient curiosity that Phillip started a urology interest group when he learned that his school did not have one. And then invited his dad to come and lecture to the new club about hypospadias and life as a urologist, telling my experiences as both an adult and pediatric urologist who knew both private and academic practice.

"It'll be great if he comes to join us some day," Bush told me, hopeful despite the long odds, because she realized the importance of that name to the practice. A name that opened doors to the various Facebook hypospadias parent groups and convinced them to provide a link to the *Impact of a Child with Congenital Anomalies on Parents* survey for their members to take, anonymously, if they wished. Which 260 of them did. Phillip collated their responses, summarized the findings, and sent the information to Bush, along with a few articles he found related to our topic.

As usual, I wrote the first draft, which Bush and my son reviewed. I also sent an abstract to the upcoming AUA meeting, confident that a report on hypospadias from the parents' perspective would find a receptive audience in this era of patient-centered care.[69] I could already envision sitting in the crowd near the stage watching my son walk up the stairs to the lectern, pull up the first slide, and introduce himself to the world of pediatric urology, much as I had done so many years earlier to announce the TIP repair.

Both Bush and I were stunned to open the email saying our abstract had been rejected. We knew the process, that abstracts are scored by a committee of pediatric urologists to select the ones to be presented at the meeting. Apparently, ours was not thought to have sufficient scientific merit or importance.

"Wow," was all I could say, leaving my disappointment unspoken.

The program would not be announced for several weeks, but we al-

---

69. *Patient-centered care* means doctors focus not only on the clinical treatments, but also take into account emotional, social, and financial perspectives.

ready knew there would not be another abstract during the entire meeting telling the specialists in hypospadias that 86 percent of parents had never heard of that birth defect before it was diagnosed in their son, and that nearly 60 percent of the mothers and 40 percent of the fathers wondered if they were to blame for it. Or that this worry increased to almost 80 percent among mothers who were given progesterone during their pregnancy. The pediatric urologists might hear some presentation about some surgical detail in some operative technique but leave the meeting unaware that one in every four parents said their explanations about surgery were not clear. More surprising, two-thirds of them still worried a great deal about their son's future even when his hypospadias repair was successful.

Phillip's last clinical rotation in medical school led him into orthopedics, where the surgeons use tools like the ones he and his brother, Will, used to tune their bikes and build the ramps they launched them from during an infatuation with BMX aerobatics. One of those was the goniometer that Phillip instantly recognized when he visited me to watch us operate and Bush asked for it to measure the bend of a penis.

"How do you know about this?" she wondered.

"We use it in the bike shop all the time," Phillip explained.

Years later he became a hand surgeon and now routinely uses the goniometer to measure angles of finger joints. He might have instead joined his father and used it every day repairing hypospadias, but the siren's call to orthopedics probably would have proven more seductive even if he had presented that abstract to pediatric urology. Dad will never know.

I polished our manuscript, "Parental Concerns of Boys with Hypospadias," and submitted it to the *Journal of Urology*. The scientific methods we used were sound and the message had already influenced my practice. So I was confident the report would be accepted this time, and then surprised, again, when it was not. "They're not even giving us an opportunity to revise it," I told Bush.

We revised it anyway, before sending the improved version to the *Journal of Pediatric Urology*. It did not matter.

"Here's something I've never seen before," I informed Bush after reading the response from that journal. "The editor is inviting us to *rewrite* the manuscript and then send it back for the reviewers to read again and decide if it's worth another formal review!"

Bush pulled up their comments on her phone.

"Well, we could add the actual Likert scores, although that won't change anything," she said with a shrug. Then she continued reading.

"Oh, this is ridiculous!" Bush declared moments later, looking up at me as she read out loud. "It is clear this population is not representative of most parents." And, "The parents who thought the surgeon did not spend enough time with them might not have been satisfied if hours were spent with them." She read on. "But here's the best. 'This information is not new and will not change the practice of pediatric urology.'

"Well, it is, and it should," Bush declared. "It certainly has ours!"

She thought of the time it would cost us to extensively rework the manuscript, and then to revise it yet again to answer new comments from the reviewers, if we were even invited to make more revisions, and all that to publish something that it seemed clear few of our colleagues would bother to read if it was finally accepted.

"The truth is, they don't like the message. I don't think it's worth the effort."

"But it's important and has never been published about hypospadias before," I countered, knowing that she was right.

We sat quietly, weighing our few options. I finally sighed, "We could send it to a different journal."

"Yeah, where even fewer people will see it," she snapped.

Then I saw a mischievous grin before Bush said, "Let's send it to an open access journal![70] That way it'll still be cited on PubMed for doctors, and parents can find it on Google and read it for free." She paused and consulted her phone. "It's going to cost us a lot, but here's a discount coupon we can use."

A few weeks later, I opened a message from the editor at Dove

---

70. Traditional academic publications are only available to subscribers or to readers willing to pay a fee. In contrast, an author pays the publisher for *open access* and then the article is available online to anyone without charge.

Press, not knowing what to expect from our first submission of a traditional manuscript to a non-traditional journal. There were three reviews.

"This is a well-written paper focusing on a very important issue of communication to parents."

"This type of study has not been conducted for this specific condition and, as such, makes a contribution to the field that deserves to be published."

"I enjoyed reading this well-written study on an important topic that deserves attention."

For once it was a pleasure for us to make the improvements these reviewers suggested, and I was proud when our article was published in 2021 listing my son as the first author.

We usually moved on to the next study after an article went into print. But that fall, when I was fully vaccinated and boosted and as the Delta wave of the coronavirus waned, I decided it would likely be safe to fly to Jackson Hole for the reopening of the PUWF cancelled the year before by the pandemic. I invited both Phillip and Will to also come ski, but that was too soon after the birth of my grandson for Will. Phillip, though, had some vacation time from residency and was excited to ski that mountain.

"It'll be fun," I agreed, "and fun for everyone who remembers you as a kid at that meeting to see you all grown up." Then I had another thought. "You can even give that parent lecture you never got to present!"

But Dad's trip cancelled when Omicron surged, and I grew uneasy thinking about the ride to the top of the mountain breathing the air inside a gondola packed shoulder-to-shoulder with other skiers. With fewer responsibilities at work, Phillip was less concerned about the virus and checked into our hotel room alone. The meeting went on as scheduled, and I Zoomed into the sessions.

Father and son reviewed the lecture before his afternoon presentation, and then I logged in to watch Phillip describe our work. He broke the ice by showing younger versions of both him and me and several of the pediatric urologists listening during the many years his dad brought the whole family to the PUWF. Then Phillip focused their attention on "What Worries Parents About Hypospadias." I could see him standing in the middle of the small conference room surrounded by my colleagues. Although the audience was only a fraction of what it would have been at the AUA, I still felt a measure of vindication, especially at the end when one of them asked Phillip for a copy of the three-times-rejected article, and then promised to share it with everyone else in the room.

I sometimes say that there is a God and He has a sense of humor, which was proven the very next morning when an email arrived coincidentally from Dove Press informing me that the paper, "had been well received" in the year since it went online, with 3,446 views. I forwarded the message to Phillip and Bush commenting, "That's almost certainly more looks than if it had been published by an academic press."

Ironically, the *Journal of Urology* had the last word several months later. When it highlighted our article, the one it once rejected, in its Urology Survey section that calls attention to "the best and most important articles published by other journals worldwide."

◀ CHAPTER 34 ▶

It's My Duty to Write This

"Look at this," I told Bush, shaking my head in disbelief as I signaled her toward my computer screen. I had just opened the program for the SPU, which planned to resume its in-person congress in September 2021.

"That's crazy!" she answered after only a glance. "How can they do a session on distal TIP and not include you . . . or at least me?" She looked at the lecture schedule again. "And why on earth would our society give Hadidi the stage to promote those old Mathieu repairs that look so ugly?"

"I have no idea," was all I could say, wondering why the program director scheduled an attack rather than a debate.

I easily imagined the lecture that was going to happen. Ahmed Hadidi, a pudgy, balding Egyptian practicing in Germany, would warn that he sees many boys with complications after TIP and say this proves the operation is flawed. He would insist that the TIP incision scars into an obstruction, rather than make a normal urethra.

I gazed back ten years to a small meeting in Cyprus, where Hadidi spoke before me and sprung an ambush of misquotes and statements taken out of context as he tried to turn my own words against TIP. An assault that crossed the line from professional debate to personal distain. Surprised, I fumbled for a slip of paper and a pen to jot notes for a rebuttal, but soon realized there would not be time to answer all the charges and still give my own lecture.

He continued that full-throated assault on TIP at HypoAlex 3, the meeting in Alexandria I declined to attend, still trying to convince surgeons to return to the Mathieu repair that most abandoned in favor of TIP.

Now the SPU was giving Hadidi a bigger stage in the US to discuss "The Weaknesses of TIP Repair." Who would counter his slander against the operation? Who would point out that meatal stenosis is uncommon and strictures are rare when Hadidi claimed the operation creates obstruction? Who would cite the many studies showing that the risk for complications is the same after TIP and Mathieu, but TIP prevails because it reliably creates a normal meatus that the Mathieu simply does not? I thought for hours planning a statement I could condense into less than a minute at the microphone during open discussion to speak even a modicum of truth to Hadidi's lecture.

But there would be no face-to-face exchange, no dramatic confrontation, when the contagion surged again and Delta forced the meeting to go virtual. Still, there was a moment of satisfaction when Hadidi asked viewers on Zoom how many had followed his advice to stop using TIP, and not a single person replied.

"That just proves how ridiculous this whole session was," Bush said, summarizing the program. "There was no reason for that slap in your face."

The matter was not settled, however, as Hadidi planned yet another strike against TIP the following year during a hypospadias conference in Brazil. This time the meeting organizer emailed me an invitation to join in a debate. But I was not yet ready to risk attending a meeting in-person while the pandemic continued, though, in a subsequent exchange of emails, we agreed that I could tape a presentation. While it would be a disadvantage to appear virtually on a screen while he stood live on the stage, I was confident that the facts on TIP would speak for themselves.

I began by reminding the audience why surgeons around the world so rapidly gave up the Matheiu flip-flaps they used for years and embraced TIP, when the new operation consistently made hypospadias into a the penis that looked normal. I told the story of how others, like Duckett, tried to fix the Mathieu, and how some, like Hadidi, were still trying. I summarized the data reported from thousands of patients worldwide that proved the TIP incision heals into a healthy urethra. I showed evidence that it is technical errors by surgeons, and not an inherent problem with the repair, that cause some to have complications. And I closed with the admonition that meetings such as this one should spend less time questioning TIP and more time helping surgeons who are having those complications do the operation better.

While I was certain my presentation countered Hadidi's accusations and his calls to return to the past, once again I spoke into the void of Zoom, my live voice filling only my office at home and not the meeting hall filled with delegates. I would not see their faces and could only wonder about their response.

Hadidi would have had a stronger argument had he focused his energies on proximal TIP, and we would have agreed that it should rarely be done. In fact, I had recently published my results to warn colleagues, again, not to use that operation when the penis is bent more than thirty degrees. A report I felt compelled to write when Bush and I continued seeing boys with complications after proximal TIPs done by other surgeons—years after I publicly declared, several times, that Snodgrass rarely did a "Long Snodgrass" anymore.

"It's easy, and that's why people still do it," Bush reminded me, which only added to the guilt that I was the one who pushed the boundary too far.

I already told the world that lifting the urethral plate to do three corporotomies underneath it followed by a proximal TIP made strictures afterward. But probably few, if any, colleagues had tried that. Instead, most straightened the curvature with plications when they did a proximal TIP, and I knew those stitches did not keep the penis straight.

I only did plications in boys I thought had mild bending, but that was in the many years before Bush found the goniometer to measure it accurately. Once we realized that I had underestimated their curvature, I wondered how many of my patients bent again afterward.

There were spare hours here and there in the summer after lockdown to look back at my entire experience with proximal TIP. I consulted the original spreadsheet that I kept current after Bush created the master file. A simple count found ninety patients, though I omitted a few because their penis was not bent at surgery or they never returned for an assessment after their repair.

Looking at the remaining rows of the spreadsheet, I saw the same inexact descriptions of curvature that Bush and I are still reading in operative notes from other surgeons. For nearly fifteen years I only placed a "+" to indicate curvature; it was not until 2008 that I started guestimating the degree of bending and entering an actual number. But those numbers were not much better than the + signs until Bush convinced us to start measuring the bend with a goniometer.

Fortunately, I had been more cautious using plications than surgeons more strongly influenced by Duckett to straighten almost any extent of curvature that way. Which made a conundrum. I expected to find less recurrent curvature than had I relied more on plications, but if I reported a low overall percentage those surgeons routinely plicating more severe bending would be reassured the risk is not very high.

"It is what it is," I sagely informed Bush when she raised this concern. "I'll just have to make it all clear in the Discussion." I saw her skepticism and answered, "It's my duty to write this."

Although the most important parts of a surgical report are the Methods that were used in the research and the Results that were found, I knew that the eyes of many readers glaze over those sections to focus on the Discussion and Conclusions. Obviously, I would have to spend most of my energy, and the allowed word count, writing those segments of the paper most likely to influence the most people.

And I remembered Bush's admonition to find good pictures to illustrate key points, and once again combed through hundreds to select a few. First, I needed to show readers how to recognize recurrent curvature in boys and chose three examples to make Figure 1 in the paper. Then I wanted a second figure with a picture of an apparently normal penis after a proximal TIP, right next to another picture of the same patient proving his penis was bent and that the whole operation had to be redone.

A review of the spreadsheet certified that one of every four of my patients had recurrent curvature resembling the picture in Figure 2. Then there were others who kept opening fistulas or dehiscing their wounds who almost certainly were also bent, but those complications were managed in a time before I rechecked artificial erections to see.

When these were added to the tally, it was likely that bending recurred in one out of every three of my proximal TIP patients.

Having submitted more than one hundred manuscripts for peer review, I knew the final polishing of this article would happen in response to comments from reviewers. I opened an email from the editor and scrolled through them.

One reviewer wrote, "I was a little surprised by the pictures the authors chose to show recurrent curvature. It looked mild in one of them, and I did not see it in the other two."

I looked back at Figure 1 and confirmed the three looked almost identical. Then I read on.

"To be sincere, I would accept these results. Does all curvature need to be corrected?"

I read that comment twice in disbelief, since the recurrent curvature I reported averaged fifty degrees!

But this was the point of peer review, and I reminded myself, yet again, that if a reviewer asked something, there were other readers who would wonder the same question. I made revisions in bold and sent the manuscript back.

Still, that reviewer was not satisfied, and countered in a harsher tone:

The figures do not add value to the manuscript.

It is not clear to me how the authors correlate the degree of curvature with clinical significance.

Is curvature that is not recognized by many pediatric urologists, or the parents, really clinically important?

I patiently typed responses to each of these new comments, cutting and pasting the reviewer's questions to my answers in a second letter to send back to the editor. But I suspected this would not end the back and forth. Not because the Methods and Results were flawed, but because the reviewer disagreed with the Discussion and Conclusions. I had papers rejected for this reason before, when a reviewer convinced the editor not to publish something simply because he did not believe it despite all the evidence placed before him. I wondered then how progress can be made if everyone has to agree before moving forward?

So, I preempted this reviewer with a detailed note of my own to the editor. I searched for an analogy to the situation, and then wrote that a cancer that a doctor fails to diagnose because he does not recognize the signs and symptoms is still very much a cancer. And I ended with a plea:

> Proximal TIP is done by many surgeons based on my earlier rec-ommendations. Now I realize it is best to limit it to the minority of patients with a straight, or nearly straight, penis, and that relying on dorsal plication to straighten greater curvature has resulted in recurrent curvature in both my patients and those of other pedi-atric urologists. Therefore, I am obligated to report this concern to our profession, and I hope you agree that the manuscript is now ready for publication.

Bush read my letter before I sent it.

"I warned you this was going to happen. How ironic that you're fighting to admit your mistakes, while Boston and CHOP kept theirs hidden for years."

CHAPTER 35

Hypospadias Matters!

My finger hovered the cursor over the trash icon, but then I changed my mind and clicked open the email. Someone wanted to arrange a call between me and the AUA TV Director, whatever that was. Something about highlighting the Hypospadias Specialty Center and my "pioneering advancements," as part of a film series produced by WebsEdge, which was something else I had never heard of. I first thought it was spam, but then I followed a suggestion to contact the AUA, which verified its support of this project.

Then I read the proposal more closely. How they chose to profile my contributions of TIP and STAG, my teaching to improve hypospadias care, my commitment to evidence-based surgery, and my goal to increase awareness of the most common birth defect that few have heard of through Operation Happenis.

"Apparently the AUA selects a few programs they consider to be at the forefront of urology to feature," I explained to Bush after forwarding her the invitation. "Which is pretty ironic considering Hadidi's lecture at the SPU last year."

She studied it, and then remembered, "We did this once before, back at the university. I think it was after we subspecialized the group, which was also something new in pediatric urology."

Now almost ten years later I was invited a second time, to focus exclusively on hypospadias. "The audience is all urologists, and mostly adult urologists," I thought out loud, and then looked back at her. "They already know about TIP from their residencies, and I don't think anyone will be interested to hear about STAG or STAC, or evidence-based surgery." I glanced back at the proposal, "Or Operation Happenis, for that matter."

Bush also pictured the AUA and its crowds of urologists moving down halls or through the product exhibit area under monitors showing these films. "We'll need something to capture their attention that they'll remember."

Which seemed to me a tall order for surgeons who do not repair hypospadias, and often discourage the few men they see with it from having anything done.

"That's true," she agreed. "So we'll title the film 'Hypospadias Matters,' and then show them why it does!"

We brainstormed that idea, wanting a message to send to both pediatric and adult urologists. *Hypospadias Matters*, because parents are afraid and feel isolated when they are told their son has a birth defect they have never heard of. *Hypospadias Matters*, because it affects the whole family, especially when surgery does not turn out as planned and one repair turns into many. *Hypospadias Matters*, because when it's not fixed, or fixed right, boys grow into men whose lives are changed by their ongoing struggle with a birth defect.

With that outline decided, we needed people other than ourselves to make each of those points. A man and two moms willing to publicly declare that they or their son has hypospadias.

"Well, isn't that part of increasing public awareness?" I asked when Bush frowned her doubt that we could find those volunteers. "Deb Smith will do it. She can tell how devastating it was when her son's distal repair didn't work."

Coming around to my point, Bush added, "Well, I spoke to a Dallas mom this week who can share the emotions she felt when she was told her son had hypospadias and she had no idea what that was."

"So that just leaves a man to talk about himself."

Then I had another thought. "Since this is what OH is about, we should have a booth at the AUA this year. I'll tell Dan to look into that."

We had no idea who he spoke to, but Dan unleashed stirred sufficient interest from the AUA Urology Care Foundation to schedule a Zoom to discuss supporting Operation Happenis's mission. Days later, he introduced us to Cynthia Duncan, the Director of Development. Once again, Bush and I sat side-by-side, this time to share our vision for Operation Happenis to increase awareness, support education and research, and promote access to the best care for hypospadias.

"That's exciting!" Cynthia declared. "And it fits hand in glove with our programs at the Care Foundation."

She extended the call another halfhour to hear more, and then offered to display postcards on their desk at the entrance to the AUA convention directing people to the Operation Happenis booth.

"We can help you do this," she closed our discussion, with a smile.

"So what's going to be happening at our booth to interest people who walk up with those postcards?" I wondered to Bush afterward. When we first agreed to pay for a cubicle, I envisioned it introducing Operation Happenis and its three great aims written large on the wall, with Dan the carnival barker ginning up enthusiasm.

"That's fine," Bush answered, without much enthusiasm. "But we'll also need stuff that people can take back home with them," meaning T-shirts and coffee mugs.

I glanced again a few weeks into the future at handfuls of urologists standing in front of our booth. Bush and I both knew that most of our colleagues would dismiss Operation Happenis as nothing more than an extension of our practice designed to attract more patients. We agreed this presence at the AUA, plus the stamp of approval from the Urology Care Foundation, might be our best opportunity to prove it can benefit everyone.

"Let's also use this meeting to announce the First International Hypospadias Awareness Day!" I said with sudden inspiration as we sat at Sunday brunch the next morning.

She grinned and reached for her phone.

"I looked into that before," Bush explained as she typed. "There's something for every day of the year." She held out her phone for me to see. "Like this Talk Like A Pirate Day!"

We continued eating while she scrolled through lists of commemorative days. I sat thinking of some designation that would encompass everyone affected by hypospadias—obviously the boys, but also the men they grow into, and the parents, and brothers and sisters, and wives, and even the surgeons who try to help.

"Maybe we call it Hypospadias Hero Day."

And there was the idea we could build into an international awareness day. An event timed to coincide with Marvel Comic's National Superhero Day, but repurposed to call attention to those who fight hypospadias rather than fictional villains. A day when boys and their parents, and men with their wives, and doctors and nurses can dress in superhero costumes to call attention to the birth defect few know about, without having to disclose if they have it.

"They can come out, or simply say they know someone with hypospadias," I smiled.

And all this organized by Operation Happenis, supported by the Urologic Care Foundation, and announced for the first time at the upcoming AUA meeting where our *Hypospadias Matters* video would also be showing.

"We'll need a logo people can press on their capes, and I'll need to design that postcard for people to find our booth," Bush told me as she considered the logistics. "We'll also want a photo booth and some masks and capes for our colleagues to get into the spirit with some pictures." Which sent her back to her phone to google superhero costumes and their costs.

We had two months to plan the video shoot and an announcement from Operation Happenis for Hypospadias Hero Day, squeezed into our already overfilled schedule operating every day and then continuing with telemeds that lasted into the evening, while somehow managing to respond to emails from new patients and parents reporting back after surgery and the occasional colleague asking a question.

WebsEdge assigned us a producer, who emailed a three-page tip sheet for organizing the shoot. We answered with a four-page outline summarizing the three patient interviews and the comments we intended to tie their stories together and prove that Hypospadias Matters. The producer sent back general instructions for us and the film crew, which Bush and I then made into a schedule of times and places for that day: when the crew should arrive, where the three interviews would take place, what B-roll they should capture showing the entrance to the building, the HSC upstairs, the ASC downstairs, and the surgeons in the operating room. We planned to film on a Friday, the day of the week we do not operate, which meant staging that scene in the OR by setting up the Mayo stand, adjusting the lights, and then gowning and gloving, draping the table, and going through the motions of an operation hoping the camera made it all look real.

Meanwhile, Bush contacted the artist who designed the logo for Operation Happenis and asked him to create one for Hypospadias Hero Day. Then she found a stock photo of a boy in a superhero costume flexing his muscles and pasted the new logo onto his chest.

"That's perfect," she decided, and imported the image onto the postcard for the Care Foundation, and onto the wall of our booth. Next, Bush posted the picture on Facebook, and within hours a surgeon in Brazil and another in Pakistan messaged they would promote the special day in their countries.

As the video shoot neared, WebsEdge sent the interviewees standard releases to show their faces, and two of the three promptly developed cold feet at the thought of several thousand urologists at the meeting, and then countless more people on YouTube, watching them talk about hypospadias.

We scrambled to salvage our plan.

"We don't have to show that first mom's face," Bush suggested. "I'm sure they can film her from behind, or something."

But persuading the man proved impossible despite our promise he could appear incognito. Desperate to find someone for this key role, I thought of Brenna Brown, one of our office staff, who moonlighted on weekends as an actress.

"I bet she can find someone to play a man with hypospadias."

"We can't do that!" Bush immediately protested. "It'll get out somehow and ruin our whole message." She thought for a few minutes and then offered a compromise. "OK, maybe we could do that if he identifies himself as an actor speaking the actual words of a man with hypospadias."

Fortunately, the man Brenna recommended proved so convincing that as soon as he assumed his role, I forgot we were filming an actor and not a real patient upset by the scars on his penis that were the legacy of surgery done when he was a child.

The first mom was shot in silhouette facing the camera, her concealed features focusing attention on the pain in her voice recounting her fear when she first heard of hypospadias.

Deb sat in full light to tell urologists there is nothing minor about surgery on the penis when something goes wrong.

"I'm amazed at the emotions you captured in those interviews," the director emailed after watching the raw footage.

A few days later she sent a rough draft of the film, which, after a few tweaks, condensed a full day's shoot into six minutes, plus an extra fifteen seconds the producer allowed to end with an announcement for the first Hypospadias Hero Day.

But few urologists saw our film at the meeting. We imagined the videos would be shown on monitors throughout the convention center, but instead found no more than a handful of TVs scattered here and there that no one seemed to watch. In fact, even though we stopped at several of these stations and watched for as long as thirty minutes each time, I happened to catch only the tail end of our video once. And no one at the scientific sessions or walking down a hallway or waiting in the line for coffee mentioned to either me or Bush that they saw *Hypospadias Matters*.

Meanwhile, our staff at the booth reported only sporadic visits from pediatric urologists. Bush and I took handfuls of postcards to hand out between presentations at the meeting, and were met with mostly blank looks when we explained in an elevator speech why it mattered to parents that hypospadias become better known.

We arrived in New Orleans filled with excitement for the opportunities this first in-person AUA in three years offered. The recognition of our practice by the American Urologic Association, the endorsement of Operation Happenis by the Urology Cares Foundation, and our professionally produced $20,000 *Hypospadias Matters* video. We left three days later discouraged, again, by how difficult it is to raise awareness and to prove, even to those who repair it, that hypospadias really does matter.

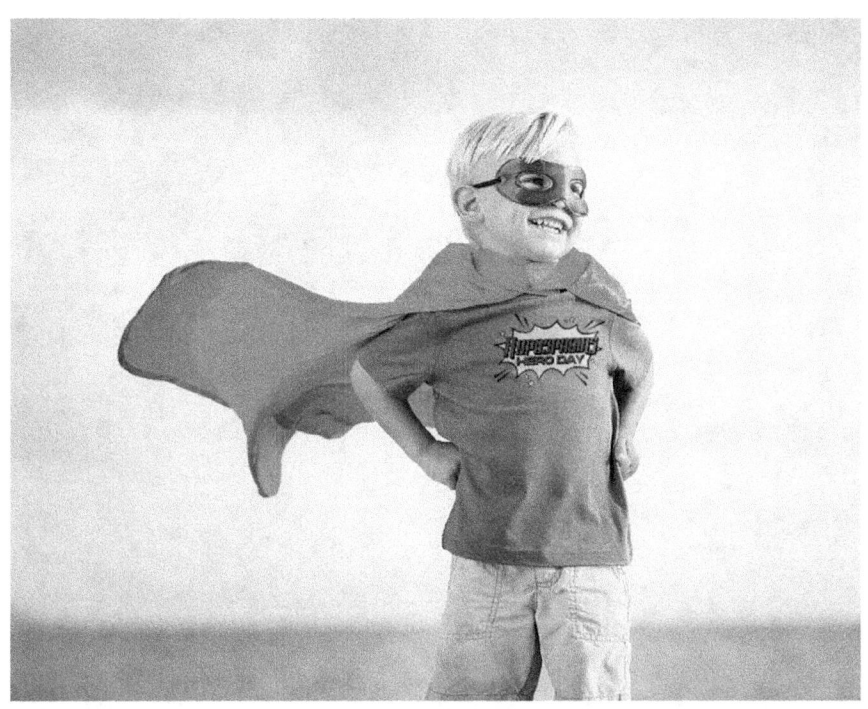

The Operation Happenis Hypospadias Hero

◀ CHAPTER 36 ▶

Dr. Bush Is More than Ready
to Do This All Herself

I have to laugh at that picture of myself. The younger version with brown hair and unwrinkled skin sporting large wireframe glasses that were the style in the mid-1980s when I finished training. I was squinting toward the sun when that photo was taken, but there is still a hint of confidence shining in my eyes. Now I am looking back through the life I never imagined when I joined my father to practice general urology. The career that hypospadias changed.

I remember how the first hypospadias repair I did made a normal penis, but the next several fell well short of that goal, leaving those penises ugly and the parents and surgeon disappointed. And how that started me on a journey that led into pediatric urology and then on to hypospadiology trying to do better.

"Wow, you looked like a typical urology nerd even back then!" Bush laughs, glancing over my shoulder at the slide as I polish my lecture.

I have to agree with her, and then explain, "I'm going to talk about what hypospadias has taught me."

That repair is more than a surgical exercise to make a urethra. That how the penis looks when the surgeon is done is just as important as how it works. How there is no mild hypospadias, and no minor operation to repair it. That it is the extent of curvature, and not the location of the meatus, that determines both the severity and the best operation for the repair. How severe hypospadias can never be successfully repaired in one step, and not often in two, but it can reliably be made into a normal penis after three corporotomies straighten the curvature and STAC makes the skin even around the shaft. That grafts are better than flaps to make the new urethra. How most complications result from errors that surgeons make.

These are among the many lessons I did not learn in training, that hypospadias had to teach me. Now I will summarize them into the admonition that these repairs are demanding, and that dissection just a few millimeters into the wrong direction can ruin the surgery and, sometimes, the penis for life. I do not know how many surgeons will listen, but there is always an audience because hypospadias repair is difficult for everyone.

My mind wanders from the slides I am writing and organizing, thinking there is so much more to discuss than surgical details; knowledge that surgeons must have to truly become experts. I did not know the fear that word *hypospadias*, so familiar to us, raises the first time parents hear their newborn son has it. I did not know the guilt they carry until someone reassures them they did not cause it to happen to their son. I did not sense the isolation that separates them from friends who innocently ask if all their baby's fingers and toes are OK, because the parents are not sure they should discuss their son's penis with others who also have no idea what hypospadias is.

I now know from their looks of surprise, their nodding agreement, the tears in their eyes when I acknowledge their fear and isolation, that they still harbor strong emotions needing a release. And the questionnaires they answered in Phillip's study told me that parents continue to worry about their son's future even when surgery to repair the hypospadias is declared a success.

Their answers also revealed that the failures of surgeons place more guilt on the shoulders of parents, who think they are somehow responsible for the complication that happened to their son. And how dread surges through them when they hear the urologist say, "This almost never happens to my patients!" because that creates even more doubt in their minds that their son will ever be right.

I had to pay a fee to publish this information on the internet when peer review in urology showed no interest. Then I paid another, far larger, fee to create the *Hypospadias Matters* video that we uploaded onto YouTube to find a bigger audience than it attracted at the AUA. Still, I must do more, adding new slides and making room in my lectures to tell surgeons who might not read our article or see our video about the worries of parents who have sons with hypospadias.

And what about the suffering of men still living with their birth defect? They, too, have important lessons to teach these experts. What it is like to live every day trying to aim their stream away from their pants and shoes. How they shied from lovers fearing they might be disappointed with their penis. Why they felt so isolated as teens, not wanting to discuss their birth defect with either friends or their parents. Those surgeons who brush off distal hypospadias as nothing more than cosmetic need to hear of their struggles too.

So we sent a manuscript to the *Journal of Urology* describing the experiences of men whose distal hypospadias was never repaired. This time the editor did not even bother to send it for peer review, but rejected it himself with the comment that the patients we see in our highly specialized practice cannot be compared to the typical men living with hypospadias. Yet, other men with, for example, prostate cancer, who go to MD Anderson or Sloan Kettering or the Mayo Clinic are apparently similar enough to those treated in less renown centers for their results to be published in that journal. And even if the men who seeks us out are somehow atypical, the potential lifelong impact of hypospadias in at least some men still deserves the attention of all urologists.

I cannot possibly mention all the lessons that hypospadias has taught me in over thirty years during the forty-five-minute lecture I am preparing. In the end I am still a surgeon, lecturing to surgeons who want to know how to repair it better. Even that is a challenge too great for my most polished speech. Because the time is always too short, and to bring others on my journey I must first retrace steps back to where most are standing now and explain that much of what they and I were taught to do is wrong. That chordee excision does not make the penis straight, plications do not keep the penis straight, and skin flaps cannot make the best urethra.

Then I can say, again, that there is no chordee, and that the best way to straighten anything more than the slightest bend is to make three incisions to lengthen the shorter side. Next, I will describe those: where, and how wide, and how deep to cut. This will be new information for some of those listening despite my articles and a textbook that published all these details, and so I will also answer before they ask how they can be sure they have straightened the curvature and rest assured they have not given the penis erectile dysfunction.

Somewhere in all this I will need to show a picture of a penis bent thirty degrees, to point out that it does not look impressive and to emphasize that is exactly why surgeons must measure, and not simply eyeball, the extent to which the penis curves. That is something that few, if any, of those watching do, and so I will click on the mouse again to superimpose a photo of a goniometer onto the bend to show how it is done.

This is a lot to say about penile curvature, but I cannot stop here. I must also tell them the consequences when they do not make the penis straight. How tension from the bent underside pulls on the urethral repair during every natural erection after surgery, tearing open fistulas and dehiscing wounds. Then, if they simply close the leak or restitch the glans and do not check an artificial erection, the complication will likely happen again. In fact, recurrent fistulas and dehiscences almost always mean the penis is bent. But they were not taught that, just as I was not.

And even if the surgery manages to heal without these complications, the boy grown into a man will worry what a lover is going to think of his bent penis, and about the struggle of making it work right during intercourse. Men have told me this, and others have also published that it is true.

I cannot narrate this section of slides in less than twenty minutes, and by then some in the audience will begin to wonder if I am ever going to move on to discuss making the urethra. So, I will conclude this opening section with a slide filled with pictures of the bent penises that come to my practice every week and say that all the surgery done so far in all these boys will have to be redone, usually in multiple stages reinforced with hyperbaric oxygen. I hope that at least some of the listeners will hear and think about their own patients.

I have to pause these preparations now, because there are telemedicines to do and emails to answer and chores around the house waiting for me. Organizing these lectures always takes many hours over several days, even if the presentation will only last minutes. My mind will keep whirling during these breaks, and pull me from bed in the early morning before the sun rises to work on it some more.

The next slide will diagram our algorithm for making the urethra, showing that Bush and I decide between TIP and STAG or STAC by the extent of curvature that artificial erection finds and the goniometer measures, and not where the meatus is. Which means I will have to say one more time that curvature is the single most important factor that determines the severity of hypospadias and the success of its repair.

Next, I will discuss distal TIP, the hit song that many in the audience have come to hear. Although it is the most common hypospadias repair done worldwide, I will still have to repeat what I have published several times, that surgeons do not need to analyze the urethral plate to choose which operation to do. Rather, they can rely on TIP to fix any and every distal hypospadias, as long as the penis is straight.

But I will have to spend precious time mentioning those contrary opinions that it does not work when the plate is narrow, or "unhealthy," because there may be some in the audience who have been persuaded to eye TIP with suspicion. I will give the alternative explanation that the fault lies not in the anatomy of the patient, or with the operation done right, but in surgeons performing it wrong. I will prove that by lifting a picture directly from one of those articles by a skeptic and projecting it next to a similar one of my own to show that the other surgeon did not make the TIP incision deep enough.

Then I will click onto the next slide covered with pictures of distal hypospadias in all its variations to say we must not return to the time of my youth when surgeons tried to describe and categorize all these different shapes and sizes to decide which operation to do.

Instead, I will tell those in the audience that I have not used a different technique to repair distal hypospadias in over thirty years. If it works for me, it can work for them too. And then I will prove that by showing meta-analyses of surgeons worldwide duplicating my success.

That leads me to proximal TIP. I will first show the early mistakes that I made adapting what I was taught for flap repairs to this new operation, and then explain how a series of technical changes steadily improved my results. The first example of the 3Ps that I will end this lecture recommending to the audience. Then I will confess that I pushed the operation too far, which hurt boys, and stress to my listeners, again, that I rarely do a proximal TIP anymore.

Now I do a STAG, or a STAC, our new operation discovered under duress. And this discussion will first loop back to the three corporotomies which straighten the penis, to say they also make it longer. Which will then introduce a new topic: the importance of penis skin, especially in boys with the most severe hypospadias who were born with too little of it on the underside of the shaft and now need even more to cover it.

I look at my slides illustrating the key steps in both these related procedures. Then I lean back in my chair and close my eyes and wonder how to better explain when to do one versus the other. Those young surgeons in Doha who surrounded me during a coffee break were confused despite my explanation, as were the Iraqis who invited me for a Zoom specifically to clarify when to STAG and when to STAC.

At first, I thought the answer was clear. STAG was done when the urethra reached beyond the three corporotomies so that the urethral graft would be placed onto a smooth surface. When it did not, STAC was better since we learned that grafts laid onto corporotomy incisions do not reliably heal.

But then we realized that the grafts in some boys still scarred after STAG, and when I looked back at the photographs taken during their first operation, I saw just how little skin each had on the underside of his penis. And that reminded me of Humby's comment that a graft needs healthy skin around it to help it heal.

Bush tried measuring the skin at the start of the operation to see if that would predict who needs a STAC. But the landmarks were not precise, and watching her I knew that others inevitably would measure it differently.

Now I study the pictures again and shake my head. "I think this is all way too complicated," I finally say to Bush. "If you and I aren't sure when the skin is good enough to place a graft, then we have to do what is most likely to work." I click back to the algorithm and erase STAG from it.

I know I will have to justify this heresy to surgeons once taught, as I was, to repair even the most severe hypospadias in one operation, and who considered it a sufficient compromise when they, like me, began doing it in two.

"We're only talking about 10 percent of boys with hypospadias, the ones who many surgeons have given up even trying to make them a normal penis," I say, overruling Bush's objection before she makes it. "By doing a three-stage STAC they can get it right."

I make a slide with a picture of a severe hypospadias before surgery next to another after the first stage of STAC showing the penis straight and covered with supple penile skin. With a click a text box appears saying this happens over 98 percent of the time.

Next, a slide of the second stage will report that nearly 95 percent of our grafts heal healthy and are easy to tubularize at the final operation. Then I will show pictures of the healed graft and the steps at the third stage to roll it into a urethra, sewing it the same way I learned while doing proximal TIPs.

The fistulas and glans dehiscences that occur after STAC add up to only a fraction of the complications that urologists encounter trying to repair proximal hypospadias every other way. Including the 100 percent complications I will once more admit to having when I used the Byars flaps that many in the audience are still doing. This will lead to several pictures of the most severe hypospadias and their final, normal, appearance after STAC.

In the last moments of the lecture I will say that this journey has been one of discovery through much trial and error, guided by recording and then reviewing my own results. The 3 Ps. Again and again I have seen that I am not as good as I thought, and again and again I have gotten better than I was. If these surgeons hear nothing else, if they forget everything I have said until now, this is the critical message for getting it right that hypospadias taught me, which everyone needs to learn.

But no matter what I say, how I say it, or how often I say it, some colleagues still insist on continuing "what works best in their hands," despite ample proof that their hands should do better. Some simply ignore me; others actively resist this message. Lately a few accuse me of questioning their abilities to repair hypospadias to convince patients to come to Dallas. But they do not realize the influence of moms advising other moms, who contact us having already decided that Bush and I will do the surgery for their sons.

I also know that all the articles Bush and I might write, all the videos we might shoot, all the lectures we might Zoom, all the visitors we might teach, all the workshops we might give, and even the most comprehensive and thoroughly illustrated edition of *Hypospadiology* we might produce, will not change the basic fact that hypospadias is a rare condition that too many surgeons try to repair.

I thought I was an expert when I left Children's, only to learn from a tsunami of patients with the most severe cases of hypospadias who came to PARC Urology, and then to the Hypospadias Specialty Center, that I was not. If those fifteen cases I did each year in a busy academic practice were not enough, what is the expectation for others who will never manage more than the national average of two a year?

"We have to grow larger," I conclude, after responding to another four new patients during the turnover between operations, and before beginning the evening consultations to meet several more.

"I cannot keep coming to work at eight in the morning, do several hard operations until late in the afternoon, and then immediately start telemeds that go on 'till eight at night!" Especially now that these long hours of meticulous operations, day after day, are making my left thumb ache and my neck painful to turn.

Bush agrees that it is nearly time, now that the pandemic is waning, our dispute with North Dallas Health is ending, and our surgery schedule is filled months into the future. "The question is how?"

Having limited our practice to hypospadias, and then pioneering the first center dedicated to treating that condition, we now must find two more surgeons who have the skills and the desire to form a second surgical team. Two more surgeons who will devote their careers to repairing hypospadias and teaching others how to do it right. Who will agree to spend several months being mentored by Bush and me after they arrive before they are assigned their own cases. Who will enter their data into the spreadsheet every day, and then study it from time to time to confirm that what they are doing and teaching is right, or to see what they have to improve.

There are so many questions. How do we assess the surgical skills of candidates before offering someone a job? Should the next team include an adult specialist to manage the men seeking out our practice? Is it possible to find another left-handed surgeon to pair with a right-handed one so that each stand on the side of the table that is the most comfortable? Should we try to hire both at the same time or one after the other, and, if we begin with one, how would the practice work with three surgeons in the interval before the fourth arrives when our model calls for two doing each operation? Will the new surgeons struggle to form a cohesive team like Bush and I did? Will we divide our own team and each work with a new surgeon? How will we pay the salaries of new surgeons until they start earning it themselves?

We attended a new all-day course at the 2022 AUA devoted to practice growth and posed these dilemmas to the faculty. John McConnell, the course director and former chairman of urology who recruited me to Dallas, listened carefully, intrigued by our unique circumstances. Then he drew on his own experience merging two healthcare systems after leaving UT Southwestern to warn me.

"Warren, whether you bring on a new team all at once or the new surgeons one at a time could well be an *existential* decision threatening all you've managed to do."

McConnell focused on the finances and team dynamics, but Bush suspects there is a greater risk to growing larger.

"The real question is whether parents will accept someone besides Snodgrass operating on their son," she insists, knowing it is not only me that they ask who will do the surgery.

But I see a different challenge that might be the greatest of all these to meet. "Will we find someone else like you to manage the skin?" I ask Bush every time the subject comes up. "You and I can't separate unless one of the new people can do the skin like you do, because I just can't and our patients have to have someone who can." What I did before Bush was certainly good, but it is no longer good enough.

We must grow bigger, while staying the same. And if we manage to do that successfully, maybe our model will someday create an even bigger center in Dallas, as well as another Hypospadias Specialty Center in the Northeast and a third on the West Coast.

Regardless, our center must live years beyond me, in a way that the practices built by Devine and Horton and Duckett and Bracka did not. A specialty center that attracts patients less by the reputation of the founder, than by an ever-evolving highest standard of care. A center for teaching the next generation of hypospadiologists to perform surgeries that are so much more technically demanding than nearly everything else a urologist does. Because repairing hypospadias will always demand the surgeon not stray millimeters into the wrong plane.

Not every surgeon is cut out for this challenge. And even fewer are obsessed, as I am, with making this birth defect right.

In the meantime, I think more parents are asking if I will still be operating when their son needs his second and third steps done. I smile at them and reassure, "I won't be retiring anytime soon." Then I sometimes add, "But if I was suddenly unable to work, Dr. Bush is more than ready to do all this herself."

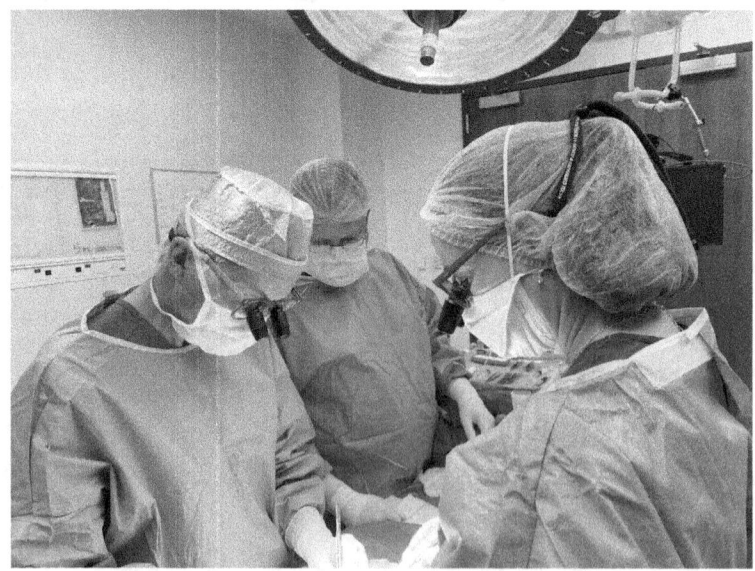

Operating with Dr. Bush in the Hypospadias Specialty Center

Afterword

The struggle with hypospadias goes on. Every day another 950 boys are born with this birth defect somewhere in the world, mostly to parents who have never heard of it before. They will join the ranks of so many others who experienced the same fears and guilt and isolation they feel now, simply because hypospadias is not better known. This must change.

Most of them will be referred to a pediatric urologist or surgeon to have it repaired and then will follow the recommendations of whichever surgeon they happen to see, not realizing that the results from the operations surgeons do can vary widely. The parents who think to ask the consultant how many complications he or she has may not realize that the answer they are told is usually not that surgeon's own results, because few surgeons know them. That, too, should change.

Those whose sons have distal hypospadias may be told by one consultant that it does not need repair, while another advises surgery. The fact that two specialists examining the same boy can give such widely varying opinions is very distressing to parents trying to decide what is best for their son. This must also change, since there are objective criteria to guide this decision which all surgeons should use.

Parents of sons born with severe hypospadias recognize this is a serious problem, and many sense that the surgeon is not confident that their boy's penis can be made normal. Some will research the matter further searching for someone who repairs proximal hypospadias often, while others will not think to do this until their son has complications they did not expect from the consultant they were referred to see. It is shocking for all of them to learn that certified pediatric urologists only do a proximal repair an average of twice a year, because proximal hypospadias is a rare condition. Nevertheless, private groups and major academic centers have not designated a surgical team to do these challenging operations, and few surgeons will refer even the most complicated case to a colleague with more experience. This too must change.

Most complications can be traced back to a mistake the surgeon made. And those technical errors were usually learned during training, from mentors who pass the wrong lessons they were taught to the next generations of surgeons. This continues because there are no standardized lessons for trainees, no performance standards to measure a surgeon's work in practice, and no expectation that surgeons review their own results. This is hard to believe.

Nearly thirty years ago, I simply told pediatric urologists there was a way to fix distal hypospadias better than what I was taught and most of them were doing. I had no idea that would open Pandora's box to reveal so many other problems affecting all aspects of the condition. It is painful to see them, but I cannot close my eyes knowing that at the center of it all are boys who suffer when surgeons do not get it right. And some of those will grow into men with scars that last their lifetime.

I do not know all the answers, and even a brief overview of my career shows how many times I have changed course because what I thought was right proved to be wrong. Meanwhile, there is so much misery in the operative reports I read after unsuccessful repairs that I am easily discouraged by the slow pace of change. All this emphasizes again how important it is for surgeons to review their work, and then to make improvements when the results could be better.

What I cannot understand are those who do this personal quality assessment, but then do not make changes to get better. Why, for example, a surgeon known for his thoughtful data analyses commented during a conference that he sewed the layers of the new urethra in the opposite way as we do, running the first layer and adding interrupted stitches in the second, even though he knew that resulted in *five times* more fistulas in his patients than ours have.

When I asked why he does not simply interrupt the first layer of stitches and then run the second layer, he replied, "I know your data. But I am satisfied with my results."

And, to my knowledge, surgeons in those three major academic centers who reported so many complications after Byars' flaps continue doing them, and teaching them to their fellows. As do many other surgeons who read those articles and concluded that expectations are simply too high for proximal hypospadias surgery, rather than asking if there is a better method to repair it.

Bush and I share the lessons we learn, but some colleagues resist our attempts to help.

An email from a pediatric urologist demanded I remove her from a mailing list informing all the training program directors about the next Hypospadias Masterclass, so they could alert their fellows to watch. "I have concerns about some of the things you propose," she wrote with no further explanation, before adding, "and about you telling parents that most of us are not qualified to repair hypospadias."

I answered that everything we teach is evidence-based, that I do not judge the abilities of other surgeons, and that nearly everyone who contacts us has already decided to come to Dallas before we exchange emails or schedule a telemedicine consultation. But she was not convinced.

Fortunately, Pandora's box also held hope, and I see that too. In the faces of the surgeons who surround me at meetings excited to ask a question. In the emails they write wanting advice for a patient. In the hundreds who come in person or join in a Zoom to hear me speak. In the abstracts such as those recently presented to the ESPU, which included an analysis of different methods to accurately measure penile curvature, and the preliminary results of STAC repair done by a young surgeon in Uzbekistan.

Hope also comes from all the surgeons around the world who have used the 3Ps to examine their own work and change. Colleagues in Mexico, Ecuador and Brazil, in Canada, in England, Denmark, the Netherlands and Italy, in Russia, in the Philippines, in Kuwait and Egypt and Israel, in India, in Japan and China, and in several centers across the US. I know this because those surgeons seek me out to tell me the same thing. "I finally looked at my own results like you said, and they weren't as good as I thought . . . but now they're getting better!"

And I also see hope in the suffering of parents and in men born with hypospadias who are ready to end the stigma of a birth defect of the penis. Soon they will rise up to demand that surgeons repairing it be held to a higher standard. I am certain that their voices will change hypospadias, just like parents and patients changed the treatment for club foot and made it better.

I originally wrote this memoir in the third person's voice because it seemed more objective, so that I could stand at arm's length to narrate the story. I did not want to fill it with I's, when it was not only about me. Bush convinced me to send the manuscript to an editor for a second opinion, and Stacey Donovan convinced me to tell it directly from my point of view.

Then a second editor said I had to decide who the readers would be, warning that the technical details in the story can be daunting. But hypospadias cannot be understood without those details, and I realize from the fact that parents and patients study the articles I wrote and the videos I shot to educate surgeons, that everyone affected by this birth defect wants to know more about it and how it can be repaired.

Everything is as true as I remember, although a few names were changed, or not mentioned, and a few stories were tweaked to make better sense.

Those who know me best will see what has been left out. The impact the move to Dallas had on my school-age children, and my marriage. The hurt that my mother rarely spoke to me after I took her grandchildren from Lubbock. The disappointment that my father was retired yet did not travel to Atlanta to hear his son's plenary lecture, before dementia ended our relationship. But this is not a story of personal tragedies.

It is also not a story of personal triumph. As I wrote in both the beginning and the end, I did not imagine this life and so I did not seek it. Rather, the wand chose the wizard, and, to this day, I have no idea why I alone saw the TIP incision when so many others could have seen it sooner. Still, it was never important that it was *me*.

This surgeon's struggle with hypospadias became easier when I found a partner to share the challenges of this demanding surgery. We both soon realized that decisions are easier to make and the steps of the operations are easier to perform as a team—a lesson that is obvious to anyone watching us work, and an example that others can follow too. As I have already said, this also needs to happen, and I am filled with hope that it will.

Because, in the end, every boy born with hypospadias wants to grow into a man with a normal penis. And so every surgeon who picks up a knife to do this surgery must continuously strive to achieve that.

March, 2023

My Bibliography of Peer-Reviewed Hypospadias Articles

Warren Snodgrass, Ross Decter, David Roth, Edmond Gonzales, Jr: Management of the Penile Shaft Skin in Hypospadias Repair: Alternatives to Byars Flaps. *Journal of Pediatric Surgery*, 1988.

Warren Snodgrass: Tubularized Incised Plate Urethroplasty for Distal Hypospadias. *Journal of Urology*,1994.

Warren Snodgrass, Martin Koyle, Gianantonio Manzoni, Richard Hurwitz, Anthony Caldamone, and Richard Ehrlich: Tubularized Incised Plate Hypospadias Repair: Results of a Multicenter Experience. *Journal of Urology*, 1996.

Warren Snodgrass, Martin Koyle, Gianantonio Manzoni, Richard Hurwitz, Anthony Caldamone, and Richard Ehrlich: Tubularized Incised Plate Hypospadias Repair for Proximal Hypospadias. *Journal of Urology*, 1998.

Warren Snodgrass: Does Tubularized Incised Plate Hypospadias Repair Create Neo-urethral Strictures? *Journal of Urology*, 1999.

Warren Snodgrass: Suture Tracts Following Hypospadias Repair. *British Journal of Urology International*, 1999.

Warren Snodgrass: Tubularized Incised Plate Hypospadias Repair: Indications and Complications. *Urology*, 1999.

Warren Snodgrass: Changing Concepts in Hypospadias Repair. *Current Opinion in Urology*, 1999.

Warren Snodgrass, Kathleen Patterson, Chadwick Plaire, Richard Grady, and Michael Mitchell: Histology of the Urethral Plate: Implications for Hypospadias Repair. *Journal of Urology*, 2000.

Warren Snodgrass and Armando Lorenzo: Tubularized Incised Plate Urethroplasty for Proximal Hypospadias Repair. *British Journal of Urology International*, 2002.

Warren Snodgrass and Armando Lorenzo: Regular Dilation is Unnecessary After Tubularized Incised Plate Repair. *British Journal of Urology International*, 2002.

Warren Snodgrass and Armando Lorenzo: Tubularized Incised Plate Urethroplasty for Hypospadias Reoperation. *British Journal of Urology International*, 2002.

Warren Snodgrass and Michael Nguyen: Current Technique of Tubularized Incised Plate Hypospadias Repair. *Urology*, 60(1): 157, 2002.

Selami Sozubir and Warren Snodgrass: A New Algorithm for Primary Hypospadias Repair Based Upon TIP Urethroplasty. *Journal of Pediatric Surgery*, 2003.

Michael Nguyen and Warren Snodgrass: Effect of Urethral Plate Characteristics on Tubularized Incised Plate Urethroplasty. *Journal of Urology*, 2004.

Michael Nguyen and Warren Snodgrass: Tubularized Incised Plate Hypospadias Reoperation. *Journal of Urology*, 2004.

Warren Snodgrass and James Elmore: Initial Experience with Staged Buccal Graft (Bracka) Hypospadias Reoperations. *Journal of Urology*, 2004.

Warren Snodgrass: Snodgrass Technique for Hypospadias Repair. *British Journal of Urology International*, 2005.

Warren Snodgrass, Martin Koyle, Lawrence Baskin, and Anthony Caldamone: Foreskin Preservation in Penile Surgery. *Journal of Urology*, 2006.

Warren Snodgrass and Rose Khavari: Prior Circumcision Does Not Complicate Repair of Hypospadias with an Intact Prepuce. *Journal of Urology*, 2006.

Warren Snodgrass and Selcuk Yucel: Tubularized Incised Plate for Midshaft and Proximal Hypospadias repair. *Journal of Urology*, 2007.

Warren Snodgrass: A Farewell to Chordee. *Journal of Urology*, 2007.

Warren Snodgrass: Management of Penile Curvature in Children. *Current Opinion in Urology*, 2008.

Warren Snodgrass: Utilization of the Urethral Plate in Hypospadias Surgery. *Indian Journal of Urology*, 2008.

Warren Snodgrass, Ali Ziada, Selcuk Yucel, and Amit Gupta: Comparison of Outcomes of Tubularized Incised Plate Hypospadias Repair and Circumcision: A Questionnaire-Based Survey of Parents and Surgeons. *Journal of Pediatric Urology*, 2008.

Warren Snodgrass and Juan Prieto: Straightening Ventral Curvature While Preserving the Urethral Plate in Proximal Hypospadias Repair. *Journal of Urology*, 2009.

Warren Snodgrass, Nicol Bush, and Nickolas Cost: Algorithm for Comprehensive Approach to Hypospadias Reoperation Using 3 Techniques. *Journal of Urology*, 2009.

Warren Snodgrass: Hypospadias Reporting—How Good is the Literature? *Journal of Urology*, 2010.

Warren Snodgrass and Nicol Bush: Tubularized Incised Plate Proximal Hypospadias Repair: Continued Evolution and Extended Applications. *Journal of Pediatric Urology*, 2011.

Warren Snodgrass, Nickolas Cost, Paul Nakonezny, and Nicol Bush: Analysis of Risk Factors for Glans Dehiscence After Tubularized Incised Plate Hypospadias Repair. *Journal of Urology*, 2011.

Warren Snodgrass, Daniel DaJusta, Carlos Villanueva, and Nicol Bush: Foreskin Reconstruction Does Not Increase Urethroplasty or Skin Complications After Distal TIP Hypospadias Repair. *Journal of Pediatric Urology*, 2012.

Nicol Bush, Michael Holzer, Song Zhang, and Warren Snodgrass: Age Does Not Impact Risk for Urethroplasty Complications After Tubularized Incised Plate Repair of Hypospadias. *Journal of Pediatric Urology*, 2012.

Nicol Bush, Daniel DaJusta, and Warren Snodgrass: Glans Penis Width in Patients with Hypospadias Compared to Healthy Controls. *Journal of Pediatric Urology*, 2013.

Warren Snodgrass, Carlos Villanueva, Candace Granberg, and Nicol Bush: Objective Use of Testosterone Reveals Androgen Insensitivity in Patients with Proximal Hypospadias. *Journal of Pediatric Urology*, 2013.

Warren Snodgrass, Candace Granberg, and Nicol Bush: Urethral Strictures Following Urethral Plate and Proximal Urethral Elevation During Proximal TIP Hypospadias Repair. *Journal of Pediatric Urology*, 2013.

Warren Snodgrass, Carlos Villanueva, and Nicol Bush: Duration of Follow-Up to Diagnose Hypospadias Urethroplasty Complications. *Journal of Pediatric Urology*, 2014.

Warren Snodgrass: Flap Versus Graft 2-Stage Repair of Severe Hypospadias with Chordee. *Journal of Urology*, 2015.

Warren Snodgrass and Nicol Bush: TIP Hypospadias Repair: A Pediatric Urology Indicator Operation. *Journal of Pediatric Urology*, 2015.

Warren Snodgrass, Carlos Villanueva, and Nicol Bush: Primary and Reoperative Hypospadias Repair in Adults—Are Results Different Than in Children? *Journal of Urology*, 2014.

Warren Snodgrass, Gwen Grimsby, and Nicol Bush: Coronal Fistula Under the Glans Without Reoperative Hypospadias Glansplasty or Urinary Diversion. *Journal of Pediatric Urology*, 2015.

Warren Snodgrass and Nicol Bush: Surgery for Primary Proximal Hypospadias with Ventral Curvature. *Current Urology Review*, 2015.

Nicol Bush, Carlos Villanueva, and Warren Snodgrass: Glans Size is an Independent Risk Factor for Urethroplasty Complications after Hypospadias Repair. *Journal of Urology*, 2015.

Warren Snodgrass and Nicol Bush: Re-operative Urethroplasty After Failed Hypospadias Repair: How Prior Surgery Impacts Risk for Additional Complications. *Journal of Pediatric Urology*, 2016.

Melise Keays, Nathan Stark, S Lee, I Bernstein, Warren Snodgrass, and Nicol Bush: Patient Reported Outcomes in Preoperative and Postoperative Patients with Hypospadias. *Journal of Urology*, 2016.

Nicol Bush, Theodore Barber, Daniel DaJusta, Juan Prieto, Ali Ziada, and Warren Snodgrass: Results of Distal Hypospadias Repair After Pediatric Urology Fellowship Training: A Comparison of Junior Surgeons with their Mentor. *Journal of Pediatric Urology*, 2016.

Warren Snodgrass and Nicol Bush: Primary Hypospadias Repair Techniques: A Review of the Evidence. *Urology Annals*, 2016.

Warren Snodgrass, Juan Blanquel, and Nicol Bush: Recurrence after Management of Meatal Balanitis Xerotica Obliterans. *Journal of Pediatric Urology*, 2017.

Nicol Bush and Warren Snodgrass: Pre-Incision Urethral Plate Width Does Not Impact TIP Urethroplasty Outcomes. *Journal of Pediatric Urology*, 2017.

Warren Snodgrass and Nicol Bush: Staged Tubularized Autograft Repair for Primary

Proximal Hypospadias with 30-Degree or Greater Curvature. *Journal of Urology*, 2017.

Warren Snodgrass and Nicol Bush: Is Distal Hypospadias Repair Mostly a Cosmetic Operation? *Journal of Pediatric Urology*, 2018.

Nicol Bush and Warren Snodgrass: Hyperbaric Oxygen Improves Oral Graft Take in Hypospadias Reoperations. *Journal of Urology*, 2019.

Warren Snodgrass and Nicol Bush: Persistent or Recurrent Ventral Curvature after Failed Proximal Hypospadias Repair. *Journal of Pediatric Urology*, 2019.

Phillip Snodgrass, Warren Snodgrass, and Nicol Bush: Parental Concerns of Boys with Hypospadias. *Dove Press*, 2021.

Warren Snodgrass and Nicol Bush: Recurrent Ventral Curvature after Proximal TIP Hypospadias Repair. *Journal of Pediatric Urology*, 2021.

Warren Snodgrass and Nicol Bush: Do New Complications Develop During Puberty After Childhood Hypospadias Repair? *Journal of Urology*, 2022.

Nicol Bush and Warren Snodgrass: Complaints of Men with Uncorrected Distal Hypospadias. *Dove Press*, 2023.

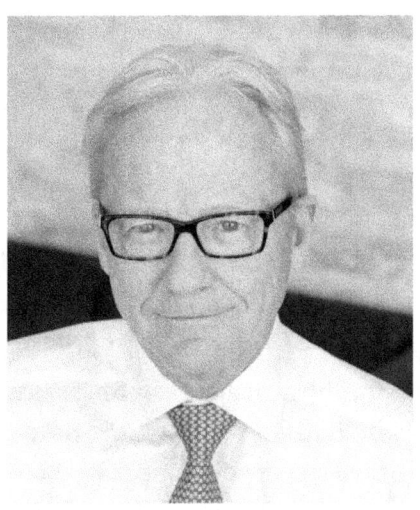

About the Author

Warren Snodgrass, MD, is an internationally recognized expert in hypospadias, who combines innovation with evidence-based decision-making to improve surgery for this common birth defect. From the beginning of his career, he has been driven not only to make the penis born with hypospadias *better*, but to make it *normal*. It was this determination that led to the TIP repair for distal hypospadias, and, eventually, the STAC repair for more severe cases when TIP should not be done. Today a surgeon can use TIP and STAC to correct all extents of the condition.

The need to document and then study his results led Dr. Snodgrass to start databases and then to keep them current by entering information as soon as an operation ends and clinic is done. It was also a key reason that he hired Dr. Nicol Bush, to organize these into a master database that could better answer the questions his growing experience posed.

And it was the need to share his discoveries with colleagues that motivated him to write his many scientific articles and book chapters and the textbook *Hypospadiology*, and sent him around the world lecturing and demonstrating the best ways he found to do this challenging surgery. Then, when Dr. Snodgrass realized that all these traditional academic methods were not enough, he and Dr. Bush started a YouTube channel to reach a younger generation of surgeons. And when they found themselves working in hospitals and surgery centers that did not have a camera to record their operations, Dr. Snodgrass created an international hypospadias email group to help keep others up to date.

Along the way he learned the truth of the maxim he heard from his chief during residency, that it takes miles and miles of ocean to turn a battleship around.

But the boys and men he saw whose penises were damaged by surgeons continuing to do older repairs when TIP and STAC are better, and still using TIP for severe hypospadias long after he warned it was the wrong operation for those, made clear towards the end of his career that Dr. Snodgrass would have to take on the risks of buying a surgical facility and creating the Hypospadias Specialty Center with Dr. Bush.

The day will come when he no longer operates. But the work to make surgery better, and hypospadias better known, will keep Dr. Snodgrass active to the end, and the Hypospadias Specialty Center busy indefinitely.

In the meantime, he is the proud father of three and grandfather of four, who looks forward to vacations skiing or scuba diving and weekends walking on the beach in Galveston with his wife and his dog, Toffee.